Foundations for Practice
in Occupational Therapy

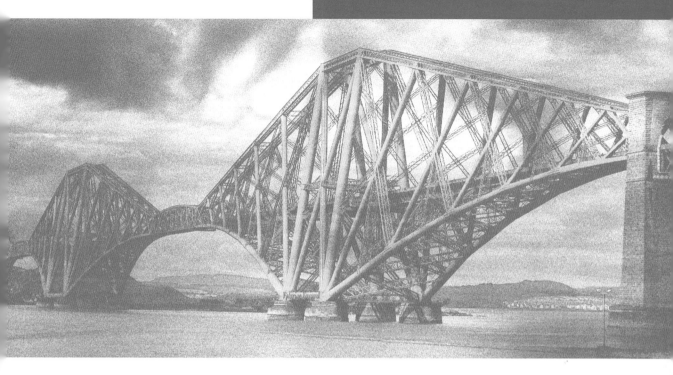

SIXTH EDITION

Foundations for Practice in Occupational Therapy

Edited by
EDWARD A.S. DUNCAN, PHD, BSC (HONS), DIP CBT

Associate Professor of Applied Health Research, Nursing Midwifery and Allied Health Professions Research Unit, University of Stirling, Stirling, Scotland, United Kingdom Honorary Advanced Clinical Practitioner, NHS Forth Valley, Scotland, United Kingdom

Foreword by
JENNY PRESTON MBE, PhD, BSc (Hons), Dip COT, FRCOT

Consultant Occupational Therapist, Clinical Lead Neurological Rehabilitation, Douglas Grant Rehabilitation Centre, Ayrshire Central Hospital, Irvine, United Kingdom

ELSEVIER   Edinburgh   London   New York   Oxford   Philadelphia   St Louis   Sydney   2021

First edition 1992
Second edition 1997
Third edition 2001
Fourth edition 2006
Fifth edition 2013
Sixth edition 2021

Notices

Practitioners and researchers must always rely on their own experience and knowledge in evaluating and using any information, methods, compounds or experiments described herein. Because of rapid advances in the medical sciences, in particular, independent verification of diagnoses and drug dosages should be made. To the fullest extent of the law, no responsibility is assumed by Elsevier, authors, editors or contributors for any injury and/or damage to persons or property as a matter of products liability, negligence or otherwise, or from any use or operation of any methods, products, instructions, or ideas contained in the material herein.

ISBN: 978-0-7020-5447-1

Content Strategist: Poppy Garraway Smith
Content Development Specialist: Fiona Conn
Project Manager: Andrew Riley
Design: Brian Salisbury
Illustration Manager: Anitha Rajarathnam
Marketing Manager: Ed Major

Printed in Scotland

Last digit is the print number: 9 8 7 6 5 4 3 2

Working together
to grow libraries in
developing countries

www.elsevier.com • www.bookaid.org

CONTENTS

FOREWORD

As an occupational therapist practicing across all four pillars of clinical, academia, research and leadership this classic occupational therapy text has played a fundamental role in my knowledge acquisition, development of my understanding of occupational therapy as a complex intervention and informing my vision and strategic direction. This latest edition does not disappoint. Editor and author Dr Edward Duncan has successfully combined tradition with the contemporary challenges facing the occupational therapy profession. Somewhat refreshingly this text openly invites readers to reflect on, debate and embrace contrasting perspectives acknowledging the importance of divergence of opinion to strengthen the profession within a more robust theoretical evidence base.

Yet this is creatively balanced with the familiarity of conceptual frameworks and case studies from previous editions. Reflecting the evolving nature of the theories underpinning occupational science and occupational therapy key conceptual frameworks have been updated within this edition by leading academics such as the CMOP-E in Chapter 7 and the PEOP in Chapter 8 reminding the reader of the contemporaneous and maturing prominence of our theoretical basis. The shift in language from previous editions such as the use of occupations in a determined move beyond the use of activities further reflects the confidence in and advancement of the vocabulary accessed within the occupational therapy profession.

Although this text is designed to be used in a variety of ways depending on your level of knowledge I would strongly urge all readers to start at the beginning of this book. The importance of the historical journey from our humble beginnings as a little known profession to a global phenomenon informing and influencing policy, delivering valued, effective and cost effective solutions to a wide range of clients is cleverly articulated within Chapter 1. Understanding this journey is paramount to recognising the challenges for occupational therapists in defining their contribution to population and global health and social challenges in different settings across the world.

This text has something to offer everyone, regardless of your knowledge and experience. It offers updated conceptual frameworks, insightful examples of application of theory to practice and intentionally stimulates discussion and debate. I thoroughly recommend this as a core text for anyone with an interest in embracing theoretically driven and evidence based occupational therapy in practice.

Dr Jenny Preston MBE

INTRODUCTION

Theory. The keystone of practice, or an unnecessary burden of occupational therapy education? It will come as no surprise that I believe that theory is indeed the keystone of practice. High-quality occupational therapy theory helps clinicians understand their scope of practice. It supports clinicians to understand the problems, challenges, strengths, opportunities and limitations of the people they are working with, as well as the opportunities and limitations of their physical and social environments. High-quality occupational therapy theory helps clinicians know how to work with the people they come into contact with, conceptualise the occupational challenges they face, measure and understand when things are getting better or worse, and know when to change direction, and stop. Occupational therapy theory can also help design intervention programmes and guide research. Crucially, however, theory should be tested and revised—challenged, evidenced or disproven. And in doing so the developing theoretical base of the profession also help clinicians, managers and commissioners of services to stop doing what is not effective.

Despite the importance and potential of occupational therapy theory, an honest appraisal of the profession must acknowledge that its universally constant use in practice remains an optional extra at best, to some appears to be perceived as an unnecessary distraction, and in some services is actively or implicitly discouraged. With the growing generations of theoretically informed occupational therapy practitioners there is, however, a steadily developing theory and evidence base for the profession. This is supported by increasing efforts by theorists to illustrate the value of evidence- and theory-based practice. There are therefore good reasons to be optimistic that theory- and evidence-based occupational therapy will become as central to practice as the values base that has traditionally guided so much of what occupational therapists do.

ABOUT ME

As a (slightly) late entrant to higher education in 1991 I remember being fascinated by my lectures on the theoretical perspectives of occupational therapy. I was fortunate to have excellent and engaging lecturers who encouraged critical thinking and appeared as enthused as I was about the academic, as well as the practice, value of occupational therapy. From the outset I recognised the two components of

theory and practice in occupational therapy as fundamentally interlinked. The importance of this theory–practice connection has guided the continued selection of a famous Scottish landmark (the Forth Bridge, a highly complicated structure linking two parts of the same landmass), as a highly appropriate symbolic image to use for the text's front cover. On graduation I worked for several years in community and forensic mental health settings, and embraced evidence- and theory-based practice. For the last 15 years I have benefitted from working in an interdisciplinary research unit for nurses, midwives and allied health professions. This has considerably broadened my research from being occupational therapy specific, to allied health, and laterally to public and global health focussed! Each of these steps has enabled me to look at and reflect on occupational therapy's theoretical developments with what feels like a more constructively critical eye than I would have managed had my research stayed solely within a purely occupational therapy domain. Conversely my exposure to public and global health has clearly illustrated the potential occupational therapy has to move beyond its traditional health care settings to influence and improve the public and global health agenda.

ABOUT THE BOOK

Foundations for Practice in Occupational Therapy is now an internationally recognised occupational therapy text. Its central worth is its potential to introduce occupational therapy students and clinicians to the key theories that explain, guide and develop contemporary occupational therapy research and practice. *Foundations* presents a range of different, and at times conflicting, perspectives. Similarities too can be drawn across seemingly different conceptual models and frames of reference. Is there one conceptual model or are all equal and is it purely down to personal preference? Some certainly have a greater evidence base; others have an intuitively attractive logic or face validity. At least one challenges the fundamental basis upon which most, if not all, of the others are based. It is a book that I hope encourages the reader to think, rather than providing a simplistic answer.

Foundations was initially published based in 1992, based on the 30 years of professional practice of Rosemary Hagedorn (its founding author). Almost 30 years later, it has evolved into its sixth edition. For the last 13 years *Foundations* has been an edited text, with a wealth of contributions from leaders across the world. A review of the fourth and fifth editions show that some chapters have come and gone. These changes are not accidental. Each edition offers the opportunity to reflect on current practice and, with an eye to the next five years or so, consider what theoretical knowledge would be of most value as the profession continues to move ahead.

This sixth edition has been substantially updated. There are new chapters and new authors of existing chapters. Chapters that were in previous editions have been updated with the latest evidence and perspectives, and all chapters have been given an even greater practice focus. It is my hope that these revisions make this edition a worthy successor to its predecessors and that the text will continue to be of value to all those who seek to enhance their understanding and implementation of evidence- and theory-based occupational therapy practice.

Edward Duncan
2018

Twitter: @easduncan

CONTRIBUTORS

The editor(s) would like to acknowledge and offer grateful thanks for the input of all previous editions' contributors, without whom this new edition would not have been possible.

Julie D. Bass PhD, OTR/L, FAOTA
Professor and Past Chair of the Department of Occupational Therapy and Founding Director of Public Health Program, St. Catherine University, Saint Paul, Minnesota, USA

Carolyn M. Baum PhD, OTR/L, MA, FAOTA
Elias Michael Director and Professor of Occupational Therapy and Professor of Neurology and Social Work, Washington University School of Medicine, Saint Louis, USA

Charles H. Christiansen BS, MA, EdD, OTR, FAOTA
Clinical Professor and Former Chair, Department of Occupational Therapy, The University of Texas Medical Branch, Galveston, USA

Jane Davis MSc, OT Reg (Ont), OTR
Lecturer, Department of Occupational Science and Occupational Therapy, University of Toronto, Toronto, Canada

Edward A.S. Duncan PhD, BSc (Hons), Dip CBT
Associate Professor of Applied Health Research, Nursing Midwifery and Allied Health Professions Research Unit, University of Stirling, Stirling, Scotland, United Kingdom; Honorary Advanced Clinical Practitioner, NHS Forth Valley, Scotland, United Kingdom

Leisle Ezekiel MRes, MRCOT
Senior Lecturer in Occupational Therapy, Faculty of Health and Life Sciences, Oxford Brookes University, Oxford, UK

Sally Feaver MSc, MA, MRCOT
Principal Lecturer in Occupational Therapy & Programme Leader BSc Occupational Therapy and MSc (Preregistration) Occupational Therapy, Oxford Brookes University, Oxford, UK

Sarah Fletcher-Shaw
PhD Candidate and Senior Lecturer in Occupational Therapy, Department of Allied Health Professionals, Sport and Exercise, School of Human and Health Sciences, University of Huddersfield, Huddersfield, UK

Kirsty Forsyth PhD, BSc, MSc
Professor of Occupational Therapy, School of Health Sciences, Queen Margaret University, Edinburgh, UK

Lou Ann Griswold PhD
Associate Professor & Department Chair, Department of Occupational Therapy, University of New Hampshire, Durham, New Hampshire, USA

Michael Iwama PhD, OT(C), MSc, BSc, OT BSc
Dean of the School of Health and Rehabilitation Sciences, and Professor in the Department of Occupational Therapy, MGH Institute of Health Professions, Boston, USA

Kee Hean Lim PhD, MSc, Dip COT, SROT
Lecturer in Occupational Therapy, Division of Occupational Therapy, Brunel University London, Uxbridge, UK

Ian R. McMillan MEd, PgDip EdRes, Dip COT, Cert Ed, MRCOT
Former Head of Occupational Therapy & Arts Therapies, School of Health Sciences, Queen Margaret University, Edinburgh, UK

Matthew Molineux JP (Qual), BOccThy, MSc, PhD, MBA
Professor and Head, Discipline of Occupational Therapy, School of Allied Health Sciences, Griffith University, Queensland, Australia

Davina M. Parker Dip COT, MSc, PhD
Former Head of Occupational Therapy, University Hospitals Birmingham NHS Foundation Trust, Birmingham, UK

Helene J. Polatajko BOT, MEd, PhD
Professor, Department of Occupational Science and Occupational Therapy, University of Toronto, Toronto, Canada

Catherine Sutherland Dip COT, MSc
Brain Injury Case Manager, The Rehabilitation Partnership Ltd, Alvechurch, UK

Carolyn A. Unsworth PhD, BAppSci (OccTher)
Professor of Occupational Therapy, School of Health, Central
    Queensland University, Melbourne, Victoria, Australia;
    Adjunct Professor, School of Rehabilitation, Jonkoping
    University, Jonkoping, Smaland, Sweden; Adjunct Professor,
    La Trobe University, Melbourne, Victoria, Australia

Gail Whiteford BAppSc, MHSc, PhD
Strategic Professor & Conjoint Chair of Allied Health and
    Community Wellbeing, School of Community Health,
    Charles Sturt University, Port Macquarie, NSW, Australia

ACKNOWLEDGEMENTS

This book would not have been possible without the generous and dedicated contribution of a range of people:

The contributors. It has been a huge privilege to work with each of the individuals who have contributed to this sixth edition of *Foundations*. Some of them have been part of the *Foundations* story since its first edited edition in 2006, and a part of my personal occupational therapy journey for considerably longer. Others have joined *Foundations* for the first time in this edition. All of them have shaped the text and my thinking. And each of them has my greatest respect for the work they do and all they give to the development of occupational therapy theory and practice.

The publishers. Elsevier have provided great support in the development of this sixth edition. Particular thanks are due to Fiona Conn and Poppy Garraway for their patience, encouragement and guidance in bringing this text to fruition.

Nursing, Midwifery and Allied Health Professions Research Unit, University of Stirling. I am highly fortunate to work in a supportive and challenging research environment. Although not contributing directly to this text, many of the staff have influenced my thinking and continually challenge and inspire me to find ways to develop high quality evidence and theory, and to bridge the theory–practice divide. Consequently, although perhaps not immediately apparent, their influence has left it imprint throughout this text.

My family. Anne, Catherine, Eleanor and Joseph have shown, yet again, their unceasing patience with me as I have worked on this edition. Their support, love and belief in me are invaluable, and more appreciated than they will ever fully realise.

ACKNOWLEDGMENTS

Introduction to the Philosophy, Principles and Practice of Occupational Therapy

Introduction

Edward A.S. Duncan

FOUNDATIONS FOR PRACTICE

Foundations for Practice in Occupational Therapy was originally published in 1992 by Rosemary Hagedorn. It was groundbreaking. Rosemary presented the first British-authored comprehensive introduction of the theoretical foundations of occupational therapy. The book was an instant success. Approaching 30 years and six editions later, *Foundations* has become an established occupational therapy core text both in Britain and internationally. The profession remains greatly indebted to Rosemary Hagedorn. In 1995, Rosemary's achievements were rightly acknowledged when she was selected to deliver the prestigious Casson Memorial Lecture at the College of Occupational Therapists' Annual Conference. In 1998 she received the honour of becoming a Fellow of the then College of Occupational Therapists.

Looking back across the different editions of *Foundations* is like reading a recent history of the profession's theoretical development. The first three editions of *Foundations for Practice* were shaped by Rosemary's personal perspective and based on her lifetime career and experience as an occupational therapist. The 4th and 5th editions formed a new perspective. This 6th edition represents another step forward for the text and reflects the changes, challenges and developments that are occurring within the profession today. This latest edition is increasingly theory and evidence based. But the focus remains on how theory and its supporting evidence can benefit practice. This is done with the aspiration that—through time—practice will become increasingly based on robust and useful theory and evidence.

THE PURPOSE OF THIS BOOK

This book is an introduction to the theoretical foundations of occupational therapy. There are differing views on the place and use of theory in practice. Great care was taken when planning the content of the book to establish a quality focus for the selected models and frames of reference, while representing a variety of differing perspectives. Each chapter has been written to provide a comprehensive introduction to its topic, setting key contemporary issues within their historical basis and focusing on their relevance to practice. Of obvious use to undergraduate occupational therapy students, the book's expanded and revised content makes it a valuable resource for therapists who wish to practice from a sound theoretical and evidence base. It will also assist nonoccupational therapists to achieve a better understanding of the scope and practice of the profession.

THE CONTENTS OF THIS BOOK

The book is arranged in four sections. Section 1 introduces the philosophy, principles and practice of occupational therapy. Key concepts concerning the philosophical and theoretical basis of the profession are defined and summarized. The section outlines some of the main external influences on the profession and places particular emphasis upon the various shifts that have occurred within occupational therapy's theoretical foundations over time. To understand the external influences that continue to shape occupational therapy clearly, this section explores the impact that various philosophical systems have had on its theory and practice.

The section then continues by concentrating on the historical and more recent internal influences that affect the development and focus of contemporary occupational therapy practice. It provides an overview of occupational therapy and outlines the practice and skills required of an occupational therapist today. This section presents a description of the processes through which occupational therapy is carried out and concludes by introducing frames of reference and conceptual models of practice, outlining their roles and mutually dependent relationships in practice.

Section 2 provides an introduction to key conceptual models of practice. Five conceptual models of practice are presented: the Model of Human Occupation (Chapter 6); the Canadian Model of Occupational Performance (Chapter 7); the Person–Environment–Occupation Performance Model (Chapter 8); the Occupational Therapy Intervention Process Model (Chapter 9); and the *Kawa* (River) Model (Chapter 10). They do not represent all the available models but have been included as conceptual models that are among the most evidence-based, reflect popular usage in practice, or are topical.

Section 3 introduces four frames of reference in occupational therapy practice. Each chapter is written by occupational therapists experienced in their theory, and direct reference is made to their application in practice. Chapters are presented on the person-centred frame of reference (Chapter 11); the cognitive–behavioural frame of reference (Chapter 12); the psychodynamic, the biomechanical frame of reference (Chapter 13); and theoretical approaches to motor control and cognitive–perceptual dysfunction (Chapter 14).

Section 4 provides an introduction to two other important areas of theory. Clinical reasoning is in many ways the 'glue' that holds together theoretical reasoning and flexibly responsive practice; Chapter 15 presents a new and engaging overview of clinical reasoning research and practice in occupational therapy. Occupational science has been a prolific focus of research and debate in occupational therapy since its inception it has been met with both enthusiasm and consternation. Chapter 16 provides an excellent introduction to the field and explores the breadth of occupational science, without shirking from the questions that surround its place in occupational therapy practice today.

ADVICE TO READERS

There are several ways in which this book can be read. For those who are particularly new to the area or who have not read about theoretical constructs in occupational therapy for some time, it is strongly advisable to work through Section 1 before moving on to other chapters. However, you may feel familiar enough with these concepts and wish to focus on a particular topic. In this situation it is possible to go directly to the chapter(s) of interest. Do not, however, assume that all your answers will always be covered in one chapter. To understand fully what each author is saying, it is often necessary to take a step away from any professional biases one may have and enter fully into the perspective of other contributors: a task that may often prove more challenging in practice than in principle. It is therefore advisable to read across chapters and evaluate differing perspectives. Throughout this process it is important to take a critically evaluative approach to the material presented.

UNDERSTANDING OCCUPATIONAL THERAPY

Occupational therapy has a broad knowledge base, derived from medical and social sciences, as well as the moral treatment and arts and crafts movements. Therapists work with all age groups and assist with a wide range of medical, social and environmental problems. Occupational therapy practice appears deceptively simple. Its focus is the doing of everyday activities; its 'complexity' is in understanding the factors that influence and shape these activities and in constructing interventions that will enable each client to achieve their goals.

THE PRINCIPAL CONCERNS OF OCCUPATIONAL THERAPY

Each person wants to participate effectively in a meaningful life and to remain healthy and happy. To achieve these goals, it is argued, a person needs a degree of personal competence in a range of culturally accepted, useful and meaningful occupations. What these occupations are will differ from person to person according to individual and societal needs and circumstances.

Occupational Therapy

- Is concerned with the key elements of occupational performance and identity: how a person identifies themselves and their future aspirations, their roles and their relationships, together with their personal capacity for fulfilling these within their physical and social environment.
- Aims to enable and empower people to be competent and confident in their daily lives, and thereby to enhance well-being and minimize the effects of dysfunction or environmental barriers.

Occupational Therapists

- Use everyday occupations and tasks creatively and therapeutically to achieve goals that are meaningful to people and relevant to their daily life.
- Encourage people to collaborate in the therapeutic process to become partners in the design and direction of therapy and the (re)enabling of their life.

COMPETENCE AND DYSFUNCTION

Occupational therapists believe that *occupational competency* in everyday activities depends on a complex interaction between the individual, the things they do and their environment. An individual's well-being is directly related to the quality of this interaction. When a person is performing, they are able to meet the demands of each task, to respond adaptively to the demands of each environment and to use the skills and knowledge they have learnt to act, interact and react appropriately in all the everyday situations that they encounter.

The opposite to occupational competence is *occupational dysfunction*. This is a temporary or enduring inability to engage in the roles, relationships and occupations expected of a person of comparable age and sex within a particular culture. Occupational dysfunction becomes apparent when a person is unable to do the ordinary everyday things they want or need to do. It is often when a person experiences occupational dysfunction that they are referred to an occupational therapist. The reasons for dysfunction are very variable and range from the simple to the extremely complex.

THE OCCUPATIONAL THERAPY PERSPECTIVE

Occupational therapists endeavour to understand the nature of a client's *occupational identity* (who they are and who they would like to be), as well as their *occupational performance* (what their physical, cognitive and social abilities are). Frequently employing a conceptual model of practice and or an appropriate frame of reference, within the context of the process of care (see Chapter 4 for further information), action is taken to reduce the impact of a client's condition (or the effect of the environment in relation to their condition) and to maximize each client's ability to engage in valued daily activities.

Occupational therapists are not, however, limited to considering the impact of health problems on a client's life, important though these may be. Occupational dysfunction is frequently associated with a failure to adapt to a changing set of circumstances that can overload one's personal capacity to respond. A client may have lost skills or never have learnt them. They may have some negative emotional reaction connected with a task. The physical environment may be badly designed, too demanding or not demanding enough. The social environment may be too stressful or insufficiently supportive. The task may be too difficult or the tools used inappropriate. The role of the occupational therapist is to intervene to help each individual to regain occupational performance where possible and (re)develop meaning and purpose in life.

Most people become dysfunctional to some extent when faced with an unfamiliar or difficult situation or when confronted by a very stressful life event. Such dysfunction is usually transient and either resolves when the stress is removed, responds to minimal advice or assistance

or disappears once the person has learnt how to cope. This type of dysfunction may also occur as a result of external factors when there is no personal impairment or health condition. One way of looking at occupational dysfunction is to describe it as a lack of balance or 'fit' between the skills of a client, the challenges of their environment and the difficulties of their required occupation.

Occupational therapists address occupational dysfunction using a range of interventions that often include adapting the demands of an everyday activity, altering the physical or social environment, teaching a client a new repertoire of skills or helping them to re-establish ones they have lost. Frequently, the kind of complex occupational dysfunction that requires intervention from an occupational therapist is persistent and will often affect many aspects of clients' lives. Unfortunately, to date, negligible research exists in several areas of occupational therapy (e.g., mental health), making it difficult to distinguish those individuals who are likely to experience persistent occupational dysfunction from those who are not. Consequently, it is possible that therapists are missing valuable opportunities for early intervention with clients who do not initially appear as if they will have enduring occupational dysfunction. Further predictive research is required in areas of complexity for occupational therapists to become more targeted and effective in their interventions. Looking to the future, occupational therapy has clear potential to become increasingly involved in public, population and global health—embracing the value of occupation to avoid or ameliorate public health and social challenges in varying different settings across the world

ACKNOWLEDGING COMPETING IDEAS

In October 2015, a disgruntled reviewer of the 5th edition of *Foundations* rated it (on a well-known online store) '1 star'. The reviewer stated that the book 'argued with itself' and was 'A book of questions, not answers!' There is some truth to this view, and yet it simultaneously missed the point completely. From source to outlet, rivers follow the path of least resistance; in wrestling with occupational theory it is tempting for therapists to do the same. This book offers no simple solutions to the use of theory in practice. Therapists should choose the most robust and appropriate theories to drive practice, not simply the easiest. Occupational therapy's theoretical and evidence base is rapidly developing, and the profession has entered an exciting new era as therapists become increasingly research-active in a variety of ways, from collaborating in clinical data collection to acting as a principal investigator. Consequently, idiosyncratic perspectives of practice are increasingly challenged, well-known conceptual models of practice and frames of reference are increasingly evaluated and new theoretical perspectives and questions arise.

Several contrasting theoretical perspectives are presented within this book. Examples of such perspectives include theorists' understanding of conceptual models of practice (see Chapter 5), their understanding of complexity (see Chapters 3, 12 and 15) and culture (see Chapters 6 and 10), and the manner in which professional knowledge is developed (see Chapters 3, 6 and 15). The debate caused by such contrasting perspectives should be embraced and not shunned, as they illustrate the challenges of developing the profession's theoretical and evidence base. Readers are encouraged to use the index and cross-references within each chapter in order to understand these issues in greater depth.

These competing ideas will, amongst others, shape the future of occupational therapy theoretical research. Through the crucible of reflection and research, clinically relevant theories will be questioned, challenged and refined. From them, practice will become ever more evidence-based, and, consequently, clients will receive a more effective and meaningful service.

A LOOK TO THE FUTURE

Delivery of effective occupational therapy is an ethical and professional imperative. Practice should be consistently effective. To reach this goal, practice needs to become increasingly theoretically and evidence-based and should be delivered in a flexibly responsive manner to meet the needs of individual clients. Each client should receive a similarly high-quality service, regardless of their location or the therapist with whom they are working. Such consistency is difficult to achieve.

It is well recognized that therapists' individual judgements, regardless of expertise, are affected by a wide range of biases and *heuristics* (mental shortcuts) (Grove & Meehl 1996, Grove et al 2000). Therapists using personal judgement alone are often much less effective than they believe. The embracing of evidence-based conceptual models of practice and frames of reference helps therapists to consider a wide range of factors and should increase their consistency and agreement. Used in this way, theoretical

frameworks enable therapists to provide comprehensive interventions with clearly definable and measurable outcomes. Some therapists may react against this suggestion and feel that using such theories places undue constraints on their practice. Perhaps some will suggest that this perspective appears to make practice fit theory instead of theory fitting practice and is therefore not client centred. This, however, is a fallacy, a false dilemma. Such a position distracts attention from the known biases of individual therapist judgements by suggesting that conceptual models and frames of reference lack perfection and this is a reason for their rejection. Although existing theoretical frameworks undoubtedly need to be enhanced, this does not justify practising from a perspective of individual judgement that is known to be flawed. Theoretically driven and evidence-based occupational therapy must be embraced in practice. The people we work with deserve no less.

SUMMARY

This chapter sets the latest edition of *Foundations* in the context of previous editions of the book. This edition continues to build on its predecessors. The book has been thoroughly updated, and new chapters are included from leading academics in the field. The theoretical basis of occupational therapy has developed over several years and has reached a very exciting stage. Several contributors to this text offer conflicting opinions about theoretical issues. Such a divergence of opinion is useful. It will, through academic debate and research, strengthen the profession and provide it with an ever more robust theoretical evidence base. Engage in the issues presented and think critically about what you read.

REFERENCES

Grove, W. M., & Meehl, P. E. (1996). Comparative efficiency of informal (subjective, impressionistic) and formal (mechanical, algorithmic) prediction procedures: The clinical/statistical controversy. *Psychology Public Policy and Law, 2*, 1–31.

Grove, W. M., Zald, D. H., Boyd, S. L., et al. (2000). Clinical versus mechanical prediction: A meta-analysis. *Psychological Assessment, 12*(1), 19–30.

2

Theoretical Foundations of Occupational Therapy: External Influences

Edward A.S. Duncan

OVERVIEW

This chapter outlines the main external influences on occupational therapy's theoretical foundation. *Philosophy* may appear to be a somewhat unrelated subject to the applied nature of occupational therapy; however, to gain a comprehensive understanding of occupational therapy theory, it is necessary to gain a conceptual understanding of the impact that various philosophical systems have had upon healthcare in general and occupational therapy in particular. This chapter commences with an overview of what theory is and the main factors that have influenced theoretical developments within occupational therapy. A particular emphasis is placed on the various shifts that have occurred within occupational therapy's theoretical foundations over time. To understand clearly the various external influences that have shaped and continue to shape the theoretical foundations of occupational therapy, this chapter dedicates a significant proportion of space to understanding the impact that various philosophical systems have had on theory and practice.

HIGHLIGHTS

- Occupational therapy's development has been shaped by the influence of a variety of external philosophical influences.
- This chapter provides an overview of key external influences and how they have shaped the profession.
- The Enlightenment and its consequent influence have led to the development of the evidence-based practice movement.
- Despite its critics, evidence-based practice will remain the dominant force in occupational therapy development over the forthcoming decade and beyond.

WHAT IS THEORY?

Put most simply, a theory is a proposition of why something occurs or does not, is or is not. Formal theories are developed, to greater or lesser extents, and should be evaluated to see if they hold up to scrutiny. In occupational therapy, these formal theories often take the form of conceptual models of practice, although occupational science also develops formal theoretical perspectives of occupational therapy practice. There are also innumerable informal theories. Known as 'folk theories', they are intuitive explanations of the world. Each of us has well-developed folk theories of how and why things happen, and what is likely to occur if a specific course of action is undertaken. Folk theories develop from our experience and from what we are told by others (Bruner 2009). The trouble with folk theories is that they are highly subjective. They can be, but are not always, deeply flawed. Despite these significant limitations, folk theories are stubborn and hard to shift, even when faced with compelling evidence that indicates they are wrong (Gelman & Legare 2011).

Occupational therapy has a number of well-developed conceptual models of practice. Several of these are introduced in this text. These formal occupational therapy theories are important because they help to define the profession and guide practice, and explain how occupations are performed, what occupational problems are and why certain participant–therapist interactions occur during therapeutic interventions (Leclair et al 2013, Taylor 2017). Such is the importance of formal occupational therapy theory that Kielhofner (2009) went as far as to suggest that without their conscious use, an occupational therapy intervention or activity that takes place is unlikely to be therapeutic (Taylor 2017).

Although formal theories have many strengths and advantages, such a strong and unsubstantiated statement is unhelpful. Practitioners who work without conscious use of occupational therapy theories know that Kielhofner's statement often does not hold up to scrutiny, and that much of what they do 'works'. Consequently, many practitioners conclude that formal occupational therapy theories are overly complicated and unnecessary. For example, in a recent survey of 783 occupational therapists in the United Kingdom (Pentland et al 2018), approximately 20% of respondents found conceptual practice models to be very helpful, while almost 40% of respondents found them to be of little or no influence or unhelpful. Other surveys of practice have found a more favourable response to the use of formal theories in practice. A survey conducted by Davis-Cheshire and colleagues (2019) of 174 occupational therapists in the United States found that 79% of respondents used a formal theory of occupational therapy in practice and 78% of participants found formal theory to be highly valuable. However, although both surveys (Pentland et al 2018, Davis-Cheshire et al 2019) used convenience samples, the Pentland survey was much larger and widely publicized, having been commissioned by the Royal College of Occupational Therapists in the United Kingdom. It is likely that the formal endorsement of the Pentland survey engaged a wider range of respondents than the Davis-Cheshire survey. The latter may also have been even more susceptible to respondent bias as it was specifically about use of formal theory in practice. It seems, therefore, that many practitioners still do not consciously use or value formal occupational therapy theory, but those who do highly value their use in practice. Therefore the argument for formal theory use in occupational therapy should not be that we cannot practice without it, but rather that it enhances practice in multiple manners: reducing individual practitioner bias and error; providing a means to evidence practice; enabling communication of complicated occupational phenomena between practitioners; and clarifying the boundaries of professional practice (Taylor 2017).

Formal theory is often viewed as being detached from practice. Indeed, there remains a prevailing tendency to view theories as part of the activities that a student undertakes at university, while practice experience is gained during fieldwork education. Implicit within this split understanding of theory and practice is the idea that theory is unimportant to practice and vice versa. This narrative has endured within occupational therapy practice for decades and regrettably forms part of its 'hidden curriculum' (Hafferty & O'Donnell 2015). This has led to an enduring theory–practice gap within occupational therapy and other allied health professions (Ryan 2001). This gap is most evident in the difficulties that practitioners have in embedding research in practice (McCluskey & Lovarini 2005). Metcalfe et al (2001) undertook a postal questionnaire study among four allied health professional groups

(dietitians, occupational therapists, physiotherapists, and speech and language therapists) within a single National Health Service (NHS) region in England; 80% ($n = 573$) of the sample responded. Although dated, the findings remain relevant for contemporary practice. Each group agreed that research (from which sound theory develops) was important; however, they also highlighted barriers to using such knowledge. These barriers included a lack of understanding of the literature, insufficient time, inadequate facilities, professional isolation and resistance from colleagues. Similar barriers have been identified in the use of routine outcome measures, which are frequently associated with conceptual models of practice (Duncan & Murray 2012). It is apparent, therefore, that when theory is viewed as a distinct reality from practice, real barriers to its use develop. Such barriers are not simple to overcome. To address this issue, theory should grow in and from practice, and be viewed as central to all that it means to be an occupational therapist. It is precisely for this reason that this book places particular emphasis on the clinical application of theories in practice. Each chapter achieves this in a different manner.

ENVIRONMENTAL INFLUENCES ON THEORY DEVELOPMENT

Professions do not exist in isolation and are therefore open to influence from the pressures and prevailing norms of other professional groups and the environment in which they exist. Occupational therapy, existing predominantly within the health and social fields of society, has been observably influenced by the environmental influences within these settings and the prevailing pressures on professional groupings within these fields. To understand the environmental influences that have shaped occupational therapy throughout the ages, it is necessary to take a historical viewpoint of the development of the profession. You might wonder how history relates to theory; however, when history is read, it becomes apparent that it is interesting not only for its own sake, but also because it facilitates an understanding of contemporary practice. Just as our personal sense of identity is rooted in our family history, our professional identity and understanding are enriched by knowing their roots (Paterson 1997). Such history, states Paterson (1997), illustrates that, although early occupational therapy intervention held a humanistic concern for individuals' well-being from the outset, it was consistently accompanied by efforts to build a theoretical understanding about the various processes involved in the work of occupational therapists.

When examining the history of occupational therapy, or at least the effect of occupation on health, it is possible to look back as far as biblical and classical periods, where the remedial and health promotional effects of occupation can easily be seen (Wilcock 2001b). Occupation came to the fore of care again in the 19th century, with the development of 'moral treatment', although the focus of occupation during this period was perhaps more for economic than therapeutic gain (Wilcock 2001a). Although this appears to be a less than positive image of occupational therapy, it is perhaps in the moral treatment movement and the vision of William Tuke, a Quaker and key proponent of moral treatment, that the enduring patient-centred philosophy of occupational therapy can find its roots (Tuke 1813). With the onset of the 20th century and the formal establishment of occupational therapy training in the United Kingdom, the environmental effects of medicine and other disciplines on occupational therapists can be seen more clearly. Such influential effects on theoretical and practice development have been described as 'paradigmatic shifts' in the profession's understanding of the who, what and why of its existence (Kielhofner 2009) (see Chapter 3 for further information).

THE INFLUENCE OF PHILOSOPHY

Further to the external environmental influences that have directly shaped occupational theory and practice, it is also important to note the influence of philosophical perceptions of 'reality' and their impact on the development of occupational theory and practice. Philosophy is defined in Chamber's Dictionary as 'the pursuit of wisdom or knowledge … the principles underlying any sphere of knowledge'. A basic understanding of the philosophical principles relating to 'truth' is important for occupational therapists to attain, as it is from these that the foundational concepts for future theoretical developments discussed in this book emanate. Fundamentally, two concepts exist within the various philosophies that are central to all theoretical understanding: *ontology* and *epistemology*. Ontology can be most easily understood as the nature of knowledge, whereas epistemology is the approach taken to knowledge (Finlay & Ballinger 2006). Both are complex. Two fundamental views of nature exist that are important to understand when considering occupational therapy's theoretical developments: *positivism* and *antipositivism*.

Positivistic and PostPositivistic Paradigms

Positivism contends that there is an absolute reality, which can be measured, studied and understood, whereas postpositivism has been described as the perspective that an absolute reality can never be understood and may only be approximated (Denzin & Lincoln 2011). Positivism emerged from the thinking of the Enlightenment, an important period of philosophical development during the 17th century in Europe. Since its emergence, positivism has been very influential within medicine and healthcare in general. This influence has assisted in the discovery of cures for many diseases and has had a significant impact on people's lives.

Influence of Positivist Thinking on Healthcare and Occupational Therapy

As discussed, positivism and the scientific approach are believed to have directly influenced occupational therapy's willing acceptance of the reductionist period, during which occupational therapists attempted to gain professional credibility through employing medical-type interventions and theoretical concepts that were not necessarily understood through an occupational framework (Pols 2002). Although the profession has moved on in itself, it continues to be externally influenced by the positivistic tendencies of healthcare in general. Most recently, this influence can be witnessed through its adoption of evidence-based practice.

Evidence-based medicine (as the term was originally known) emerged from the McMaster medical school in Canada during the 1980s (Taylor 2000). However, the origins of the concept can be traced to the mid-19th century and Paris, and to Charles Alexandre Louis, considered a founding father of modern medical statistics (Hadjiliadis 2004). Sackett and colleagues (1996, p.71) defined evidence-based medicine as 'the conscientious, explicit and judicious use of current best evidence in making decisions about the care of individual patients'. Best evidence in this context is information that has been researched using quantitative methods such as randomized controlled trial and metaanalysis, both procedures that embrace the objective/positivistic nature of knowledge. Evidence-based practice is not, however, a purely objective pursuit. Sackett (1996) also emphasized that evidence-based practice is only part of the clinical decision-making process. Taylor (2000, p.2–3) reinforced this, stating, 'Evidence is gathered conscientiously but is used judiciously so that the experience of the occupational therapist, the needs of the patients/ client, the demands of the system and the up to date best evidence are weighed together in order that the best care is given'. Evidence-based practice has proven to be more than a passing trend. Despite the original emphasis on individual experience, as outlined in the quotation from Sackett, evidence-based practice has well-developed hierarchies of evidence that place greatest importance on objective studies such as metaanalyses and randomized controlled trials, with least emphasis given to clinical experience. Such studies have not always been universally accepted as appropriate methods to be used in occupational therapy and their use or potential use was the subject of great debate within British occupational therapy literature (Bannigan 2002, Copley 2002, Hyde 2002, Hyde 2004, Legg & Walker 2002, MacLean & Jones 2002, Bryant 2004, Eva & Paley 2004). However, with some exceptions (see later), the debate has largely moved on in recent years and high quality studies of the effectiveness of occupational therapy interventions are becoming more commonplace and generally well accepted (see for example Garvey et al 2015, Ikiugu et al 2017, Sackley et al 2015, Whitehead et al 2018).

AntiPositivistic Paradigms

Not everybody, however, agrees with the suppositions of positivistic and postpositivistic thinking. Some theorists view such structures as fundamentally restrictive and ignorant of alternative perspectives. This has led to the development of, amongst others, constructivist, interpretive and critical theory paradigms of nature. The fundamental basis of such approaches is that they propose multiple constructed realities, as different people are likely to experience the world in differing ways. This, in turn, leads to 'radical scepticism' regarding the possibilities for knowledge and a belief that research and, consequently, theoretical developments are only interpretations of multiple realities (Henwood & Nicholson 1996). Antipositivism is not therefore a single set of beliefs, but a set of approaches, each of which places a particular emphasis on the way that people may experience and understand the world. Such theories often appear initially attractive for occupational therapy, as the profession has frequently tried to define itself separately from the more traditional medical positivistic approach to healthcare. However, these philosophical approaches, although useful in delivering an alternative perspective of reality, are often unhelpful in a health economic era where finances are often restricted and scarce resources are dedicated to interventions that have a known efficacy (Duncan & Nicol 2004). There are too many antipositivistic philosophies to describe in this text and it is suggested that the interested reader should consult the bibliography and beyond for further information. Some antipositivistic theories are, however, of particular importance or have been increasingly used in occupational therapy research; three of these theories are introduced later as a primer for further reading.

Phenomenology

Developed by the German philosopher Edmund Husserl (1859–1938), phenomenology focuses on describing personal experiences and interpreting these experiences for individuals without developing overarching theories of truth (Schwartz 1994). The fundamental theory that forms phenomenology is that 'meaning can only be understood by those who experience it' (DePoy & Gitlin 1998). As we each experience life in differing ways, we will each therefore also make sense and find meaning in differing ways. Occupational therapy literature is increasingly influenced by phenomenological thought. This influence stems from its roots in 'moral treatment' and the arts and craft movement (Mattingly & Fleming 1994).

From a phenomenological perspective, illness or disease is not viewed simply as a matter of physiological dysfunction, but is understood through the effect that it has on the broader social place of the person in society (Mattingly & Fleming 1994). Several occupational therapy studies have explicitly used a phenomenological approach in their research (e.g., Colaianni et al 2015, Zafran et al 2017, Drolet & Désormeaux-Moreau 2016).

Because occupational therapists are often interested in viewing a person holistically, it is easy to see where phenomenological thought resonates with occupational theory and practice. An interest in the phenomenological approach to engaging with clients naturally leads occupational therapists to encourage clients to discuss their experiences of illness or disability and to develop meaningful life stories. This technique is known as using a narrative approach. A specific occupational therapy assessment has also been developed from this perspective (Kielhofner et al 1998).

Feminism

Feminism is a global term referring to a range of activities, movements and ideologies that aim to establish sexual equality. Fundamentally, feminism can be explored through three perspectives: liberal feminism, which focuses on the impact of socialization into gender roles; radical feminism, which posits that existence within a patriarchal society subordinates women; and Marxist feminism, which focuses on the exploitation of the capitalist class and its consequential effects on women (Hartery & Jones 1998). Occupational therapy's gender imbalance is believed to have had a considerable impact on its development and position in society. Wilcock (2001a, 2001b) acknowledges the overwhelming dominance of female occupational therapists during the early years of the profession. Although this appears to have been initially unquestioned and indeed related to caring roles previously associated with females (e.g., nursing and infant teaching), its potentially negative impact has more recently been considered. Taylor (1995) used a feminist approach to reflect on the impact of being a predominantly female profession. She highlights how occupational therapy has developed under the mantle of medicine, a profession that is dominated by men and is said to espouse the patriarchal values of society (Hugman 1991). Taylor (1995) relates this relationship to the distancing of the profession from its original connections with the arts and crafts movements and consequential move toward objective science. MacWhannell and Blair (1998, p.64) continue this theme, stating that 'a recurring issue within occupational therapy literature is a concern with the development of standardised assessment [a consequence of the patriarchal influence]. If the features that draw people to the profession are associated with engaging people in a process that moves toward growth and personal change and are not measurable or directly open to standardised outcome measures, the profession is in a conceptual conundrum. It is torn between one set of values and another'.

The impact of the profession's gender imbalance on occupational therapy's development is unquestionable; it has affected both the profession's value base and its position within society. Taking a single stance on the impact of gender on the profession is, however, unlikely to be beneficial in the long term and leaves one open to bias. A nonoccupational therapy example of how such bias can affect the theoretical and research basis of a subject is evident in two studies of therapeutic interventions with women who self-harm and are resident in secure units in England. Liebling and Chipchase (1996) describe a therapeutic group intervention for women who self-harm. Instead of taking a cognitive behavioural approach (see Chapter 12), which is widely used with this client group, Liebling and Chipchase (1996) employed feminist group therapy (Burstow 1992). The authors initially used a range of outcome measures, but these were abandoned, apparently because of resistance. Taking a feminist theory perspective, the authors interpreted this as a rejection of control. Low et al (2001), working with the same client group in a similar environment, carried out a similar study using a broadly cognitive behavioural approach. Unlike Liebling and Chipchase, Low employed a range of psychometric assessments without apparent detrimental impact. Although the studies are now relatively old, this example of differing outcomes based on opposing philosophical foundations still highlights the dangers of adhering to one perspective and the impact that this can have on research and practice, without considering one's own personal biases in influencing the interpretation or outcome of an event.

Kelly (1996, p.6), a male occupational therapist, acknowledged the continuing existence of the feminist principle within occupational therapy, but suggested that 'any system based upon the feminine principle or the masculine principle alone will not be sufficient; they must merge and actualise in the practice of occupational therapy'. More recently a study of occupational therapists in the United States surveyed participants' perceptions of the issues and factors around male occupational therapy practitioners (Maxim & Rice 2018). Although differences by gender of respondents were evident on issues such as the positive and negative impacts of therapists' gender, they expressed shared perspectives on job satisfaction, their contribution to society and sense of job security.

Pragmatism

Pragmatism is a philosophical tradition that originated in the United States in the late 19th century. The origins of pragmatism are attributed to American philosophers including William James, John Dewey and George Mead. Another important figure in the development of pragmatism, and in particular the application of its principles, was Jane Addams (1860–1935), who was also highly involved in the founding of occupational therapy in the United States (Morrison 2016). In essence, pragmatism values an idea on how useful it is or can be applied; it emphasizes action over thought and raises practical action to a higher level than abstract thinking. This approach to knowledge is in sharp contrast to more abstract idealistic philosophies that preceded its development. Hooper and Wood (2002) argue that some occupational therapists' rejection of evidence-based practice is essentially due to the differences between the objective and measurable perspective of structuralism, that lies evidence-based practice, and the pragmatic philosophical approach to practice that can been found within contemporary occupational therapy and was fundamental to its origins. Certainly, the practical nature of pragmatism and its near contemporaneous development with the founding of occupational therapy in the United States and the United Kingdom led to pragmatism having a strong influence on the development of the profession. In fact, the close relationship of pragmatism to occupational therapy led Breines (1986) to suggest that pragmatist philosophy was introduced into healthcare via occupational therapy. The relationship between occupational therapy and pragmatism is therefore clear. Characteristics of the profession, such as its emphasis on providing a holistic approach, its advocacy for social inclusion, and its recognition on social inclusion barriers occurring in society, not the individual, all have their roots in the profession's application of pragmatism (Morrison 2016), and a novel analysis of occupational therapy and pragmatic literature by Ikiugu and Schultz (2006) concluded that the assumptions, values and principles of occupational therapy are directly compatible with pragmatist philosophy.

PostModernism

Postmodernism is not an easy concept to grasp. It has affected a wide range of disciplines, from the arts to the sciences, and architecture to technology. It is not therefore surprising that occupational therapy has also been evaluated from a postmodernist perspective (Weinblatt & Avrech-Bar 2001). Postmodernism rejects the modernist proposal that truth can be controlled and explained through scientific analysis (Weinblatt & Avrech-Bar 2001). Webber (1995, p.439), in explaining the postmodernistic rejection of objectivity, states that 'there is nothing to be gained from past "explanatory systems" but that there is a real danger in generalising or universalising since each individual or event is unique'. Postmodernism, therefore, directly challenges the concept of objectivity and suggests that, if reality can be described at all, it is as a process of continual change that focuses on the local rather than the universal. Such concepts are attractive to occupational theorists and practitioners, as they appear to validate professional values such as the worth of an individual or the uniqueness of each moment and activity.

Within occupational therapy's theory development, Webber (1995) aligns with postmodernism in their rejection of scientific objectivity and the use of standardized assessments and outcome measurements in practice. Many occupational therapists' rejections of objectivity, universal conceptual models of practice and standardized assessments can find a philosophical basis within postmodernistic thinking.

The limitations of positivistic thinking in occupational therapy practice are evident. However, outright rejection of objective theories and philosophical foundations requires careful consideration. Occupational therapists work predominantly in generally positivistic systems (such as healthcare) and are required to demonstrate their value within such environments. It is unlikely, therefore, that a purely postmodernistic stance will greatly affect the philosophical basis of healthcare and may in fact lead to great professional isolation for occupational therapists in an increasingly evidence-based context. However, healthcare environments are evolving and moving from a purely positivistic understanding of reality. This is perhaps most starkly evident in the prominence given to the experience and voice of service users in healthcare today. What, then, is the way forward for occupational therapy and theory development?

Traditionally, positivism and antipositivism have been viewed as too conceptually conflicting to merge in any meaningful manner. However, the complex nature of developing meaningful and transferable theories on which to enhance individuals' level of care and intervention requires the employment of a variety of approaches.

Realism

Realism is the philosophical position that reality exists independent of how we perceive it and of how we think it functions, but recognises that our understanding of reality is always partial (Maxwell 2012). Within social science, realism is most closely associated with the work of Roy Bhaskar, who developed critical realism (Archer et al 2013). Critical realism offers a resolution to the dilemmas faced by the contrasting arguments of positivism and postmodernism. From Bhaskar's original work several other forms of realist understanding have developed (Archer et al 2013). One form of realist understanding is 'subtle realism' (Hammersley 1990). Its proponents state that all knowledge involves subjective perceptions and observations, and concede that various individuals will produce different pictures of the reality under study. Hammersley (1990) and Kirk and Miller (1986), however, propose that these subjective perceptions and observations do not preclude the existence of independent phenomena, and that objects, relationships and experiences can therefore be studied and understood. The subtle realist understands that there is no manner in which an individual can claim to have absolute certainty regarding a phenomenon. Rather, 'the objective should be the search for knowledge about which we can be reasonably confident. Such confidence will be based upon judgements about the credibility and plausibility of knowledge claims' (Murphy et al 1998, p.69). This concept has been criticised as having no true ontological basis (Seale 1999), despite others (Smith & Heshusius 1986) arguing that subtle realism is a postpositivist/realist approach. Despite such criticisms, the realist approach is increasingly being embraced in healthcare and supported as a positive advancement for theoretical and research development in healthcare. The challenges in developing occupational therapy theory 'reach to the ontological and epistemological roots of knowledge' (Duncan 2004). Subtle realism offers a philosophical foundation that embraces the complexity of knowledge and of occupational therapy within the intricacies and realities of its working environments and provides a useful alternative perspective for future research and theoretical development. It is now over 15 years since I first wrote about the application of subtle realism in occupational therapy (Duncan 2004). During this time I have worked as an applied health researcher and grappled with issues of truth, evidence and complexity. I have found no better explanation of how to approach reality in practice. Subtle realism is a pragmatic solution, which appeals to my occupational therapy education, reflects my understanding of the world and enables me to make sense of occupational therapy in both research and practice.

Marxism

Marxist thought is undoubtedly best known for its effect on politics and sociology during the 20th century. Most people, on hearing the word Marxist, think of the historical communist regime of the Eastern Bloc (Wilcock 2001a). Such was the impact of Marx's political thinking that his founding philosophies of the centrality of occupation remain relatively unknown. This is, in part, caused by the fact that the majority of his early writings were not published in English until the mid-20th century (Wilcock 2001a). The inclusion of a section on Marx may surprise some readers, yet he could be described as an early occupational scientist (Wilcock 2001a) (see Chapter 18 for an introduction to occupational science). Fundamentally, Marx (1964) developed the concept of 'alienated labour', which he viewed as an inevitable consequence of capitalist societies. Although Marx believed that occupations should be uplifting and socially involving, he also believed that in general individuals' productive occupations were developed to produce commodities (Corrigan 2001). In essence, Marx argued for a more socially just way of living: one that recognized that individuals require satisfaction in what they do, as well as adequately meeting life's requirements. Marx viewed the difficulties that faced individuals in life as largely being a result of the imposition of social organization rather than naturally occurring (Hartery & Jones 1998). Such a vision of occupation suggests that occupational therapists should focus on being agents of social change rather than a part of the process that maintains social conformity. Indeed, Corrigan (2001, p.204) suggests that 'the profession's need to maintain credibility within other discourses inadvertently diminishes its capacity to act socially'. In other words, it could be suggested that in occupational therapy's determination to become accepted within the systems in which it works, it has to a certain extent limited its potential to become a social agent for change. Increased recognition of the impact of society on the individual's occupational potential has, however, redressed this balance to some extent, and occupational therapists are increasingly adding their voice as agents of social change. Bryant (2016), in her Casson Memorial Lecture, convincingly argued that there is direct line from Marx to current occupational therapy theory and practice, such as that by Creek (2010), Gerlach (2015) and Godoy-Viera et al (2018).

Culture

The nature of culture is complex and is not easily defined. Culture refers to shared meanings through which individuals interact and the specific beliefs, values and norms that shape the everyday behaviour of individuals and groups of people. The breadth of occupational therapy practice is now international, and multicultural societies are commonplace within Western societies (Dyck 1998). It is appropriate, therefore, to question whether the philosophical foundations of the profession and the professional frames of reference and models of practice that have developed from them (which have been developed in Western society) are relevant to substantial populations with whom occupational therapists interact. Occupational therapy is recognized as a profession that embraces Western values (e.g., independence) and the maintenance of a 'healthy' life-role balance between work, leisure and self-care. Such concepts may, however, be of less importance to people of other cultures. These issues have led to the presentation of alternative philosophical constructs of occupational therapy that are based on Eastern philosophies (Jang 1993, Dawson 2000) (see Chapter 5 for further discussion on cultural issues in conceptual models of practice and Chapter 10 for information about the Kawa [River] model that has roots within Japanese culture). However, cultural incompatibility of Western-based occupational therapy models should not be assumed. Despite legitimate cultural concerns, evidence for the compatibility of Western-based models of practice (such as the Model of Human Occupation, see Chapter 6) with culturally diverse environments, such as that of African traditional healers (Kelly 1995) and other cultures, suggests that it is possible for such approaches to have resonance with culturally diverse populations.

Consideration of the societal culture in which occupational therapy is practiced and the cultural groupings of an individual within any given environment are of the utmost importance to occupational therapy practice. An individual's cultural background, whether at a macro level (e.g., country or religion) or at a micro level (e.g., an individual's family, work and social background), will undoubtedly affect their belief in self, habits and routines and the social and physical environment in which they exist. This should, in turn, affect the manner in which the occupational therapist relates to an individual and the nature of their collaboration. The precise impact of employing a Western-based cultural model of practice with individuals from other cultural backgrounds, however, remains uncertain.

SUMMARY

Occupational therapy has been shaped by a wide variety of philosophies throughout the course of its history to the present day. These theories form the foundation of the profession's current theoretical developments. It is possible to see how each of the philosophies has moulded the profession through its paradigmatic shifts and how each of them provides lenses through which the profession and an individual's professional practice can be understood today. Each reader is invited to reflect on the discussions presented in this chapter, and to consider where their philosophical life perspectives place them and the impact these have on their practice as an occupational therapist.

✳ REFLECTIVE LEARNING

- What philosophical perspectives influence how you live your life and what your values are?
- How do these perspectives affect your practice?
- Do you have any philosophical beliefs or values that may ethically affect your practice? If yes, how do you avoid this occurring? If no, what sort of philosophical beliefs could affect your practice?
- What role do you think culture has in how occupational therapists practice?

REFERENCES

Archer, M., Bhaskar, R., Collier, A., Lawson, T., & Norrie, A. (2013). *Critical realism: Essential readings*. Routledge.

Bannigan, K. (2002). EBP, RCTs and a climate for mutual respect. *British Journal of Occupational Therapy*, 65(8), 391–392.

Breines, E. (1986). *Origins and adaptations: A philosophy of practice*. Lebanon, NJ: Geri-Rehab.

Bruner, J. S. (2009). *Actual minds, possible worlds*. Harvard University Press.

Bryant, W. (2004). Numbers in evidence. *British Journal of Occupational Therapy*, 6(2), 99–100.

Bryant, W. (2016). The Dr Elizabeth Casson Memorial Lecture 2016: Occupational alienation – A concept for modelling participation in practice and research. *British Journal of Occupational Therapy*, 79(9), 521–529.

Burstow, B. (1992). *Radical feminist therapy*. Newbury Park: Sage.

Davis-Cheshire, R., Davis, K., Drumm, L., Neal, S., Norris, E., Parker, M., Prezzia, C., & Whalen, C. (2019). The perceived value and utilization of occupational therapy models in the United States. *Journal of Occupational Therapy Education*, 3(2), 11.

Colaianni, D. J., Provident, I., DiBartola, L. M., & Wheeler, S. (2015). A phenomenology of occupation–based hand therapy. *Australian Occupational Therapy Journal*, 62(3), 177–186.

Copley, J. (2002). RCTs: Continuing the debate. *British Journal of Occupational Therapy*, 65(7), 346–347.

Corrigan, K. (2001). Doing time in mental health: Discipline at the end of medicine. *British Journal of Occupational Therapy*, 64(4), 203–205.

Creek, J. (2010). *The core concepts of occupational therapy: A dynamic framework for practice*. Jessica Kingsley Publishers.

Dawson, F. (2000). The three-dimensional model of self: A Japanese model of practice. *British Journal of Occupational Therapy*, 63(7), 340–342.

Denzin, N. K., & Lincoln, Y. S. (Eds.). (2011). *The Sage handbook of qualitative research*. Sage.

DePoy, E., & Gitlin, L. N. (1998). *Introduction to research* (2nd ed.). St Louis: Mosby.

Drolet, M. J., & Désormeaux-Moreau, M. (2016). The values of occupational therapy: Perceptions of occupational therapists in Quebec. *Scandinavian Journal of Occupational Therapy*, 23(4), 272–285.

Duncan, E. A., & Murray, J. (2012). The barriers and facilitators to routine outcome measurement by allied health professionals in practice: A systematic review. *BMC Health Services Research*, 12(1), 96.

Duncan, E. A. S., & Nicol, M. (2004). Subtle reasoning and occupational therapy: An alternative approach to knowledge generation and evaluation. *British Journal of Occupational Therapy*, 67(10), 453–456.

Dyck, I. (1998). Multicultural society. In D. Jones, et al. (Ed.), *Sociology and occupational therapy: An integrated approach*. Edinburgh: Churchill Livingstone.

Eva, G., & Paley, J. (2004). Numbers in evidence. *British Journal of Occupational Therapy*, 67(1), 47–50.

Finlay, L., & Ballinger, C. (Eds.). (2006). *Qualitative research for allied health professionals: Challenging choices*. John Wiley & Sons.

Garvey, J., Connolly, D., Boland, F., & Smith, S. M. (2015). OPTIMAL, an occupational therapy led self-management support programme for people with multimorbidity in primary care: A randomized controlled trial. *BMC Family Practice*, 16(1), 59.

Gelman, S. A., & Legare, C. H. (2011). Concepts and folk theories. *Annual Review of Anthropology*, 40, 379–398.

Gerlach, A. J. (2015). Sharpening our critical edge: Occupational therapy in the context of marginalized populations: Aiguiser notre sens critique: L'ergothérapie dans le contexte des populations marginalisées. *Canadian Journal of Occupational Therapy*, 82(4), 245–253.

Godoy-Vieira, A., Soares, C. B., Cordeiro, L., & Campos, C. M. S. (2018). Inclusive and emancipatory approaches to occupational therapy practice in substance-use contexts. *Canadian Journal of Occupational Therapy*, 85(4), 307–317.

Hadjiliadis, D. (2004). *Early clinical statistics. Internet web presentation*.

Hafferty, F. W., & O'Donnell, J. F. (Eds.). (2015). *The hidden curriculum in health professional education*. Dartmouth College Press.

Hammersley, M. (1990). *Reading ethnographic research*. New York: Longman.

Hartery, T., & Jones, D. (1998). What is sociology? In D. Jones, et al. (Ed.), *Sociology and occupational therapy: An integrated approach*. Edinburgh: Churchill Livingstone.

Henwood, K., & Nicholson, P. (1996). Qualitative research. *The Psychologist*, 3, 109–110.

Hooper, B., & Wood, W. (2002). Pragmatism and structuralism in occupational therapy: The long conversation. *American Journal of Occupational Therapy, 56*(1), 40–50.

Hugman, R. (1991). *Power in caring professions.* London: Macmillan.

Hyde, P. (2002). RCTs: Legitimate research tool or fancy mathematics? *British Journal of Occupational Therapy, 67*(2), 89–93.

Hyde, P. (2004). Fool's gold: Examining the use of gold standards in the production of research evidence. *British Journal of Occupational Therapy, 67*(2), 89–93.

Iklugu, M. N., & Schultz, S. (2006). An argument for pragmatism as a foundational philosophy of occupational therapy. *Canadian Journal of Occupational Therapy, 73*(2), 86–97.

Ikiugu, M. N., Nissen, R. M., Bellar, C., Maassen, A., & Van Peursem, K. (2017). Clinical effectiveness of occupational therapy in mental health: A meta-analysis. *American Journal of Occupational Therapy, 71*(5) 7105100020p1–71051000 20p10.

Jang, Y. (1993). Chinese culture and occupational therapy. *Journal of the Occupational Therapy Association of the Republic of China, 11*, 95–104.

Kelly, G. (1996). Feminist or feminine? A feminine age. *British Journal of Occupational Therapy, 59*(7), 345.

Kelly, L. (1995). What occupational therapists can learn from traditional healers. *British Journal of Occupational Therapy, 58*(3), 111–114.

Kielhofner, G. (2009). *Conceptual foundations of occupational therapy* (4th ed.). Philadelphia: FA Davis.

Kielhofner, G., Malisson, T., Crawford, C., et al. (1998). *A user's manual for the occupational performance history interview (V2) (OPHI II).* Chicago: University of Illinois.

Kirk, J., & Miller, M. (1986). *Reliability and validity in qualitative research.* Newbury Park: Sage.

Leclair, L. L., Ripat, J. D., Wener, P. F., et al. (2013). Advancing the use of theory in occupational therapy: A collaborative process/Promouvoir l'application de la theorie en ergotherapie: Un processus de collaboration. *Canadian Journal of Occupational Therapy, 80*(3), 181–193.

Legg, L., & Walker, M. (2002). Let us use randomized control trials. *British Journal of Occupational Therapy, 65*(3), 149.

Liebling, H., & Chipchase, H. (1996). Feminist group therapy for women who self harm: An initial evaluation. *Issues in Criminological and Legal Psychology, 25*, 24–29.

Low, G., Jones, D., & Duggan, C. (2001). The treatment of deliberate self harm in borderline personality disorder using dialectical behaviour therapy: A pilot study in a high security hospital. *Behavioural and Cognitive Psychotherapy, 29*, 85–92.

MacLean, F., & Jones, D. (2002). RCTs: Need for wider debate. *British Journal of Occupational Therapy, 65*(6), 294–295.

MacWhannell, D., & Blair, S. E. E. (1998). Sex, gender and feminism. In D. Jones, et al. (Ed.), *Sociology and occupational therapy: an integrated approach.* Edinburgh: Churchill Livingstone.

Mattingly, C., & Fleming, M. H. (1994). *Clinical reasoning: Forms of inquiry in a therapeutic practice.* Philadelphia: FA Davis.

Maxim, A. J., & Rice, M. S. (2018). Men in occupational therapy: Issues, factors, and perceptions. *American Journal of Occupational Therapy, 72*(1) 7201205050p1–72012050 50p7.

Maxwell, J. A. (2012). What is realism, and why should qualitative researchers care. *A Realist Approach for Qualitative Research*, 3–13.

McCluskey, A., & Lovarini, M. (2005). Providing education on evidence-based practice improved knowledge but did not change behaviour: A before and after study. *BMC Medical Education, 5*, 40.

Metcalfe, C., Lewin, R., Wisher, S., et al. (2001). Barriers to implementing the evidence base in four NHS therapies: Dieticians, occupational therapists, physiotherapists, speech and language therapists. *Physiotherapy, 89*(8), 433–441.

Morrison, R. (2016). Pragmatist epistemology and Jane Addams: Fundamental concepts for the social paradigm of occupational therapy. *Occupational Therapy International, 23*(4), 295–304.

Murphy, M. K., Black, N. A., Lampling, D. L., et al. (1998). Consensus development methods and their use in clinical guidelines development. *Health Technology Assessment, 2*(3), 1–88.

Paterson, C. (1997). An historical perspective of work practice services. In J. Pratt, & K. Jacobs (Eds.), *Work practices: International perspectives.* Oxford: Butterworth–Heinemann.

Pols, V., 2002. The phoenix, staff and serpent. In: Wilcock, A. (Ed.), *Occupation for health. Vol. 2. A journey from prescription to self health.* London: College of Occupational Therapists.

Pentland, D., Kantartzis, S., Giatsi Clausen, M., & Witemyre, K. (2018). *Occupational therapy and complexity: Defining and describing practice.* London: Royal College of Occupational Therapists.

Ryan, S. (2001). Breaking moulds – shifting thinking. *British Journal of Occupational Therapy, 64*(11), 252.

Sackett, D. L., Rosenberg, W. M. C., Gray, J. A. M., et al. (1996). Evidence-based medicine: What it is and what it isn't. *British Medical Journal, 312*, 71–72.

Sackley, C. M., Walker, M. F., Burton, C. R., et al. (2015). An occupational therapy intervention for residents with stroke related disabilities in UK care homes (OTCH): Cluster randomised controlled trial. *British Medical Journal, 350*, h468.

Schwartz, C. (1994). Chambers, Dictionary. Chambers, Edinburgh.

Seale, C. (1999). Quality in qualitative research. *Qualitative Inquiry, 5*, 465–478.

Smith, J., & Heshusius, L. (1986). Closing down the conversation: The end of the quantitative-qualitative debate among educational enquirers. *Educational Researcher, 15*, 4–12.

Taylor, J. (1995). A different voice in occupational therapy. *British Journal of Occupational Therapy, 58*(4), 170–174.

Taylor, M. C. (2000). *Evidence-based practice for occupational therapists.* Oxford: Blackwell Science.

Taylor, R. R. (2017). *Kielhofner's research in occupational therapy: Methods of inquiry for enhancing practice.* FA Davis.

Tuke, S. (1813). *Description of the retreat: An institution near York for insane persons for the society of friends containing an account of its origin and progress, the modes of treatment and a statement of cases*. York: W Alexander.

Webber, G. (1995). Occupational therapy: A postmodernist perspective. *British Journal of Occupational Therapy*, 58(10), 439–440.

Weinblatt, N., & Avrech-Bar, M. (2001). Postmodernism and its application to the field of occupational therapy. *Canadian Journal of Occupational Therapy*, 68(3), 164–170.

Whitehead, P. J., Golding-Day, M. R., Belshaw, S., Dawson, T., James, M., & Walker, M. F. (2018). Bathing adaptations in the homes of older adults (BATH-OUT): Results of a feasibility randomised controlled trial (RCT). *BMC Public Health*, 18(1), 1293.

Wilcock, A. A. (2001a). *Occupation for health: A journey from prescription to self-health*. London: College of Occupational Therapists.

Wilcock, A. A. (2001b). *Occupation for health: A journey from self-health to prescription*. London: College of Occupational Therapists.

Zafran, H., Mazer, B., Tallant, B., Chilingaryan, G., & Gelinas, I. (2017). Detecting incipient schizophrenia: A validation of the Azima battery in first episode psychosis. *Psychiatric Quarterly*, 88(3), 585–602.

3

Theoretical Foundations of Occupational Therapy: Internal Influences

Edward A.S. Duncan

OVERVIEW

The focus of this chapter is on the internal influences that shape the development of occupational therapy. The chapter commences with a historical overview of the foundations of occupational therapy. The wealth and importance of the historical foundations of occupational therapy are not always appreciated. Readers are encouraged not to skip this section (as can often be so tempting), but to read it and reflect on the relevance of the profession's pioneers for practice today. Having briefly reviewed the biographical and philosophical history of the profession, the chapter continues with an evaluation of the theoretical influences that have shaped it. The chapter then progresses to describe and evaluate contemporary approaches to knowledge development within the profession.

 HIGHLIGHTS

This chapter
- provides a historical context to the development of occupational therapy
- gives a clear introduction to the central paradigm shifts that have occurred through the development of occupational therapy
- highlights the importance of using knowledge exchange mechanisms to ensure the rapid transfer of knowledge between research and practice
- provides an introduction to the concepts of complexity, complex interventions and complexity theory.

HISTORICAL PERSPECTIVES

The only way of knowing where we are going is knowing where we have come from.

Llobera 1998

The historical basis for health through occupation can be traced back to the biblical times of the Old Testament and the Classical period of the Ancient Greeks and Romans (Wilcock 2001a, p.74). The focus of occupation in health came to the fore in Western society, however, during the development of moral treatment, which is recognized as providing a central philosophical basis for occupational therapy. That occupational therapy has both a philosophical and a theoretical basis and that the philosophical basis came first place it in a unique position amongst health professions (Schwartz 1994). Understanding this historical basis helps us to understand the tensions occupational therapists may perceive when they share their view of a person with other professionals, who view the person from a completely different philosophical perspective. The history of occupational therapy, therefore, 'can provide insight on how to face new clinical challenges and reshape the profession itself' (Hall 2013, p.389).

American Founders

Occupational therapy as we know it today emerged at the beginning of the 20th century. Although occupation programmes are known to have been developed from the very beginning of the 20th century (Wilcock 2001b), it was in 1917 that the National Society for the Promotion of Occupational Therapy (which later became the American Occupational Therapy Association) was founded (Schwartz 1994). This group was formed by several individuals who came from various professional backgrounds:
- William Rush Dunton—a psychiatrist
- George Edward Barton and Thomas Bessell Kidner—architects
- Eleanor Clarke Slagle—social service background
- Susan Cox Johnson—a teacher of arts and crafts
- Susan Tracy—a nurse (Schwartz 1994).

The broad nature of the professional backgrounds is noteworthy. This group of individuals had a significant impact on the early conceptualization of occupational therapy. Their individual contributions to the field are not of particular interest in this text, however, and the interested reader is directed to other publications that have described this group in great depth (Schwartz 1994).

Another individual who had considerable effect on the transatlantic development of occupational therapy was Dr Adolf Meyer. Meyer (1866–1950) was born in Switzerland but spent the majority of his professional career in the United States, eventually as the director of the Johns Hopkins University Medical School. Meyer can be looked on as the father of American psychiatry. Meyer visited the United Kingdom on several occasions and acknowledged the effect that these visits had on his development, when he expressed 'a real personal indebtedness to British medicine and British Psychiatry' (p.435). Perhaps one of the most influential of these visits was his first, while on a travelling scholarship, when Meyer attended a conference in Edinburgh at which he heard William James, the American pragmatist philosopher and psychologist, give a talk.

Meyer described himself as a 'mental hygienist' and assisted in the foundation of the (American) National Committee of Mental Hygiene (Wilcock 2001b). The mental hygiene movement held the following objectives:

- To work for the conservation of mental health
- To promote the study of mental disorders and mental effects in all their forms and relations
- To obtain and disseminate reliable data concerning mental disorders and effects
- To help raise the standard of care and treatment (Henderson 1923).

These apparently philanthropic aims are, however, tainted by an aspect of Meyer's life that is less well known and has had little mention in occupational therapy literature. Meyer, like many others involved in the mental hygiene movement, was also a proponent of eugenics. Eugenics is the proposed improvement of the human species by encouraging or permitting reproduction of only those individuals with genetic characteristics judged desirable. The mental hygiene movement was permeated with eugenic thought, a philosophy most notoriously and extremely supported by the Nazis during the Second World War. From Meyer's perspective, eugenics provided an opportunity to eradicate mental illness through the prevention of reproduction by people with mental illness. It has since been strongly discredited. Eugenic organizations do, however, continue to exist to the present day and Meyer's membership and espousal of such a philosophy provides a different perspective of the man who is credited as providing the first conceptual model of occupational therapy (Meyer 1922, Reed & Sanderson 1999).

During his career, Meyer recognized the impact of instincts, habits and interests, as well as experiences, on people's lives and because of this developed an interest in the effect of occupation with his patients (Wilcock 2001b). Indeed, such was his interest in this that he employed Eleanor Clarke Slagle, following her early occupational therapy training. During this period, Dr David Henderson, a young graduate from Scotland, came to work with Meyer. Henderson saw Slagle's work within her institution and was impressed by the effect she had on the patients with whom she worked (Wilcock 2001b). On his return to Scotland, it was Dr Henderson, inspired by the time he had spent with Meyer and Slagle, who opened the first occupational therapy department in the United Kingdom, at Gartnavel Royal Hospital, Glasgow, in 1919. In 1922, the first 'occupational therapist', Dorothea Robertson, was appointed in the same department.

British Founders

Although Dr Henderson was the first individual to introduce occupational therapy to the United Kingdom and Dorothea Robertson the first appointed occupational therapist, two other key figures require presentation to understand more fully the introduction of occupational therapy to the United Kingdom; they are Margaret Barr Fulton and Elizabeth Casson. Margaret Fulton was the first qualified occupational therapist in the United Kingdom. Born in Scotland and raised in England, Margaret Fulton trained to be an occupational therapist while in the United States. On her return she was put in contact with Dr Henderson; however, as he was unable to appoint, she was employed by the Aberdeen Royal Asylum. Although Margaret Fulton did not write or present a great deal on her philosophy of practice, her work stood out and gained her high office. In 1937, while working in Aberdeen, she met Alfred Adler, one-time colleague of Sigmund Freud and founder of individual psychology (Wilcock 2001b). He was later to comment, 'I was particularly struck with the Occupational Therapy department and with the high degree of interest which is shown in psychological problems' (Aberdeen Press and Journal 1937). Fulton's capabilities were also apparent from her election to the position of first president of the World Federation of Occupational Therapists (Wilcock 2001b).

Another key British founder of occupational therapy was Elizabeth Casson. Born in 1881, Elizabeth was brought up in a family with various artistic talents, so it is not surprising that the young Elizabeth was noted to be good with her hands, demonstrating practical as well as academic talents (Wilcock 2001b). Following an initial period of secretarial work, Casson worked with Octavia Hill (1838–1912), a remarkable woman who is credited with the foundation of several organizations and professions, including the open space movement, the National Trust, and housing management and social work (Wilcock 2001a). Hill is believed to have had a considerable effect on Casson during their period together at the Red Cross Hall, where Hill employed Casson as a secretary (Wilcock 2001b). Casson became very involved in the practical activities of the tenants, for whom she organized a variety of educational and recreational activities. Casson then surprised those closest to her by announcing to everyone that she intended to study medicine. Graduating in 1929 as the first female doctor from the University of Bristol, Casson herself stated that her 'real introduction' to occupational therapy came through reading a description of Henderson's work in Glasgow. Casson's medical training and intrigue, coupled with her personal and family talents and social commitment, naturally fostered a profound interest in occupational therapy. This interest culminated in her establishing the first British occupational therapy school at Dorset House, Bristol (Wilcock 2001b). Casson's importance to the development of occupational therapy in Britain today is honoured by the Royal College of Occupational Therapists annual Casson Memorial Lecture.

This partial overview of some of the historical developments of occupational therapy within the United States and Britain is provided to demonstrate the very real connections between the external influences on the early development of the profession and the foundations of the profession as we know it today. Further descriptions of the development of the profession in these two countries are available for the interested reader (Paterson 2010, Quiroga 1995). The history of occupational therapy is a rich tapestry. Accounts of the history of the profession in Australia (Anderson & Bell 1988), Canada (Friedland 2011) and Ireland (Pettigrew et al 2017) have also been published. While these accounts are rich and valuable, the methods used to develop some of them are either unclear or have been critiqued as being open to bias (Dunne et al 2016). To counter these limitations, Dunne et al (2016) argue that rigorous historical documentary research methods should be used to provide a transparent understanding of the development of occupational therapy.

PARADIGM SHIFTS IN OCCUPATIONAL THERAPY

Having reviewed the philosophical basis and some of the influential individuals who were responsible for the foundation of the profession, it is important to examine the theoretical developments of occupational therapy. Such developments are perhaps best understood through the concept of paradigms and paradigm shifts. Kuhn (1970)

understood that members of a profession were bound by a shared vision of what it meant to be. Paradigms represent the shared consensus regarding the most fundamental beliefs of a profession. Paradigm shifts, therefore, are the moments in which the shared vision and understanding of a field changes and a new consensus on the fundamental beliefs of the profession is adopted. Understandably, as paradigms represent the core of a profession, such shifts are both rare and traumatic to the field. The concept of paradigms has been developed by a variety of individuals, including Tornebohm (1986) and MacIntyre (1980). Tornebohm (1986) viewed a profession's paradigm as the defining feature of a profession and believed that within it can be found a profession's vision of practice. MacIntyre (1980) argued that paradigms provide professions with their values and concerns for practice.

Within occupational therapy, it is the work of Professor Gary Kielhofner (2009) that is most closely associated with the paradigmatic conceptualization of occupational therapy's professional development. Kielhofner (2009) developed the work of Kuhn (1970), Tornebohm (1986) and MacIntyre (1980) in his understanding of the paradigmatic content of occupational therapy, and suggested that the occupational therapy paradigm consists of three elements: core constructs, focal viewpoints and integrated values. 'Core constructs' of the profession address the issues of the profession's service provision. Core constructs relate to the need for the profession, the problems it focuses on and the manner in which it addresses such problems. The 'focal viewpoint' of a paradigm is interested in the way in which a profession views, understands and interprets the world. The focal viewpoint of a profession will also influence the knowledge that is deemed important within the profession. Finally, 'values' highlight the level of importance that a profession places on issues from its own perspective (Kielhofner et al 2004).

Kielhofner (2009) outlined three different paradigms that have existed in occupational therapy since its inception (Table 3.1): the occupational paradigm, the mechanistic paradigm and the contemporary paradigm. The original paradigm (the occupational paradigm) arose from the work of the profession's founders and was based on their core constructs, views and values. During the 1940s and 1950s, occupational therapy was placed under increasing pressure from the medical profession to become objective and create an empirical basis for its intervention (Kielhofner et al 2004). In search of professional acceptance, occupational therapy increasingly focused on biomedical explanations for practice; thus the mechanistic paradigm period of occupational therapy was born. During this period, occupational therapists became increasingly competent at measuring and attempting to objectify their practice. However,

TABLE 3.1 Paradigmatic Shifts in Occupational Therapy			
The Nature of Paradigms	**Core Constructs**	**Focal Viewpoint**	**Integrated Values**
Paradigm of occupation (1900s–1940s)	Occupation is essential to life and influences people's health. Occupation includes thinking, acting and existing, and requires each of these elements to be balanced in daily life. Mind and body are intrinsically linked. Occupation can be used to regain function.	Focusing on both personal motivation and the effect of the environment on performance.	Human dignity is realized through performance of occupation. Occupation is important for health. Holism.
Crisis	Occupational therapy is placed under increasing pressure from medicine to become objective. Occupational therapy seeks professional recognition through the adoption of biomedical explanations and approaches to dysfunction.		
Mechanistic paradigm (1960s–1970s)	Performance is dependent on the functioning of inner systems: intra-psychic, nervous and musculoskeletal. Damage to any of the above systems causes dysfunction. Functional performance is regained through addressing or compensating for deficits in these systems.	This period focused on the internal mechanisms described in the above core constructs.	In-depth knowledge of inner systems. Objectivity. Use of occupation to address and measure disordered inner systems precisely.
Crisis	The acceptance of reductionism and focus on inner systems were recognized as incomplete. Prominent occupational therapy figures called for a return to occupation, with a focus on the importance of occupation to health.		
Contemporary paradigm (1980s onwards)	Occupation has a central role in human life; it provides motive and meaning to life. Lack of access (or restricted access) to occupations may have a negative effect on health and quality of life. The use of occupation to address impacts on health or quality of life is the core of occupational therapy.	This person focuses on a return to occupation and a focus on the whole, rather than its component parts	Respect for the value of human life. The importance of individuals' empowerment and engagement in occupation. The integration of individuals into life through meaningful occupation.

such developments caused the profession to lose sight of its roots and the original impetus for the profession's birth. The initial call for the profession to return to its original vision came from Mary Reilly, a highly influential scholar in the history of modern occupational therapy (Kielhofner et al 2004). Reilly's original call for the return of occupational therapy's focus on occupation came in her Eleanor Clarke Slagle Lecture in 1961. During this keynote speech to the annual conference of the American Occupational Therapy Association, she gave a poetic (but from our current perspective, completely unevidence-based) vision of the impact of occupation on health, stating that 'man through the use of his hands, as they are energized by his mind and will, can influence the state of his own health'

(Reilly 1962, p.1). Through this clarion call to the profession, a new crisis emerged as practitioners sought to return once again to being occupationally focused, while retaining the developments in objectivity and professional status they had gained during the mechanistic period. This return to occupation heralded the contemporary paradigm, in which occupation is understood in a new and more complex manner and the importance of occupation in health has once again been established.

Professional paradigms are dynamic in nature. Although whole-scale paradigm shifts are relatively rare, occupational therapy is constantly evolving and developing. This process, while perhaps not quite as traumatic as a paradigm shift, can nonetheless be painful and challenging.

Contemporary debates regarding approaches to theoretical development within occupational therapy constitute one such challenge. What Kielhofner termed the *contemporary paradigm* remains generally well accepted; however, some people are beginning to call for a shift for occupation to focus on health, wellbeing and quality of life in a public health context (Pizzi & Richards 2017). This call comes at a time of increased attention being placed on the importance of public health in general, and so the intertwined relationship between the external influences discussed in the preceding chapter and the internal evolution of occupational therapy continue. Time will tell if these developments herald a new paradigm shift for occupational therapy or not.

The Importance of Healthy Professional Scepticism

Wilcock (1998, p.203) recognized at an early stage that the developing complexity of occupational therapy theory would lead to 'heated debate' between professionals. Despite stating that 'heated debate about the profession's foundation is not part of occupational therapists' tradition', she felt that such debate was important and would ultimately benefit the profession. Wilcock was right on both counts. There is an ongoing reluctance within the profession to engage in constructive critical argument and debate. Bannigan (2001) recognized occupational therapists' reluctance to argue but supported the requirement of professional argument to develop a robust knowledge base and pursue excellence in practice. Several years later Duncan et al (2007, p.200) noted that 'robust academic argument is new to occupational therapy: [and that] to date, there has been a notable lack of scholarly articles presenting counter arguments to theoretical ideas'. That assessment remains largely accurate today. A respectful professional scepticism is invaluable to the development of a profession and its ideas. As Whalley Hammell (2009, p.11) stated, 'Much of what we believe and assume about occupational therapy's theories may be justifiable. However, fostering a culture of healthy scepticism within our profession will enable us to challenge the veracity of our assumptions, contest the universality of their application, and insist on a supportive evidence base for our theories that is derived from a broad range of perspectives. This will inform more relevant and inclusive theory, and more relevant and inclusive practice'. Readers are encouraged to adopt this attitude in all that they read in this and other professional texts.

THEORETICAL DEVELOPMENTS WITHIN OCCUPATIONAL THERAPY

Possibly the first elucidation of the theoretical (as opposed to the philosophical) basis of occupational therapy was

in 1940, with the publication of a text entitled *Theory of Occupational Therapy for Students and Nurses* (Haworth & Macdonald 1940). Although theoretical developments have emerged throughout each of the profession's paradigms, it is during the period of the contemporary paradigm that occupational therapy research and theoretical developments have truly gathered pace. These developments are the natural evolution from the paradigm of occupation that has now emerged and established itself as the central focus of occupational therapists' concern (Kielhofner et al 2004).

> Theory *is a term that is readily used in our everyday conversations (e.g., 'In theory I could do this but …');* however, within occupational therapy, theoretical approaches are not always as easily articulated. Mitcham (2003, p.65) describes a scenario that will still be recognised by many students and practitioners. Discussing the complexity of theory in practice, she states, 'we panic when a keen, bright eyed student asks us in the clinic one day, "which theoretical approach guides your practice?" We stumble and mumble a response along the lines of, "Oh, I haven't touched that theory stuff since I graduated", or "I'm eclectic, I use a little of everything"'.

Such a scenario is commonly recounted by students undertaking fieldwork placements. Although the reasons for a practitioner's inability to justify their practice theoretically may be various, such a response in effect perpetuates the theory–practice divide and suggests to the practitioners of the future—in a form of hidden curriculum—that theory is not important in practice. This is not the case. The aim of this text is to demonstrate the importance of theory to practice, to assist students and practitioners to make sense of theory in practice, and to develop understanding of how theory can be developed and implemented in practice.

So, what is theory? Reed (1997, p.521) defined it as 'an organized way of thinking about given phenomena … It attempts to:
- define and explain the relationships between concepts or ideas related to phenomena of interest;
- explain how these relationships can predict behaviour or events; and
- suggest ways that phenomena can be changed or controlled'.

Kielhofner (2009, p.8) offers another definition, stating that theory is 'a network of explanations that provides concepts that label and describe phenomena and postulates that specify relationships between concepts'.

Creek (2002, p.46) defines theory as a 'conceptual system or framework used to organize knowledge. A theory consists of a description of a set of phenomena, an explanation of how and under what circumstances they occur, and a demonstration of how they relate to each other'.

Various definitions of theory have been offered and agreement is clear between authors cited.

Theory and Practice

The relationship of theory to practice varies in different professions. Radiology, for example, draws heavily upon knowledge that has been developed in the fields of chemistry, physics, anatomy and physiology. Radiography places less emphasis on the social sciences than occupational therapy. Furthermore, unlike occupational therapy, radiography has not developed its own theoretical understandings to guide practice. Each of these issues can help us understand why some professions do not appear to have a theory–practice dilemma, whilst others, such as occupational therapy, do (Mitcham 2003). The issue of the theory–practice gap and the manner in which theory is built, tested, understood and applied to practice form the basis for an important and current debate in occupational therapy. This debate is core, as it presents conceptually differing approaches to theory and knowledge development.

Basic Science. Basic sciences emerged from the development of logical positivism (see Chapter 2). The focus of basic research is the development of pure theory. No consideration is given to its potential application. Basic research can certainly be influential in applied settings. Nuclear magnetic resonance (which was discovered in 1938) was integrated into radiography practice several decades later to assist in the early detection of diseases. While the time taken to integrate these research findings into practice was considerable, it could be argued that the delay in application was a result of having to wait for technology to catch up, before such basic science could be applied. The study of the therapeutic effects of aspirin, however, highlights that even when research can be easily applied with life-saving effects, considerable delays can occur in the transference of knowledge (Esdaile & Roth 2003). Aspirin's role in preventing heart attacks first emerged in 1948. Dr Lawrence Craven, a general practitioner in California, undertook a small study of 400 men whom he placed on an aspirin regimen. Over a period of 2 years, no participants suffered a heart attack. The initial study was expanded, and in 1956 it was reported that a study of 8000 men found that those who took one or two aspirin tablets daily did not suffer heart attacks. In 1988 Harvard University undertook a study of 22 000 male doctors and found that those who took one 325 mg aspirin tablet every second day had 44% fewer heart attacks than those who did not. The study had been scheduled to last 8 years, but the researchers found the results so positive that ethically

they did not feel they should withhold aspirin's benefits from the control placebo group (Steering Committee of the Physicians' Health Study Research Group 1988). Further studies have amended the dosage of aspirin required to prevent a heart attack and identified the populations who would most benefit from such usage; however, aspirin continues to be underused for conditions in which its efficacy is well established (Reilly & Fitzgerald 2002). It would appear, therefore, that basic research can influence practice, but that there may be a time delay and the influence of such research on practice can be accidental or unplanned. One well-cited study (Morris et al. 2011) has quantified the time delay between a basic science discovery and its application in practice as being 17 years. However, this claim relates to studies that have laboratory-based basic science discoveries at their root. The vast majority of research that takes place within an occupational therapy context is more accurately described as applied health research. Although the challenges of implementing applied health research are still significant, the time lag between applied health research and implementation is often much less protracted.

Occupational Therapy's Relationship with Basic Science. Mosey (1992) distinguished theory that explains phenomena (basic science) from the integration of such research into practice (application). Mosey (1992) argues that occupational therapy's remit is solely within the application of theory to practice and suggests that such theory can be found in the scientific disciplines of biology, sociology, philosophy and so on. In doing so, Mosey (1992) supported the separation of theory from practice and the basic science approach to knowledge generation. Mosey (1992) supported the application of existing knowledge to support occupational therapy. Others have argued, however, that it is necessary to create a basic science of occupation. This approach, known as occupational science (Clark et al 1991), is discussed in greater depth in Chapter 16.

Basic science is based on the premise of technical rationality (Schon 1983). Technical rationality assumes that knowledge that is generated in basic research will naturally lead to applications of knowledge in practice (Fig. 3.1). Viewed from this perspective, knowledge is seen as hierarchical in nature, with the highest position given to the developers of knowledge, whilst lower positions are occupied by problem-solving and other applications (Schon 1983). The transference of such knowledge into practice, however, is not as linear as the technical rational perspective suggests. A major criticism of the basic science approach to integrating theory into practice is that it does not provide either evidence or applications that are directly

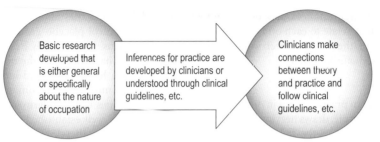

Fig. 3.1 The application of basic science to practice.

applicable in practice (Taylor et al 2002). In recent years a whole field of research, known as implementation science, has emerged that focuses on improving the implementation of science into practice (Brownson et al 2018).

It is increasingly recognized within the allied health professions that the development of clinically relevant knowledge is a truly collaborative process. Occupational therapists, amongst others, must strive to develop the highest quality of evidence-based theories, relevant to the individuals receiving the service and demonstrably effective in practice. These cannot be developed in isolation. Collaborations between academics, practitioners and service users, as equal partners in the development, evaluation and implementation of theory into practice, are essential.

Scholarship of Practice

The scholarship of practice is a method of knowledge generation that has gained momentum in occupational therapy practice (Lyken-Segosebe 2017). Schon (1983) is widely credited with developing the concept of scholarship in practice. As with other areas of theory and knowledge development, the term *scholarship of practice* is understood by differing theorists in different ways. Esdaile and Roth (2003, p.161) describe a scholarship of practice 'in terms of an integrated model in which basic research from both the physical and social sciences informs practice, and practice generates further questions for research'. From Esdaile and Roth's (2003) perspective, the focus of scholarship of practice is on

- discovery—not only of research, but also of practice observations, often achieved in collaboration between academics and clinicians
- integration—including information from other disciplines; crucially, integration is seen as the process through which academics and practitioners are linked
- application—using evidence-based techniques and models or frames of reference on practice
- teaching—continuous professional development and the sharing of knowledge with peers, students, clients and carers.

Scholarship of Practice Within the Model of Human Occupation. In occupational therapy, the term *scholarship of practice* is most closely associated with the process of knowledge development in the Model of Human Occupation. In this model, scholarship of practice is described as a dialectic (that is, a discussion or debate) between theory and practice (Hammel et al 2002, Kielhofner et al 2004). Furthermore, Forsyth et al (2005b, p.260) describe the scholarship of practice as a partnership between academia and practice 'in which theoretical and empirical knowledge is brought to bear on the practical problems of therapeutic work and in which the latter raise questions to be addressed through scholarship'. This scholarship of practice approach focuses on

- research that is carried out and contributes directly to *practice*
- partnerships that are developed outside academic institutions; such partnerships provide new research, *practice* and educational opportunities
- the creation of effective collaborations that advance both academia and *practice* (Forsyth et al 2005b) [emphasis added].

To develop effectively as a 'practice scholar' (Forsyth et al 2005b) who builds and implements knowledge directly relevant to practice, an alternative approach to research, other than the technical rational approach of basic research described above, must be considered. It is necessary to create equal partnerships, between clinicians, academics and the recipients of services, in knowledge development: partnerships that reflect true collaboration and power sharing so that 'all participants may have a degree of responsibility, voice and decision-making about all aspects of knowledge generation' (Kielhofner 2005).

Scholarship of practice recognizes the strengths of all approaches that support the development of practice-related research. However, to engage in a scholarship of practice approach to knowledge development, Kielhofner (2009) advocates for the development of an 'engaged scholarship' (Boyer 1990) that examines alternative ways of addressing and resolving the everyday life difficulties of people and society. Although positivistic approaches can achieve this (Gitlin et al 2001), engaged scholarship requires a re-evaluation of how knowledge is best developed. An alternative method for developing knowledge, used within this scholarship of practice approach, is 'participatory action research' (Chevalier & Buckles 2019). Participatory action research is incorporated within the scholarship of practice approach, as it provides an alternative method of knowledge generation that supports partnership working and leads to change within the practice setting (Forsyth et al 2005a, Kielhofner et al 2004).

Kurt Lewin (1890–1947) is credited with coining the phrase 'action research', an approach that he initially used to study intergroup relations and issues of minority groups in the United States (Meyer 2000). Action research is a cyclical process that intertwines action, reflection and research. Key elements of action research include the clear definition of phases of the study, a clear description of everyone involved, and consideration of the local context throughout the study and the nature of the relationship between the researchers and participants (Waterman et al 2001). Action research has been recognized as a solution to the theory–practice gap (Meyer 2000).

Participatory action research has been advocated for use within an occupational science framework (Wilcock 1998). However, its use within this scholarship of practice approach is focused on research that is centred on practice. Moreover, the adoption of participatory action research within an engaged scholarship approach does not require a total dismissal of previous research approaches. Kielhofner (2009) recognized the importance of preserving the positive components of traditional methods of knowledge generation, while engaging with contemporary approaches (such as participatory action research) that are more suited to creating theories that both are global and have a concurrent practical utility. Therefore scholarship of practice supports the development of a knowledge-creating system (Senge & Scharmer 2001). This system integrates research and theory development, capacity-building among professionals and practical utility, through the development of tools for practice, into a single process of combined strength. In this manner, the divide of knowledge development and application found in basic science is removed (Kielhofner et al 2004) (Fig. 3.2).

Kielhofner's approach to the scholarship of practice, whilst originating from the USA, has spread throughout the international occupational therapy community. Forsyth and colleagues (2005b) described how a forensic occupational therapy service in Scotland had developed a scholarship of practice approach to research and practice. More recently the scholarship of practice approach has been used within dementia care (Forsyth et al 2015) and primary care (Killian et al 2015). Although the scholarship of practice approach has been used for several years in practice, it is only one type of knowledge exchange that occurs in occupational therapy (Bannigan 2009).

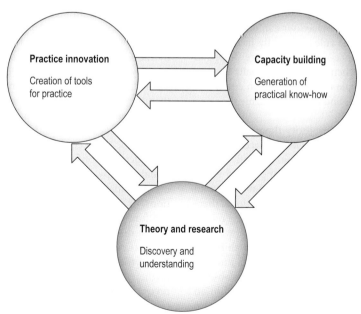

Fig. 3.2 A Knowledge-Creating System. (From Kielhofner G. (2005). Scholarship and practice: bridging the divide. *American Journal of Occupational Therapy* 59(2), 231–239.)

COMPLEXITY

The word 'complexity' has lay and technical meanings. In practice, clinicians will often refer to the 'complexity' of practice; however, more often than not this is using a lay definition of the term. Just because something appears complex in a general sense does not necessarily mean (and mostly will not mean) that it is also complex in the technical sense of the word. The technical senses of 'complexity' are, well, complex!

Complexity theory is one technical explanation of complexity. It explores how complex systems (such as humans) sometimes behave in the real world and how complex systems can generate simple outcomes. Complexity theory views all living creatures as complex adaptive systems (Lewin 1993). Such complexity is easy to witness. Consider the sight of a flock of geese flying south (in the northern hemisphere) in a 'V' formation in the autumn or a murmur of starlings that twist and turn in harmony in the dusk of a city landscape. Such sights are truly wondrous. Complex adaptive systems are also observable in humans at a multitude of levels. Consider the complexity of getting out of bed in the morning and getting yourself to university or work. Such complexity is then magnified when we consider the systems in which such an activity occurs (e.g., the other people you meet on your way to university, the environment in which you live, etc.). Humans do not exist in isolation and complexity theory acknowledges the importance of understanding the interconnectedness of nature. Despite such complex interactions, complexity scientists have discovered that complex behaviour can emerge from the existence of a few simple rules. Geese fly in the manner that causes least resistance—their bodies are shaped to decrease wind resistance when they fly diagonally to each other. Starlings have a simple rule of staying an equal distance from their fellow birds and flying in roughly the same direction.

A further component of complexity theory is the recognition of small changes that potentially lead to larger effects. This is commonly known as the 'butterfly effect', as it has been shown that a butterfly flapping its wings in India can cause changes in air currents that lead to an eventual windstorm in Chicago. Within occupational therapy, it could be argued that Reilly's (1962) call for a return to occupation-focused activity sparked a similar wave of effects that resulted in a professional paradigm shift and influenced the practice of occupational therapists internationally. Within occupational therapy practice, it is observable that a small positive action or interaction within an occupational therapy session can have significant effects on the whole of a person's functioning. Similarly, provision of a simple piece of adaptive kitchen equipment can lead to

someone returning to previously valued occupations and life roles—small changes can have a big effect on the whole system. It is not, therefore, surprising that complexity theory has gained attention within healthcare research.

Another related but separate issue is that of complex intervention. Complex interventions have many different components, and it can at times be hard to tell which of them are the most important or 'active ingredients'. Just having an intervention with many components does not mean that the components interact with each other according to complexity theory. Indeed, there may be a very simple interaction between the elements (and thus it is a complex intervention); the only way truly to tell is by conducting research into the action of the intervention. The Medical Research Council (MRC) of the United Kingdom has recognized the importance of complexity interventions in healthcare. In 2000 it published its first guide to developing and evaluating complex interventions (Medical Research Council 2000). This was later substantially updated (Medical Research Council 2008), and a further revised version is due at the time of writing. Creek (2003) used the original MRC framework to study occupational therapy as a complex intervention, viewing it as a complex intervention that meets the MRC definition of comprising 'a number of separate elements which seem essential to the proper functioning of the intervention although the "active ingredient" of the intervention that is effective is difficult to specify' (Medical Research Council 2000, p.1). Creek's work focused on the establishment of the theoretical basis and 'modelling' that represents an attempt to separate occupational therapy's component parts and illustrates how they interrelate. This document was published by the College of Occupational Therapists (COT). More recently, Creek (2009) conducted an overview of the use of the document. Interestingly, her definition of occupational therapy as a complex intervention has not been used for its original purpose (research) but has instead been used and misused by academics and practitioners trying to explain or describe the occupational therapy process (Creek 2009). Considerable confusion has arisen over whether occupational therapy is a complex intervention, whether some occupational therapy interventions are complex interventions, or whether in fact some occupational therapy interventions can be better understood by complexity theory. A robust discussion occurred in the literature on these very issues (Creek et al 2005, Duncan et al 2007, Lambert et al 2007); the interested reader is guided to these articles for further information and consideration. In 2009, a 5-year review of Creek's original (2003) document was published (Creek 2009). Undertaken by the original document's author, it highlighted that the document (Creek 2003) had created a considerable impact on how occupational therapists understood the world in which they practiced. Although the review found that the definition of occupational therapy as a complex intervention was being used and cited a range of reasons for this, it appeared it was not being used in research; the purpose for which it was originally conceived. Furthermore there is neither rebuttal or acknowledgement of any of the preceding criticism of the original document. In 2016 the Royal College of Occupational Therapists commissioned a revision of the original complex interventions document, by Pentland et al (2018). What emerged was a considerably expanded document that presents a theoretically and empirically informed understanding of contemporary occupational therapy. Interestingly, the Pentland document also sidesteps the academic arguments that had arisen following the publication of the original document.

SUMMARY

This chapter has provided an overview of the internal influences on the theoretical foundations of occupational therapy. These influences were first placed within their historical context. Following this, an overview of the various contemporary influences on theory development within occupational therapy was given. The challenges of the issues presented and multiple uses of similar terms are often disheartening for students and practitioners who are trying to grapple with the theoretical influences of the profession. There can be a temptation either to look for a single theoretical answer or to give up and conclude that theory is not important. Both views are erroneous. Theory and knowledge are vital to practice, and practice is the crucible in which new theories are developed and evaluated. Without a theoretical basis, the profession will crumble. The multiplicity of views and debate within the profession serves only to progress our theoretical understanding of the effect of occupation on health. Debate fosters development and this would not occur if a single perspective was consistently taken. Furthermore, without knowledge and understanding of the theoretical basis for practice, a practitioner's intervention may be viewed as unethical. How can a professional work in an ethical way without knowing the theoretical basis for such intervention? It is important, therefore, to grapple with the literature and engage in the debate surrounding theory development and its application in practice.

This review of the internal influences on theory development is, by necessity, partial. Other themes are picked up on in subsequent chapters and debated more fully. Having read and reflected on the issues raised in this chapter, readers are encouraged to explore internal influences discussed by other authors in this text and beyond and to explore the issues in greater depth.

REFERENCES

Aberdeen Press and Journal. (1937). Welfare Work in Aberdeen. *Professor Adler pays tribute*. Aberdeen Press and Journal.

Anderson, B., & Bell, J. (1988). *Occupational therapy: Its place in Australia's history*. Sydney: New South Wales Association of Occupational Therapists.

Bannigan, K. (2001). Use argument to deliver excellence. *British Journal of Occupational Therapy*, 64(3), 113.

Bannigan, K. (2009). Knowledge exchange. In E. A. S. Duncan (Ed.), *Skills for practice in occupational therapy* (pp. 231–248). Edinburgh: Elsevier/Churchill Livingstone.

Boyer, E. (1990). *Scholarship reconsidered: Priorities of the professorate*. Princeton: Carnegie Foundation for the Advancement of Teaching.

Brownson, R. C., Colditz, G. A., & Proctor, E. K. (Eds.). (2018). *Dissemination and implementation research in health: Translating science to practice*. Oxford: Oxford University Press.

Chevalier, J. M., & Buckles, D. J. (2019). *Participatory action research: Theory and methods for engaged inquiry*. Abingdon: Routledge.

Clark, F. A., Parham, D., Carlson, M. E., et al. (1991). Occupational science: Academic innovation in the service of occupational therapy's future. *American Journal of Occupational Therapy*, 45(4), 300–310.

Creek, J. (2002). The knowledge base of occupational therapy. In J. Creek (Ed.), *Occupational therapy and mental health*. Edinburgh: Churchill Livingstone.

Creek, J. (2003). *Occupational therapy defined as a complex intervention*. London: College of Occupational Therapists.

Creek, J., Ilott, I., Cook, S., & Munday, C. (2005). Valuing occupational therapy as a complex intervention. *British Journal of Occupational Therapy*, 68(6), 281–284.

Creek, J. (2009). Occupational therapy defined as a complex intervention: A 5-year review. *British Journal of Occupational Therapy*, 72(3), 105–115.

Duncan, E. A. S., Paley, J., & Eva, G. (2007). Complex interventions and complex systems in occupational therapy. *British Journal of Occupational Therapy*, 70(5), 199–206.

Dunne, B., Pettigrew, J., & Robinson, K. (2016). Using historical documentary methods to explore the history of occupational therapy. *British Journal of Occupational Therapy*, 79(6), 376–384.

Esdaile, S. A., & Roth, L. M. (2003). Creating scholarly practice: Integrating and applying scholarship to practice. In G. Brown, S. A. Esdaile, & S. E. Ryan (Eds.), *Becoming an advanced healthcare practitioner*. London: Butterworth–Heinemann.

Forsyth, K., Duncan, E. A. S., & Summerfield-Mann, L. (2005a). Scholarship of practice in the United Kingdom: An occupational therapy service case study. *Occupational Therapy in Health Care*, 19(1–2), 17–29.

Forsyth, K., Summerfield-Mann, L., & Kielhofner, G. (2005b). Scholarship of practice: Making occupation focused, theory driven, evidence based practice a reality. *British Journal of Occupational Therapy*, 68(6), 260–268.

Forsyth, K., Melton, J., Raber, C., Burke, J. P., & Piersol, C. V. (2015). Scholarship of practice in the care of people with dementia: Creating the future through collaborative efforts. *Occupational Therapy in Health Care*, 29(4), 429–441.

Friedland, J. (2011). *Restoring the spirit: The beginnings of occupational therapy in Canada, 1890–1930*. Montreal: McGill-Queen's Press.

Gitlin, L. N., Corcoran, M., Winter, L., et al. (2001). A randomized control trial of a home environmental intervention. Effect on efficacy and uptake in caregivers and on daily function of persons with dementia. *Gerontologist*, 41, 4–14.

Hall, J. (2013). Histories of work and occupational therapy—and occupational therapists as historians? *British Journal of Occupational Therapy*, 79(6), 376–384.

Hammel, J., Finlayson, M., Kielhofner, G., et al. (2002). Educating scholars of practice: An approach to preparing tomorrow's researchers. *Occupational Therapy in Health Care*, 15(1–2), 157–176.

Haworth, N. A., & MacDonald, E. M. (1940). *Theory of occupational therapy for students and nurses*. London: Bailliere, Tindall and Cox.

Henderson, D. K. (1923). Mental hygiene. *Glasgow Medical Journal*, 99(6), 337–360.

Kielhofner, G. (2005). Scholarship and practice: Bridging the divide. *American Journal of Occupational Therapy*, 59(2), 231–239.

Kielhofner, G. (2009). *Conceptual foundations of occupational therapy* (4th ed.). Philadelphia: FA Davis.

Kielhofner, G., Hammel, J., Helfrich, C., et al. (2004). Studying practice and its outcomes: A conceptual approach. *American Journal of Occupational Therapy*, 58, 15–23.

Killian, C., Fisher, G., & Muir, S. (2015). Primary care: A new context for the scholarship of practice model. *Occupational Therapy in Health Care*, 29(4), 383–396.

Kuhn, T. (1970). *The structure of scientific revolutions*. Chicago: University of Chicago.

Lambert, R., Harrison, D., & Watson, M. (2007). Complexity, occupational therapy, unpredictability and the scientific method: A response to Creek et al (2005) and Duncan et al (2007). *British Journal of Occupational Therapy*, 70(12), 534–536.

Lewin, R. (1993). *Complexity: Life on the edge of chaos*. London: Phoenix.

Llobera, J. (1998). Historical and comparative research. In C. Seale (Ed.), *Researching society and culture*. London: Sage.

Lyken–Segosebe, D. (2017). The scholarship of practice in applied disciplines. *New Directions for Higher Education*, 2017(178), 21–33.

MacIntyre, A. (1980). Epistemological crisis, dramatic narrative, and the philosophy science. In G. Gutting (Ed.), *Paradigms and revolutions: Appraisals and applications of Thomas Kuhn's philosophy of science*. Notre Dame: Notre Dame Press.

Medical Research Council. (2000). *A framework for the development and evaluation of RCTs for complex interventions to improve health*. London: Medical Research Council.

Medical Research Council. (2008). *Complex interventions guidance*. London: Medical Research Council.

Meyer, A. (1922). Philosophy of occupation therapy. *Archives of Occupational Therapy*, 1(1), 1–10.

Meyer, J. (2000). Using qualitative methods in health related action research. *British Medical Journal*, 320, 178–181.

Mitcham, M. D. (2003). Integrating theory and practice: Using theory creatively to enhance professional practice. In G. Brown, S. A. Esdaile, & S. E. Ryan (Eds.), *Becoming an advanced healthcare practitioner*. London: Butterworth–Heinemann.

Morris, Z. S., Wooding, S., & Grant, J. (2011). The answer is 17 years, what is the question: understanding time lags in translational research. *London: Journal of the Royal Society of Medicine*, 104, 510–520.

Mosey, A. C. (1992). *Applied scientific inquiry in health professions*. Rockville: American Occupational Association.

Paterson, C. F. (2010). *Opportunities not prescriptions: The development of occupational therapy in Scotland 1900–1960*. Aberdeen: Aberdeen History of Medicine Publications.

Pentland, D., Kantartzis, S., Giatsi Clausen, M., & Witemyre, K. (2018). *Occupational therapy and complexity: Defining and describing practice*. London: Royal College of Occupational Therapists.

Pettigrew, J., Robinson, K., Dunne, B., & O'Mahoney, J. (2017). Major trends in the use of occupation as therapy in Ireland 1863–1963. *Irish Journal of Occupational Therapy*, 45(1), 4–14.

Pizzi, M. A., & Richards, L. G. (2017). Promoting health, well-being, and quality of life in occupational therapy: A commitment to a paradigm shift for the next 100 years. *American Journal of Occupational Therapy*, 71(4), 7104170010p1–7104170010p5.

Quiroga, V. A. M. (1995). *Occupational therapy: The first 30 years 1900 to 1930*. Bethesda, MD: American Occupational Therapy Association.

Reed, K. L. (1997). Theory and frame of reference. In M. E. Neistadt, & E. B. Crepeau (Eds.), *Willard and Spackman's occupational therapy*. Philadelphia: Lippincott Williams & Wilkins.

Reed, K. L., & Sanderson, S. N. (1999). *Concepts of occupational therapy*. Philadelphia: Lippincott Williams & Wilkins.

Reilly, M. (1962). Eleanor Clarke Slagle Lecture. Occupational therapy can be one of the great ideas of 20th century medicine. *American Journal of Occupational Therapy*, 16, 1–9.

Reilly, M., & Fitzgerald, G. (2002). Gathering intelligence on antiplatelet drugs: The view from 30000 feet. *British Medical Journal*, *324*, 59–60.

Schon, D. (1983). *The reflective practitioner*. New York: Basic.

Schwartz, C. (1994). *Chambers dictionary*. Edinburgh: Chambers.

Senge, P., & Scharmer, O. (2001). Community action research. In P. Reason, & H. Bradbury (Eds.), *Handbook of action research: Participatory inquiry and practice*. London: Sage.

Steering Committee of the Physicians' Health Study Research Group. (1988). Findings from the aspirin component of the ongoing Physicians' Health Study. *New England Journal of Medicine*, *318*, 262–264.

Taylor, R., Braveman, B., & Forsyth, K. (2002). Occupational science and the scholarship of practice: Implications for practitioners. *New Zealand Journal of Occupational Therapy*, *49*(2), 37–40.

Tornebohm, H. (1986). *Caring, knowing and paradigms*. Goteborg: University of Goteborg.

Waterman, H., Tillen, D., Dickson, R., et al. (2001). Action research: A systematic review and guidance for assessment. *Health Technology Assessment*, *5*(23).

Hammell, K. W. (2009). Sacred texts: A sceptical exploration of the assumptions underpinning theories of occupation. *Canadian Journal of Occupational Therapy*, *76*(1), 6–13.

Wilcock, A. A. (1998). *An occupational perspective of health*. Thorofare, NJ: Slack.

Wilcock, A. A. (2001a). *Occupation for health: A journey from self health to prescription*. London: British College of Occupational Therapists.

Wilcock, A. A. (2001b). *Occupation for health: A journey from prescription to self health*. London: British College of Occupational Therapists.

4

Skills and Processes in Occupational Therapy

Edward A.S. Duncan

OVERVIEW

This chapter focuses on the theoretical foundations of what occupational therapists 'do' and how they reason. Specifically, it examines how both doing and reasoning are simultaneously combined in practice. Describing occupational therapy, which focuses on individuals within the context of their physical and social environments, is not, therefore, quite as simple as it may at first appear. This chapter commences with a brief summary of the historical search for a coherent definition of occupational therapy. Over the years, there has been considerable interest within occupational therapy literature regarding the nature of practice and the skills of an occupational therapist. To address this, the focus of this chapter is on the unique core reasoning skills and context-dependent shared and specialist practice skills of an occupational therapist. The chapter concludes with an overview of the central occupational therapy process.

◎ HIGHLIGHTS

This chapter
- discusses the evolving nature of occupational therapy definitions
- highlights occupational therapy core reasoning skills, and context-dependent shared and specialist practice skills
- outlines the occupational therapy process and its cyclical nature
- examines issues arising in assessment, goal setting and evaluation.

DEFINING OCCUPATIONAL THERAPY

Definitions are important. Defining something provides clarity and vision and delineates its scope. Defining occupational therapy, however, has proven an elusive pursuit. In part this is as a result of the multi-faceted and complicated (sometimes, even complex [Pentland et al 2018]—see Chapter 3) nature of occupational therapy practice. This makes sense. Try defining what a medical doctor/physician does. Any overarching definition is so broad as to be largely meaningless. However, it is relatively simple to define what a particular specialist medical doctor/physician does. So too with occupational therapy. It is much easier to define what an occupational therapist does in any given context than to define what an occupational therapist is and does more generally. But, arguably, occupational therapy has a further challenge: it has a well-recognized problem with language (Creek 2010) and is known to struggle to develop meaningful taxonomies (Paley et al 2006). Despite significant efforts to develop a comprehensive taxonomy of occupational therapy terms (e.g., Creek 2010, Fisher & Marterella 2019), an agreed and stable taxonomy remains elusive. This ever-evolving nature of occupational therapy terminology is not all negative. It may in fact reflect a more powerful underlying reality that is largely out of the profession's control: that the developing nature of terminology over the years was—and still is—highly influenced by occupational therapy's professional evolution within whatever prevailing socio-political context it finds itself in (Turner & Alsop 2015). Early terminology reflected the profession's romantic, pragmatic roots; later terminology reflected the more mechanistic and evidence-based reality in which occupational therapy found itself located. Most recently, the profession's association of its practice as a complex intervention (Creek 2003, Pentland et al 2018) is directly attributable to intervention development and evaluation more generally within healthcare, and in the United Kingdom in particular (Craig et al 2013).

The World Federation of Occupational Therapists (WFOT) describes occupational therapy as

'a health discipline which is concerned with people who are physically and/or mentally impaired, disabled and/or handicapped, either temporarily or permanently. The professional qualified occupational therapist involves the patients in activities designed to promote the restoration and maximum use of function with the aim of helping such people meet the demands of their working, social, personal and domestic environment, and to participate in life in its fullest sense' (World Federation of Occupational Therapists 2003).

WFOT (2003) provides a further 37 definitions of occupational therapy that have been developed by its national member associations. There is substantial consensus of opinion on the definition of occupational therapy. National differences appear more reflective of the differing layers of complexity considered rather than significant differences of opinion. A critique of these existing definitions, however, suggests that they are likely to become limited or outdated in years to come. Through concepts such as occupational justice (Durocher et al 2014) and community-based rehabilitation (Grandisson et al 2014), occupational therapy has become increasingly interested and involved in public, population and global health theory and practice. Current definitions of occupational therapy practice, and much of this textbook, remain focused on individual-level therapeutic interventions. These will require to evolve in future if occupational therapy theory and practice developments in public, population and global health continue to grow. The current definitions of the profession are already stretching at their seams.

WHAT ARE THE SKILLS OF AN OCCUPATIONAL THERAPIST?

Turner and Alsop (2015) undertook a critical review of the unique core skills of an occupational therapist. Their paper, a combination of rigorous critical literature review and in-depth reflective analysis by two distinguished UK emerita professors of occupational therapy, provides important insights into what they described as occupational therapists 'hidden assets': the combination of a central philosophy, unique core-reasoning skills and context-dependent practice skills. The central philosophy of the profession has been presented in Chapters 2 and 3. This section, therefore, will provide an introduction to the unique reasoning skills of an occupational therapist (see Chapter 15 for a comprehensive overview of clinical reasoning in occupational therapy), present some of the skills that occupational therapists share with other professionals, and provide an introduction to some of the specialist areas of practice that exist and can be a source of professional development for occupational therapists.

Occupational Therapy Reasoning Skills

Although previous literature, including previous editions of this text, have focused on the unique core skills of an occupational therapist, Turner and Alsop (2015, p.746) convincingly argue that the contemporary consensus is that, "the unique core skills of occupational therapists comprise the processing and integrating, through reasoning, of the unique knowledge and theories of occupation into professional practice executed with each individual service user." While this understanding may need to be expanded over time to account for occupational therapy in population, public and global health, it does provide an insightful manner in which to understand the unique contribution of occupational therapists, wherever they may be. Turner and Alsop (2015) describe the profession's unique contribution as identifying and analyzing occupational needs; in co-operation with service users; facilitating occupational performance/engagement; and evaluating, reflecting and acting upon occupational outcomes.

Identifying and Analyzing Occupational Needs

Analysis and adaptation of occupations. The analysis of occupations and their use in therapy has been long recognized as a central skill of the occupational therapist (Hagedorn 2001). Analyzing and adapting occupations and activities have two purposes:

- to understand the challenges experienced by clients in all aspects of their everyday life—these are frequently classified as work, leisure and self-care challenges
- to adapt existing or planned tasks so that a client is able to address existing or foreseeable occupational performance difficulties.

Analyzing occupations and activities involves breaking them down into their component parts (tasks) and sequence, looking at their stable and situational components and evaluating their therapeutic potential. Occupational therapists analyze occupations and activities to

- consider the kind(s) of performance needed to achieve the desired goal
- consider the degree of complexity of the occupation or activity
- consider their social or cultural associations

- define the component tasks of which the occupation or activity is composed
- analyze the sequence of task performance and whether this is fixed or flexible
- define the tools, furniture, materials and environment required for completion of the occupational form
- define and consider safety precautions or risk factors.

There are a variety of approaches to analyzing occupations and tasks. Some are theory-based (Kielhofner & Forsyth 2009), others are atheoretical but logical approaches to analyzing the activity or occupation required. One such approach is the in-order-to analysis approach (Paley et al 2006). In this analytical approach the therapist starts with a particular activity or occupation in a particular context. They then ask themselves a series of questions, chaining backwards or forwards (whichever appears easier) to understand the component parts of the activity or occupation required for completion (Fig. 4.1). If the client is able to complete a larger component (e.g., selecting ingredients) of an activity or occupation without difficulty there is no need to analyze it further. However, where it is clear that a client will have difficulty with a component part of an activity or occupation, then a further detailed analysis of that specific component will be required to understand the actual source of the challenge they face. With that analysis complete, they are then able to locate the source of the client's difficulties and use their clinical reasoning—in conjunction with the client's preferences—to understand whether it is necessary to work with the client to attempt to overcome the identified challenge(s), or whether an adaptation of the occupation, activity or environment is required.

Environmental analysis and adaptation. Occupational therapists recognize that both physical and social environments can have important beneficial or detrimental effects on the individual. Environmental analysis may provide information on the causes of problems for the individual, explanations for behaviour or ideas or suggestions for therapeutic adaptation.

An occupational therapist may suggest adapting, removing or adding to elements of the physical environment—for example, physical features of buildings, access, sound, colour, lighting level, temperature, decor, furniture, information content—to remove obstacles to performance or to enhance the opportunities for performance, learning or development. Occupational therapists should also consider adapting the social environment (i.e., the groups of people that a person is involved with in their environment), as these can also positively or negatively affect the client in achieving their goals.

The way in which an environmental analysis is carried out depends on both the needs of the client and the conceptual model/frame of reference within which the therapist is working, as these will alter the significance of the components that are observed.

In general terms, the occupational therapist will observe and accurately record the physical environment (e.g., buildings, interiors, heat, light, sound) and the social environment (e.g., How many people are in the environment? What is the nature of the relationships? How supportive are they? and so on) that contribute to or detract from a client's performance and positive occupational identity.

Why Assess? Assessment is the gathering of relevant information that informs the prioritization, development and evaluation of clinical goals for intervention. All assessment procedures require a basis of theoretical knowledge,

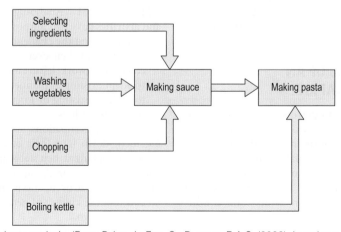

Fig. 4.1 An in-order-to analysis. (From Paley, J., Eva, G., Duncan, E.A.S. (2006). In-order-to analysis: An alternative to classifying different levels of occupational activity. *British Journal of Occupational Therapy, 69*(4), 161–168.)

practical experience and expertise. There are several basic skills required to carry out effective assessments:
- clinical judgement of what is to be assessed
- decision-making about the most appropriate assessment methods to use
- objectivity
- good observation skills
- production of consistent, accurate and, where possible, replicable results
- communication of results clearly to others
- sensitivity to client and carer hopes and expectations.

Assessment is a means to an end—identification of the problem; definition of a starting point for intervention; measurement of progress; and evaluation of outcome. As well as assessing an individual's ability, it is also important to assess the context in which they are carrying out the task—the environment.

How do you assess? Assessments can be carried out in either a structured or an unstructured manner; depending on their aim, both can be valid (Forsyth 2017). Using either structured or unstructured procedures, assessment information can be gathered through a variety of methods:
- observation, for example, of a client performing an *occupational form*
- interview, for example, with the client or relevant others
- self-report or checklists, for example, to provide a client perspective
- performance tests, for example, of physical or cognitive ability
- measurement techniques, for example, of physical performance.

In practice, a combination of these methods is often used; observation may be combined with interview, a structured assessment with an unstructured assessment. Therapists may interview a client, watch them carry out a task or occupational form, and ask them to complete a checklist or self-report instrument. Frequently, some of these assessments will be unstructured. The Model of Human Occupation (see Chapter 6) has developed some structured assessments that use a combined method of assessment. These assessments are not the only ones available, but they form a substantial bank of theory-based occupational therapy assessments, and are appropriate for a wide variety of situations and requirements.

Unstructured assessment. Unstructured assessments are also referred to as informal, ad hoc or nonstandardized. Many unstructured assessments are constructed by occupational therapists who developed them to meet local needs. Although unstructured assessments can never provide the reliability of structured assessments, several reasons exist that can justify their use:
- lack of an appropriate structured assessment

- lack of acceptability of structured assessments to a client
- use of unstructured assessments to add to information previously gained through structured assessment
- lack of time to complete a structured assessment
- structured assessments not available at an unforeseen opportunity to gather more information (Forsyth 2017).

Structured assessment. Structured or standardized assessments are tools that have been rigorously developed over a period of time and are designed to be dependable. Two specific issues are of particular importance in the development and appraisal of a structured assessment: validity and reliability.

Validity. Validity concerns whether the assessment actually deals with matters that are appropriate to the situation and measures the right things. There are various forms of validity (Heale & Twycross 2015):
- *Face validity.* Does the assessment look as if it does the things it is supposed to?
- *Construct validity.* Does the assessment measure what it is intended to?
- *Content validity.* Does the assessment gather all relevant information?
- *Criterion validity.* Is the measure related to other assessments that measure the same thing?

Depending on the focus of the assessment, a structured assessment may require more than one form of validity to be evaluated in its development and appraisal. Furthermore, an assessment's validity grows with each study that develops its evidence base.

Reliability. Reliability means that you can be sure that, each time the test is used, the findings can be depended upon. There are different types (or attributes) of reliability (Heale & Twycross 2015):
- *Homogeneity.* The extent to which all the items of an assessment are measuring the same thing.
- *Stability.* The extent to which, if an assessment is repeated, it will get the same result.
- *Equivalence.* The assessment is repeated by different therapists, or different versions of the same assessment are used, with the same result.

Analyzing and Prioritizing Occupational Need in Co-Operation with Service Users

The Therapeutic Use of Self. The therapeutic use of self is arguably one of the most important skills a therapist has. Mosey (1986) described an occupational therapist's use of self as a conscious therapeutic tool and suggests that there is a difference between a spontaneous interaction that is unplanned and a planned interaction that, whilst appearing spontaneous, is guided and informed.

Occupational therapists can adopt various theoretical frames of reference that assist in the development of the therapeutic use of self in differing ways. These include the client-centred and the cognitive–behavioural (see Chapters 11 and 12 for further information). Taylor (2008) stresses that the use of self in occupational therapy is distinct from a purely psychotherapeutic approach. Whereas within psychotherapy the interpersonal relationship is the primary focus of the intervention, in occupational therapy the central focus of the therapeutic interaction is engagement in occupation. Taylor (2008) presents a comprehensive occupational therapy intentional relationship model that has been designed to sit alongside conceptual models of practice, and explains how the therapist–client relationship exists and is enacted in occupational therapy encounters. Therapists can enable their therapeutic use of self in at least six different ways (modes) of relating: advocating, collaborating, empathizing, encouraging, instructing and problem-solving (Taylor 2008).

Each of us has natural preferred ways of interacting. It is worth reflecting on which of these therapeutic modes we are most naturally inclined to adopt. The reflexive and skilled therapist is able to dynamically consider which relational mode is suitable to each therapeutic encounter. Doing this we adapt our ways of interacting accordingly, changing mode during the same clinical contact if required. However, achieving this can be challenging. And it is easy to fool yourself with a belief that you have good people person skills, without engaging in critical reflection of how good you actually are in each moment. For this reason it is worth taking time to personally reflect and regularly consider in supervision how you relate to your clients, which ways are easiest, when and with whom do you find it difficult, and what, if anything you could do to respond in more nuanced and person-centred manner.

Goal Setting. Having assessed the client and formed a professional perspective of a person's priorities and needs, it is vital to understand the client's views of what they wish to achieve; that is, what their goals are. 'Goals are targets that the client hopes to reach through involvement in occupational therapy' (Creek 2002, p.129). Developing goals is a vital component of the occupational therapy process. However, practice of occupational therapy goal setting varies across teams (Scobbie et al 2015) and, as Wade (2009 p.291) states, while 'setting goals with patients and monitoring their achievement is a core practice within much of rehabilitation, … the evidence base behind this practice is patchy'. However, goal setting research in occupational therapy has progressed in recent years, particularly in the United Kingdom: Dr Niina

Kolehmainen has developed and evaluated a goal setting intervention with paediatric populations (Kolehmainen et al 2012, Kolehmainen et al 2013, Gilmore et al 2015), whereas Dr Lesley Scobbie has developed a goal setting and action-planning framework (G-AP) for stroke rehabilitation (Scobbie et al 2013, Scobbie et al 2015, Scobbie & Dixon 2014). The research supporting G-AP was then extended by Dr Sally Boa, a speech and language therapist, for use within palliative care settings (G-AP PC) (Boa et al 2014, Boa et al 2018). Although each of these goal setting approaches is distinct, they share core behavioural goal setting theory in common, and have each been co-constructed with therapists and clients within their distinct clinical areas. Key stages of goal setting that appear to be important across these areas of practice are discussed in the following section.

Negotiating and agreeing goals. Involvement of clients in the decision-making process surrounding setting goals is crucial. Neistadt (1995) found that clients who participated in the development of their goals made statistically and clinically significant gains in their performance ability. Negotiating goals requires the therapist and client to discuss what they see as the problems that exist, and from what may be an initial long list, agree a specific goal that is important to the client (Scobbie et al 2015).

Developing action plans. Action plans describe in detail what will be done, by whom and when. These plans should be specific enough to be able to return to them at a later date to evaluate whether or not they have been achieved. Many studies suggest setting SMART goals (specific, measurable, realistic and timed) (Bovend'Eerdt et al 2009, Page et al 2015) to achieve this. There is evidence that at least a few services use this approach (Scobbie et al 2015). However, SMART goals can have unintended consequences and may result in the setting of goals that are achievable and measurable, rather than actually what is desired by the client. It can also be very difficult to meaningfully predict what a client will be able to achieve. These difficulties make the SMART process challenging in practice.

Reviewing progress and deciding next steps. Reviewing progress is central to the goal-setting process. Although there is no set time at which reviewing should occur, it makes sense to have a conversation together at the end of each action plan to see how things have gone and consider next steps. Positive progress can be motivating for clients to recognize when progress is reviewed. Lack of progress can be discouraging for clients; however, a therapist's therapeutic relationship with the client can be used to encourage and motivate them to keep going, or—when necessary—open up discussions about alternative options when it looks like the goal will not be achieved.

Facilitating Occupational Performance/Engagement. Therapy, treatment and intervention are largely synonymous terms; however, each suggests certain philosophical beliefs about the position and role of the client in relation to the therapist. For example, the term *treatment* suggests a largely passive experience where a person is done to instead of done with. The term *intervention* is preferred in this text, as it recognizes the intrusion (however welcome) in a person's life and indicates a broadly based form of service provision. Within occupational therapy, the form of the intervention is occupation based. In one of the UK's earliest theoretical texts on occupational therapy, it was suggested that the range of occupations that could be used for therapeutic intentions was infinite. Of greater importance was the aim of their use and whether this was suitable and achievable (MacDonald 1960). This perspective remains as true today as it did then.

Application of occupation as therapy. The selection of an occupation as a therapeutic intervention requires that a balance be achieved between the needs and interests of the client, the personal repertoire of skills possessed by the therapist, and the requirements of the conceptual model or frame of reference within which the therapist chooses to work. Occupations should be specifically selected for the individual client in respect of the developed goals.

Occupations may be used casually for recreation or as pastimes; such use is perfectly valid in the right context; however, their use in this way is diversional occupation, not occupational therapy.

Adapting occupation. Occupations may be presented in an unadapted manner or may be adapted to meet the specified goals. Types of adaptation that may be required to assist the client to achieve their goals include
- *environmental*, for example, location, setting, milieu
- *equipment*, for example, quantity of tools/materials, adaptation to tools
- *social*, for example, number of people, degree of interaction
- *physical*, for example, position, strength, range of movement
- *cognitive*, for example, complexity, sequence, need for instructions
- *emotional*, for example, interest, meaning, self-expression
- *temporal*, for example, duration, repetition
- *structural*, for example, order of tasks, omission of non-essential tasks.

The amended factors of an occupation can then be graded over time to increase the client's occupational performance and development of a positive occupational identity.

Environmental context of interventions. Interventions can occur in a client's natural environment (such as their home or community), in proximate environments (such as a group home/hostel or a local community near their current residency) or in artificial environments (such as hospitals or prisons). Within these settings, interventions may take place in various forms of group setting (whether naturally occurring groups such as a football team, or artificial groups such as an on-ward cooking group) or individually.

Specific interventions are shaped and influenced by the frames of reference and conceptual models of practice that guide them. Interventions from each of these theoretical constructs are described in detail in the following chapters.

Evaluating, Reflective and Acting on Occupational Outcomes

Evaluation. Evaluating the effectiveness of occupational therapy is an ethical and professional imperative.

Individual evaluation. Evaluation is the method by which the client, therapist and other relevant individuals (such as carers) or bodies (such as the multi-disciplinary team) know if the agreed goals have been met. Although evaluation is an ongoing process throughout therapy, it is the final evaluation that is often most significant. Measuring 'success' is often achieved using the same assessment measures employed at the initial and ongoing assessment, looking for significant changes in the desired direction. Evaluation can also be measured by examining whether the specified goals have been met and by discussing the client's perspective of the situation.

Shared/Context-Dependent Practice Skills. Occupational therapists have a variety of shared skills. Whilst shared, these skills are no less essential to practice. Occupational therapists also draw on the wealth of assessments and interventions that have not been developed by occupational therapists, but facilitate the development of occupational performance and assist in the creation of a greater occupational self-identity. The use of interventions that are not occupational therapy-specific is a contentious topic, as the profession becomes ever more deeply occupation-focused. Do nonoccupational therapy-specific interventions have a place in the profession today? Several of the chapters in this book address this issue, either directly or indirectly. It would be challenging to list all the shared skills occupational therapists possess. Examples of key shared skills are as follows:

Leadership and Management. Often placed together, leadership and management are two important but distinct skills.

Management. Occupational therapists have to manage services, a caseload, an academic department or research team resources. The therapist needs to set standards, monitor quality and audit performance. These findings need to be communicated within the profession and to others. The therapist must be critically aware of their own performance, seeking regular supervision and evaluating and updating personal knowledge. Management is not, therefore, a skill that is the remit of the head of a service, but the responsibility of all staff, albeit in differing ways. Furthermore, as well as managing externally, therapists must also be able to manage themselves. Self-management consists of the actions and strategies we use to direct our own activity and ensure that we remain fit for purpose at work and at home. Bannigan (2009) describes the importance of self-management and the development of professional resilience in the face of the many challenges that arise in the workplace.

Leadership. Leadership is different from management. Whilst management has been defined as the 'bottom line … how can I best accomplish things', leadership has been defined as knowing 'what are the things I want to accomplish' (Covey 1989, p.101). Leaders in occupational therapy develop innovative approaches to intervention, work with clients in new ways, spot opportunities and develop services. The historical view of management and leadership as components of the same role is increasingly recognized as ineffectual. Indeed, the roles of consultant and clinical specialist occupational therapists (within the UK) appears to recognize that certain career pathways offer and require particular leadership qualities. Managing a service is an alternative professional pathway. Therefore, the leader of an occupational therapy team is not necessarily the manager, but may be a senior clinician with the vision and skills to move the service forwards. Developing as a leader, however, is more than merely a professional skill; it is a personal and professional quality.

An awareness of one's need for continuous self-improvement and openness to others' perspectives of our own leadership qualities is essential. Although everyone will have their own leadership style, lots can be learnt from other people. Often the best way to start developing this quality is to observe leaders you admire (both within and outside the profession), taking a bird's-eye view of their practice/life. What do they do that makes you admire them? How do they deal with other people? How do they deal with themselves? What is their vision? How do they maintain their integrity in difficult situations? Conversely, the same exercise can be carried out with individuals whose practice you may not like to emulate! Reflect on these observations and consider any lessons that can be learnt. What would you wish to integrate into your practice/life?

As well as observation, a lot can be learnt from the wealth of literature that is available on this subject (e.g., Covey 1989, Goleman et al 2002). Christiansen (2009) has written on leadership with direct reference to leadership in occupational therapy and Tempest and Dancza (2019) have recently promoted the idea of occupational therapists as social leaders: leading from behind in a quiet, yet determined way, to bring people together to co-create meaningful change in communities. Social leaders, they argue, need not been senior personal, but are born when a person brings a community of people together to work for change. Ultimately, regardless of the type of leadership approach, leadership qualities are lived, developed and refined over a lifetime.

Research. Research is a central component of occupational therapy practice (Ilott & White 2001) and the emphasis on research is arguably the single most significant development that has occurred in occupational therapy in the last 25 years (Duncan 2009). Every occupational therapist is required to use skills in research. This does not mean that every occupational therapist must carry out independent research, but at the very least everyone should be effective and critical consumers of research (Ilott & White 2001). The skills required to do this include

- information and communication technology skills, to search and locate the literature
- critical appraisal skills, to evaluate research
- development of a personal evaluative perspective, to challenge custom and practice
- ability to integrate research into practice, to deliver consistently the highest quality of service available.

Specialist Skills. Specialist skills are skills that cannot be expected of a competent clinician without further training, supervision and expertise (Duncan 1999). Occupational therapists can develop specialist skills that are either an extension of their core skills, such as specialist assessments (e.g., the Assessment of Motor and Process Skills (AMPS), Fisher 2003), or an extension of their shared skills, such as undertaking advanced splinting or psychotherapy training (Duncan 1999).

DEFINING THE OCCUPATIONAL THERAPY PROCESS

The occupational therapy process is the term given to the series of actions a therapist initiates to provide services to their client. This process is clearly not unique to occupational therapy. It is a form of problem analysis and solution that has been used by various healthcare professionals. There have been several representations of the process in occupational therapy, each differing a little from the others in accordance with each author's personal concept of the sequence. Generally, there is close agreement on the basic format. This involves gathering information concerning the client, their situation and challenges, carrying out assessments, identifying and formulating the problem or need, setting goals, setting consequent priorities for action, deciding on how to achieve these, implementing action and evaluating the outcome. Creek (2003) illustrates this process in a linear model (Fig. 4.2). Hagedorn (2001) uses similar points but illustrates the process's cyclical nature (Fig. 4.3). In practice, the occupational therapy process is often not linear (Creek 2003) or even cyclical. Frequently, these activities occur in synchrony and as part of a dynamic process repeated at various stages of therapy (Pentland et al 2018). The process is therefore circuitous, with overlapping and interwoven aspects of the process occurring throughout.

A simplified version of this process is illustrated in Figure 4.3. A referral is received by the therapist. This starts the intervention sequence. The therapist will then enter the cycle of information gathering and problem analysis, decision-making, implementation of action and review of outcome, which is repeated until intervention is judged to be completed.

Throughout this process, the occupational therapist employs the unique combination of knowledge, skills and values that form the practice of occupational therapy. The way in which this happens is often informed and directed by conceptual models of practice and frames of reference, several of which are outlined in Chapters 5 to 14.

SUMMARY

This chapter has introduced the skills and process of occupational therapy. It introduced the notion of the uniqueness of occupational therapists' reasoning skills, what occupational therapists 'do' and how they do things in practice. The evolving nature of occupational therapy definitions was presented. This continual evolution is a response to the changing demands of health, social, public, population and global care in which occupational therapy is either currently or increasingly situated. Future years are likely to see definitions of the profession continue to evolve.

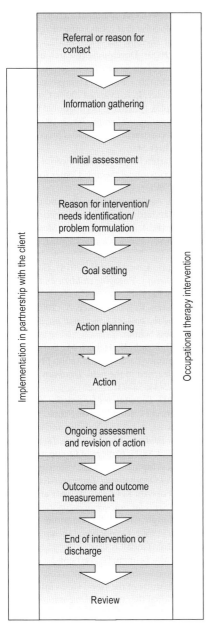

Fig. 4.2 The occupational therapy process viewed linearly. (Reproduced with permission of the College of Occupational Therapists from Creek 2003.)

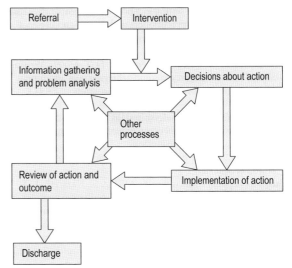

Fig. 4.3 The occupational therapy process viewed cyclically.

Occupational therapy's apparent simplicity is both its strength and its greatest challenge. This chapter's brief review of an occupational therapist's skills and the component parts of the occupational therapy process illustrates that, whilst occupational therapy interventions are not always complex in the technical sense of the word (Duncan et al 2007), they can certainly be multi-factorial and challenging to describe. Perhaps it is for this reason that the challenging nature of delivering sophisticated occupational therapy interventions is not always immediately apparent to those who do not appreciate the processes at work.

✳ REFLECTIVE LEARNING

- What do you consider to be the key skills and processes you use in practice? How aware of them are you when you use them?
- How do you choose which method of assessment to use with a client?
- Have you seen or do you use goal setting in practice? What are its strengths and limitations?
- How do you evaluate your practice?

REFERENCES

Bannigan, K. (2009). Management of self. In E. A. S. Duncan (Ed.), *Skills for practice in occupational therapy* (pp. 231–248). Edinburgh: Churchill Livingstone.

Boa, S., Duncan, E. A., Haraldsdottir, E., & Wyke, S. (2014). Goal setting in palliative care: A structured review. *Progress in Palliative Care*, 22(6), 326–333.

Boa, S., Duncan, E., Haraldsdottir, E., & Wyke, S. (2018). Patient-centred goal setting in a hospice: A comparative case study of how health practitioners understand and use goal setting in practice. *International Journal of Palliative Nursing*, 24(3), 115–122.

Bovend'Eerdt, T. J., Botell, R. E., & Wade, D. T. (2009). Writing SMART rehabilitation goals and achieving goal attainment scaling: A practical guide. *Clinical Rehabilitation*, 23(4), 352–361.

Christiansen, C. (2009). Leadership skills. In E. A. S. Duncan (Ed.), *Skills for practice in occupational therapy* (pp. 313–322). Edinburgh: Churchill Livingstone.

Covey, S. (1989). *The 7 habits of highly effective people*. London: Simon & Schuster.

Craig, P., Dieppe, P., Macintyre, S., Michie, S., Nazareth, I., & Petticrew, M. (2008). Developing and evaluating complex interventions: The new Medical Research Council guidance. *BMJ*, 337, 1655.

Creek, J. (2002). Treatment planning and implementation. In J. Creek (Ed.), *Occupational therapy in mental health* (3rd ed.) (pp. 119–138). Edinburgh: Churchill Livingstone.

Creek, J. (2003). *Occupational therapy defined as a complex intervention*. London: College of Occupational Therapists.

Creek, J. (2010). *The core concepts of occupational therapy: A dynamic framework for practice*. London: Jessica Kingsley Publishers.

Durocher, E., Gibson, B. E., & Rappolt, S. (2014). Occupational justice: A conceptual review. *Journal of Occupational Science*, 21(4), 418–430.

Duncan, E. A. S. (1999). Occupational therapy in mental health: It is time to recognise that it has come of age. *British Journal of Occupational Therapy*, 62(11), 521–522.

Duncan, E. A. S. (2009). Developing research in practice. In E. A. S. Duncan (Ed.), *Skills for practice in occupational therapy* (pp. 279–292). Edinburgh: Churchill Livingstone.

Duncan, E. A. S., Paley, J., & Eva, G. (2007). Complex interventions and complex systems in occupational therapy. *British Journal of Occupational Therapy*, 70(5), 199–206.

Fisher, A. (2003). *Assessment of motor and process skills* (5th ed.). Fort Collins: Three Star.

Fisher, A. G., & Marterella, A. (2019). *Powerful practice: A model for authentic occupational therapy*. Center for Innovative OT Solutions, Ft. Collins, CO.

Forsyth, K. (2017). Assessment: Choosing and using standardized and nonstandardized means of gathering information. In R. R. Taylor (Ed.), *2017. Kielhofner's Model of Human Occupation: Theory and application*. Philadelphia: Wolters Kluwer.

Gilmore, R., King, G., Law, M., et al. (2015). *Goal setting and motivation in therapy: Engaging children and parents*. London: Jessica Kingsley Publishers.

Goleman, D., Boyatzis, R. E., & McKee, A. (2002). *Primal leadership: Realizing the power of emotional intelligence*. London: Harvard Business School.

Grandisson, M., Thibeault, R., Hébert, M., & Templeton, A. (2014). Community-based rehabilitation programme evaluations: Lessons learned in the field. *Disability, CBR & Inclusive Development*, 25(1), 55–71.

Hagedorn, R. (2001). *Foundations for practice in occupational therapy*. Edinburgh: Churchill Livingstone.

Heale, R., & Twycross, A. (2015). Validity and reliability in quantitative studies. *Evidence-based Nursing*, 18(3), 66–67.

Ilott, I., & White, E. (2001). College of Occupational Therapists research and development strategic vision and action plan. *British Journal of Occupational Therapy*, 64(6), 270–277.

Kielhofner, G., & Forsyth, K. (2009). Activity analysis. In E. A. S. Duncan (Ed.), *Skills for practice in occupational therapy* (pp. 91–104). Edinburgh: Churchill Livingstone.

MacDonald, E. M. (1960). *Occupational therapy in rehabilitation*. London: Baillière, Tindall & Cox.

Kolehmainen, N., MacLennan, G., Ternent, L., et al. (2012). Using shared goal setting to improve access and equity: A mixed methods study of the Good Goals intervention in children's occupational therapy. *Implementation Science*, 7(1), 76.

Kolehmainen, N., MacLennan, G., Ternent, L., et al. (2013). Multi-level case studies in development of complex interventions: An example of the good goals intervention. *Trials*, 14(1), P5.

Mosey, A. C. (1986). *Psychosocial components of occupational therapy*. New York: Raven.

Neistadt, M. E. (1995). Methods of assessing clients' priorities: A survey of adult physical dysfunction settings. *American Journal of Occupational Therapy*, 49, 428–436.

Page, J., Roos, K., Bänziger, A., et al. (2015). Formulating goals in occupational therapy: State of the art in Switzerland. *Scandinavian Journal of Occupational Therapy*, 22(6), 403–415.

Paley, J., Eva, G., & Duncan, E. A. S. (2006). In-order-to analysis: An alternative to classifying different levels of occupational activity. *British Journal of Occupational Therapy*, 69(4), 161–168.

Pentland, D., Kantartzis, S., Giatsi Clausen, M., & Witemyre, K. (2018). *Occupational therapy and complexity: Defining and describing practice*. London: Royal College of Occupational Therapists.

Scobbie, L., & Dixon, D. (2014). *Theory-based approach to goal setting. Rehabilitation goal setting: Theory, practice and evidence*. Boca Raton: CRC Press, 213–236.

Scobbie, L., McLean, D., Dixon, D., Duncan, E., & Wyke, S. (2013). Implementing a framework for goal setting in community based stroke rehabilitation: A process evaluation. *BMC Health Services Research*, 13(1), 190.

Scobbie, L., Duncan, E. A., Brady, M. C., & Wyke, S. (2015). Goal setting practice in services delivering community-based stroke rehabilitation: A United Kingdom (UK) wide survey. *Disability and Rehabilitation*, 37(14), 1291–1298.

Taylor, R.R., 2008. The intentional relationship: Outpatient therapy and use of self. FA Davis. Philadelphia.

Tempest, S., & Dancza, K., (2019). Embracing the leadership potential of occupational therapy in the social age: Time for a silent revolution. *British Journal of Occupational Therapy*, 82(10), 601–603.

Turner, A., & Alsop, A. (2015). Unique core skills: Exploring occupational therapists' hidden assets. *British Journal of Occupational Therapy*, 78(12), 739–749.

Wade, D. (2009). Goal setting in rehabilitation: An overview of what, why and how. *Clinical Rehabilitation*, 23, 291–295.

5

An Introduction to Conceptual Models of Practice and Frames of Reference

Edward A.S. Duncan

OVERVIEW

This chapter provides an introduction to frames of reference and conceptual models of practice in occupational therapy. It commences by exploring the rationale for having theoretical constructs in practice. It continues by examining the challenges that theoretical terminology has posed occupational therapists, before defining key terms used in this text. The proliferation of frames of reference and conceptual models of practice is then discussed and a guide for future theoretical development and evaluation presented. Following this, the relationship between conceptual models of practice and frames of reference in this text is explained. The cultural assumptions and implications embedded within the development of conceptual models of practice are discussed.

KEY POINTS

This chapter
- introduces conceptual models of practice and frames of reference
- emphasizes the importance of language and understanding theoretical terminology
- discusses the development of theory in occupational therapy
- examines the stages of theoretical development of conceptual models of practice.

WHY HAVE FRAMES OF REFERENCE OR CONCEPTUAL MODELS OF PRACTICE?

Imagine the following scenario. After a few weeks of feeling unwell, you consult your doctor, who decides that you should go to see a consultant surgeon. Your consultation goes as follows:

You: Doctor, I haven't felt well for several weeks. My stomach's upset. I've lost my appetite and some weight, and I don't feel that I have the same energy and get up and go that I normally have.
Consultant surgeon: I see. Well, I tell you what … why don't I do some tests?
You: What are you testing for?
Consultant surgeon: Not sure, really. I have a few personal favourite tests that I've used a lot. Did I tell you I've been qualified for over 20 years? So I think I'll use those and see what they show up. I reckon I know what I'm going to do anyway.

How would you feel leaving this consultation? It probably would not engender much confidence that your health was being considered in a structured, evidence-based manner.

It is difficult to come up with 'answers' in healthcare, and all the more so in professions such as occupational therapy that have inherently broad aims. However, it is known that professionals' individual perspectives are highly vulnerable to a range of biases and heuristics when making clinical judgements (Gilovich et al 2002), regardless of their clinical 'expertise'. It is also true that experience and 'time served' as a practitioner have fairly consistently shown to have no effect on improving clinical judgements (Grove & Meehl 1996, Grove et al 2000). Knowledge of such inherent limitations of individual perspectives supports the acceptance and development of evidence-based decision-making approaches to therapeutic interventions. Frames of reference and conceptual models of practice are an ideal way in which clinicians can use theory, in a structured manner, to conceptualize clients' difficulties, shape intervention and evaluate success. Using a well-developed frame of reference and/or conceptual model of practice encourages therapists to consider a whole range of options that they would per-haps be less likely to do if left to their own devices.

In her review of the history of occupational therapy in the United Kingdom, Wilcock (2001) attributes the first use of the terms *frame of reference* and *model* to McClean, an American occupational therapist working as a lecturer in England (McClean 1974). McClean's rationale for the development of a structured theory to underpin occupa-tional therapy practice was financial. Hospital manage-ment, McClean (1974) argued, was no longer willing to tolerate therapeutic interventions for reasons of enjoyment alone. The requirement to demonstrate the value of prac-tice had dawned and the development of theories, McClean suggested, would enable the evaluation of practice and research to be undertaken (McClean 1974). In today's world of clinical governance and evidence-based practice, finance remains a dominant driver in the development of theory. It is certainly true, now more than ever, that the demonstration of effectiveness is of vital importance—not only for the good of the patients who receive the service, but also for the good of the profession as it faces increas-ingly probing questions about its worth in a financially challenging climate.

Structured theories develop out of a desire to explain the function and mechanisms of impact of occupational therapy, and help explain why a person is experiencing a particular problem, what a potential solution could be and why a particular intervention works. Structured theories provide explanations and describe the relationship between different aspects of a person (Kielhofner 2009). Theories also identify occupational therapy's unique contribution to health and assist in defining professional boundaries (Feaver & Creek 1993b).

Supporting the use of structured theory in practice does not negate the requirements for occupational therapists to use their judgement. Occupational therapists have to decide which conceptual model provides the best evidence base and supporting structure for the setting in which they work. Sometimes this will be self-evident; it is highly unlikely that a psychodynamic frame of reference would be a useful *primary* frame of reference in an orthopaedic ward; the occupational therapist is more likely to use a biome-chanical frame of reference and an associated conceptual model of practice. At other times, however, the case may not be so clear and a careful appraisal of the available evi-dence is required to inform theoretical decisions and the directions of practice.

Defining and Understanding Theoretical Terminology

Having articulated the rationale for having a structured theoretical basis for practice, it is important to consider the challenge of developing a clear understanding of the key terms that are used to articulate them. This is not as straightforward as it first sounds, basically because 'differ-ent writers use them [theoretical terms] in different ways and their meaning is modified by the context in which they are used' (Feaver & Creek 1993a, p.4).

The description of occupational therapy theory has rapidly evolved since the mid-1980s. During the early years of theory development, the language that described theory developed and terms such as *paradigm*, *model*, *frame of reference* and *approach* were often used interchangeably and with different meanings by vari-ous authors (e.g., Reed 1984, Mosey 1986, Creek 1992, Kielhofner 1992, Young & Quinn 1992, Hopkins & Smith 1993). Such variation added considerably to the confusion of clinicians, students and academics who tried to understand and evaluate contrasting concep-tual foundations of practice. Hagedorn (2001) likened the struggle to understand the various uses of terminol-ogy in occupational therapy to the following discourse between Alice and Humpty Dumpty (Lewis Carroll, *Alice Through the Looking Glass*). Despite the passing of years it remains as relevant today as when she first pub-lished her analogy:

> 'There's glory for you!'
> 'I don't know what you mean by "glory",' Alice said.
> 'I meant, "there's a nice knock-down argument for you!"'
> 'But "glory" doesn't mean "a nice knock down argu-ment",' Alice objected.
> 'When I use a word,' Humpty Dumpty said in a rather scornful tone, 'it means just what I choose it to mean—neither more nor less.'

For a while it seemed that this terminological debate may have abated. However, more recent arguments have been made that suggest that occupational therapists con-tinue to fail in providing a consistent description of terms to describe what they do and how they do it (Fisher 2014). One solution to this is the development of internationally recognized standard definitions of theoretical terms and concepts. However, whilst this is a tempting proposal, it is questionable whether it could be meaningfully achieved. The ongoing nature of this debate (over 30 years and count-ing!) gives little hope that it will be resolved anytime soon. Consequently, it is important to remain mindful that spe-cific terms are used by different people in different ways. Differences in definitions of terminology are not simply semantic; they frequently expose an author's conceptual bias. By way of example, two contemporary definitions of 'models', developed by theoretical leaders in the field, are provided here. Creek (2003, p.55) defines a model for practice as a '*simplified representation* of the structure and content of a phenomenon or system that describes or explains certain data or relationships and integrates elements of theory and practice', whilst Forsyth (see Chapter 6, page 18) highlights how 'the strength and application of MOHO [a well-known conceptual model of practice] is *neither simple nor formulaic*. Instead it aims to understand important multiple dimensions of each client's unique experience and bring a sophisticated understanding to bear on the life issues facing each client in practice' (author's emphasis added).

These contrasting definitions of models of practice illustrate
* the reason why a universally defined shared terminology is unlikely to work, and
* the continuing importance of truly understanding the perspective of an author(s) when reading and appraising literature relating to occupational therapy theory and practice.

Although theory should never be presented as unnecessarily complicated, neither should its inherent complexity be watered down towards an unachievable simplicity. Theoretical terminology is important; it defines key terms, enables the succinct communication of complex ideas, and supports the testing of theoretical hypothesis in research and practice. However, terminology can require effort to understand. It is easy to become disheartened when grappling with a massive amount of new theoretical 'language'. As a result, some students and clinicians venture no further with such texts than is required (e.g., to pass their assignments). This elective loss of knowledge is not simply a personal issue; it means that an individual's professional capacity is also diminished through a lack of engagement with the profession's rich knowledge base. I encourage students, clinicians and academics therefore to overcome their frustration (if they have any) and engage with theoretical terminology where it exists, in both this text and others. The investment of time and reflective thought, as well as discussions with peers and colleagues, will all assist in further understanding the concepts that are being communicated. These days there are ever more opportunities to develop your understanding through discussion with others. Social media events such as weekly Twitter chats (e.g., #otalk www.otalk.co.uk), specialist Facebook pages and so on, all provide opportunities to engage with peers, even when you may be professionally isolated in your practice. If you sustain your engagement with the theoretical occupational therapy literature, through individual study and group discussions, you will encounter a wealth of knowledge that you would otherwise have left undiscovered. As a consequence your practice will be enriched with a greater understanding of what you are doing, how you do what they do and why you are doing it (Fisher 2014).

Theoretical Definitions Used in this Book

To give meaning to the structure of this book and to assist the reader in following the arguments and propositions contained within, it is necessary to define some key theoretical terms. Where possible, these definitions have been adhered to throughout the text. In defining theoretical terms, consideration has been given to lessening confusion by providing clear and (hopefully) uncontroversial taxonomy. Some terminology has already been introduced in the preceding chapter; however, it is repeated here for clarity.
* *Paradigm.* The shared consensus regarding the most fundamental beliefs of the profession.
* *Frame of reference.* Theoretical or conceptual ideas that have been developed outside the profession but which, with judicious use, are applicable within occupational therapy practice.
* *Conceptual model of practice.* Occupation-focused theoretical constructs and propositions that have been developed specifically to explain the process and practice of occupational therapy.

OCCUPATIONAL THERAPY'S THEORETICAL PROLIFERATION

The development of formalized theory came relatively late in the genesis of occupational therapy. Whilst its development is welcomed, the manner in which it has occurred has, perhaps, not always been helpful. One example of this is the variance in theoretical depth of some of the profession's 'models' of practice.

In 2001, Hagedorn outlined 11 person–environment–occupational performance models (Hagedorn 2001). Some of these were based on ongoing research; others represented the perspectives of an individual or a small group of occupational therapists at a particular moment in time. Although the publication of scholarly debate on occupational therapy's theory base is invaluable, the ongoing proliferation of personal perspectives shaped as nascent conceptual models of practice does not meaningfully support the development of occupational therapy's knowledge base and can increase confusion amongst clinicians and students in an already complex field.

Conversely, occupational therapy should not necessarily be limited to the few conceptual models or frames of reference that have an established evidence base. The profession's theoretical development would be poorer if the above call for rationalization of personal conceptual models was understood as an attempt to stifle novel ideas and innovations.

New conceptual models of practice/frames of reference, which recognize or perceive limitations in existing theories or practice and aim to address these, should be welcomed. They will enhance the knowledge base and encourage greater debate and understanding within the profession. However, these developments should contain sound theoretical arguments and vision of future development.

Kielhofner (2009) suggested that sustained development of a conceptual model of practice is required to ensure that its theoretical constructs are valid and useful. Furthermore, as well as providing a theoretical structure, a conceptual model of practice should also develop appropriate assessments and technology (e.g., intervention protocols) for use in practice (Kielhofner 2009). As such developments require to be gradually developed and tested, it is perhaps useful to consider what the developmental stages of a conceptual model of practice should be.

Proposed Stages of Theoretical Development

The following stages are based on a review of conceptual models to date and outline a proposed developmental sequence that illustrates the required developmental stages of contemporary conceptual models of practice. Frames of reference, as applied knowledge, are likely to have undergone a similar process within their original knowledge base. The process of integrating frames of reference is therefore different and is referred to throughout this text (see Chapters 6–10).

Although the developmental stages of conceptual models of practice suggest a general progression, it is acknowledged that some of these stages may occur simultaneously (Kielhofner 2009).

Develop Initial Conceptual Ideas
- Why is a new theoretical construct necessary?
- Form a basis for a new theoretical perspective.
- What are the factors that differentiate this construct from existing conceptual models?

Refine Conceptual Ideas
- Present the conceptual model to the occupational therapy community.
- Work with others (academics, clinicians and clients) to refine ideas and understandings.
- Continue to present refinements for critical appraisal and debate.

Test Theory in Practice
- This can be achieved through the use of a variety of research methods to examine the validity of the developing theory's claims in practice situations.

Develop Tools for Practice (Technology for Application)
- Develop self-report assessments, interview schedules, observation measures and so on.
- Develop protocols that support the clinician to enable them to use the information they gain using the model and associated tools to assist the client.

Increase the Evidence Base for the Conceptual Model
- Refine the theoretical arguments and understanding based on research carried out in clinical settings.
- Build the evidence base for the validity, reliability and utility of the conceptual model and its associated tools for practice.

Verify the Conceptual Model and Associated Tools for Practice Externally
- Theoretical constructs are rigorously tested by people with no personal bias as regards their success or failure.
- The tools for practice are evaluated by people with no personal bias as to their success or failure.
- Publications from independent research support the conceptual model's theoretical basis and utility in practice settings.

THE RELATIONSHIP BETWEEN CONCEPTUAL MODELS OF PRACTICE AND FRAME OF REFERENCE

Developed and evidence-based conceptual models of practice provide a rigorous organizational structure that avoids personal biases and heuristics. In doing so, such models also ensure that interventions remain occupation focused. Frames of reference are useful supports to conceptual models of practice and bring with them additional knowledge, tools and priorities. Frequently, occupational therapists will use one or more frames of reference in conjunction with their selected conceptual model of practice. The frames of reference should be selected before the assessment and goal setting commence because they may shape and influence the information that is gathered and the interventions that are employed to meet a client's goals (Fig. 5.1).

Selection of Frames of Reference and Conceptual Models of Practice in this Book

Amongst other theoretically important chapters, this book provides a detailed introduction to four frames of reference and five conceptual models of practice. Their selection was not arbitrary, but was based on their

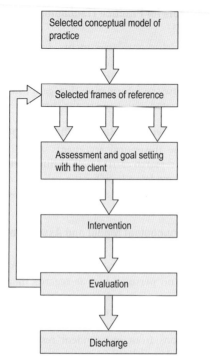

Fig. 5.1 The relationship between conceptual models of practice and frames of reference.

prominence within the literature, developing evidence base or commonality of use in practice. This sixth edition of *Foundations* has seen some frames of reference that were in previous editions omitted and new conceptual model chapters added. Not all the models and frames of reference presented in this text have equal evidence to support their practice.

PHILOSOPHICAL CHALLENGES TO THE DEVELOPMENT OF CONCEPTUAL MODELS OF PRACTICE IN OCCUPATIONAL THERAPY

The vast majority of occupational therapy conceptual models of practice have been developed in and from a Western societal perspective. Hammell (2011) contests that this has resulted in what Mann (1995) describes a form of *theoretical imperialism*, which privileges their own perspectives over the views and perspectives of others. From this perspective, assumptions that underpin many of the conceptual models of practice presented in this book are viewed as culturally and class specific, as they have all been developed primarily within predominantly white middle class Western cultural contexts and lack a wider evidence base (Hammell 2009, Hammell

2011). Hammell (2015) states that such developments have led to fundamental theoretical deficiencies in occupational therapy, which will remain until their proponents embrace the wisdom and diversity found in global cultures. An exception to this perspective, included in this text, to bring balance and completeness to the occupational therapy theoretical landscape, is the Kawa (River) Model (Iwama 2006). The Kawa (River) Model (see Chapter 10) challenges the nature of evidence-based practice (Iwama 2006). The Kawa model conceptualizes occupation and the relationship between occupation and well-being differently to other established occupational therapy conceptual models. In doing so it places greater emphasis on the inter-connectedness of people's lives to the past and to others in the present. A person defending the development and practice of the more established conceptual models would cite their successful use and the use of their associated assessments in non-Western settings and with non-Western participants (e.g., Chan & Lee 1997, Yamada et al 2010) as evidence of their wider applicability, beyond the confines in which they were originally developed. This argument has validity. However, the multiple contributions of Dr Karen Whalley Hammell (Honorary Professor in the Department of Occupational Science and Occupational Therapy at the University of British Columbia, Vancouver, Canada) challenge the fundamental philosophical positioning of most theoretical developments in occupational therapy, and display a level of intellectual rigour often lacking within the profession (Whalley Hammell 2015). Future conceptual model and frame of reference development is likely to require to—at least— take greater explicit account of the differing personal and cultural contexts from which their clients come and in which they live. Individuals who are interested in learning more about Whalley Hammell's perspectives would do well to watch her inspiring 2018 World Federation of Occupational Therapy plenary lecture (https://www.youtube.com/watch?v=9WipUPXx_Kk).

SUMMARY

This chapter has introduced the importance and use of frames of reference and conceptual models of practice in occupational therapy. Their importance in assisting structured clinical decision-making has been highlighted. The chapter explains the relationship between conceptual models and frames of reference, underlines the importance of their continued development, and introduces the rationale for the selection of the frames of reference and conceptual models of practice introduced in this text.

☀ REFLECTIVE LEARNING

- In your own words, describe what a conceptual model of practice and a frame of reference are.
- Imagine you are explaining the importance of conceptual models of frames of reference to someone in your family. What would you say?
- What basis would you use when considering which conceptual model and/or frame of reference to use in practice?
- Choose one of the conceptual model or frames of reference and consider the cultural considerations and/or implications of its development and core assumptions.

REFERENCES

Chan, C. C., & Lee, T. M. (1997). Validity of the Canadian occupational performance measure. *Occupational Therapy International, 4*(3), 231–249.

Creek, J. (1992). *Occupational therapy and mental health.* Edinburgh: Churchill Livingstone.

Creek, J. (2003). *Occupational therapy defined as a complex intervention.* London: College of Occupational Therapists.

Feaver, S., & Creek, J. (1993a). Models for practice in occupational therapy: Part 1. Defining terms. *British Journal of Occupational Therapy, 56*(1), 4–6.

Feaver, S., & Creek, J. (1993b). Models for practice in occupational therapy: Part 2. What use are they? *British Journal of Occupational Therapy, 56*(2), 59–69.

Fisher, A. G. (2014). Occupation-centred, occupation-based, occupation-focused: Same, same or different? *Scandinavian Journal of Occupational Therapy, 20,* 162–173

Gilovich, T., Griffen, D., & Kahneman, D. (2002). *Heuristics and biases: The psychology of intuitive judgement.* Cambridge: Cambridge University Press.

Grove, W. M., & Meehl, P. E. (1996). Comparative efficiency of informal (subjective, impressionistic) and formal (mechanical, algorithmic) prediction procedures: The clinical/statistical controversy. *Psychology, Public Policy, and Law, 2,* 1–31.

Grove, W. M., Zald, D. H., Lebow, B. S., Snitz, B. E., & Nelson, C. (2000). Clinical vs mechanical prediction: A meta analysis. *Psychological Assessment, 12,* 19–30.

Hagedorn, R. (2001). *Foundations for practice in occupational therapy.* Edinburgh: Churchill Livingstone.

Hammell, K. W. (2009). Self-care, productivity, and leisure, or dimensions of occupational experience? Rethinking occupational "categories". *Canadian Journal of Occupational Therapy, 76*(2), 107–114.

Hammell, K. W. (2011). Resisting theoretical imperialism in the disciplines of occupational science and occupational therapy. *British Journal of Occupational Therapy, 74*(1), 27–33.

Hopkins, H., & Smith, H. (1993). *Willard and Spackman's occupational therapy* (8th ed.). Philadelphia: Lippincott.

Iwama, M. (2006). *The Kawa Model. Culturally relevant occupational therapy.* Edinburgh: Elsevier.

Kielhofner, G. (1992). *Conceptual foundations of occupational therapy.* Philadelphia: FA Davis.

Kielhofner, G. (2009). Introduction to the model of human occupation. In G. Kielhofner (Ed.), *Model of human occupation: Theory and application* (4th ed.) (pp. 1–7). Philadelphia: Lippincott Williams & Wilkins.

Mann, H. S. (1995). Women's rights versus feminism? Postcolonial perspectives. In G. Rajan, & R. Mohanram (Eds.), *Postcolonial discourse and changing cultural context: Theory and criticism* (pp. 69–88). Westport, CN: Greenwood Press.

McClean, H. (1974). Towards developing a frame of reference and defining a treatment model in occupational therapy as applied to psychiatry. *British Journal of Occupational Therapy, 37*(11), 196–198.

Mosey, A. C. (1986). *Psychosocial components of occupational therapy.* New York: Raven.

Reed, K. L. (1984). *Models of practice in occupational therapy.* Baltimore: Williams & Wilkins.

Whalley Hammell, K. (2015). Respecting global wisdom: Enhancing the cultural relevance of occupational therapy's theoretical base. *British Journal of Occupational Therapy, 78*(11), 718–721.

Wilcock, A. A. (2001). *Occupation for health: A journey from prescription to self health.* London: College of Occupational Therapists.

Yamada, T., Kawamata, H., Kobayashi, N., Kielhofner, G., & Taylor, R. R. (2010). A randomised clinical trial of a wellness programme for healthy older people. *British Journal of Occupational Therapy, 73*(11), 540–548.

Young, M., & Quinn, E. (1992). *Theories and practice of occupational therapy.* Edinburgh: Churchill Livingstone.

Conceptual Models of Practice

6

The Model of Human Occupation
Embracing the Complexity of Occupation by Integrating Theory Into Practice and Practice into Theory

Kirsty Forsyth

OVERVIEW

Every day, occupational therapists must answer questions such as
- What are the occupational needs of this client?
- How do I best support the client to engage in this activity?
- What goals does this client want and need to achieve?
- How can I assist in the achievement of these goals?

To answer these and other practice questions, occupational therapists need comprehensive ways of understanding the client situation.

Evidence suggests that, worldwide, occupational therapists use the Model of Human Occupation (MOHO) more than any other framework to address these types of practice questions (Law & McColl 1989, Haglund et al 2000, National Board for Certification in Occupational Therapy 2004, Lee et al 2009, Taylor et al 2009). Widespread use of this model reflects the fact that MOHO has the concepts, evidence and practical resources to enable occupational therapists to plan and implement high-quality, evidence-based, client-centred and occupation-focused practice.

This chapter will first take an overview of how and why MOHO was developed. It will then introduce its major concepts and note their relevance to understanding clients and to therapy. Following this, the chapter discusses some of the available resources for using MOHO in practice. Finally, the use of MOHO will be illustrated through a case example.

⊚ HIGHLIGHTS

- MOHO is a client-centred, occupation-focused, evidence-based conceptual model of practice
- MOHO provides a way of embracing the complexity of clients' occupational needs
- MOHO provides specific occupationally focused outcomes measures to measure occupational participation
- MOHO provides a range of therapeutic intervention options
- MOHO has been applied successfully across cultures and used extensively internationally.

WHY AND HOW MOHO WAS DEVELOPED

From the 1960s onward, there was a recognition that occupational therapy had become too concerned with addressing impairment and needed to recapture its original focus on occupation (Reilly 1962, Shannon 1970, Kielhofner & Burke 1977). The Model of Human Occupation (MOHO) was the first occupation-focused model to be introduced in the profession (Kielhofner 1980a, Kielhofner 1980b, Kielhofner & Burke 1980, Kielhofner et al 1980). It was developed by three occupational therapy practitioners who wanted to organize concepts that could guide their delivery of occupation-focused practice. In the three decades since MOHO was first formulated, numerous practitioners and researchers throughout the world have contributed to its development. Today, literature of approximately 500 published works supports this model, making it the most evidence-based, occupational-focused model in the field.

The developers of MOHO have always sought to ensure that its concepts and tools are relevant and useful in practice. MOHO has been developed through an approach called 'the scholarship of practice'. This approach emphasizes the importance of an ongoing dialogue between theory/research and practice (Taylor et al 2002). Consequently, the scholarship of practice represents a commitment to scholarship, which supports occupational therapy practice, as well as a commitment to partner clinicians who are involved in the application of MOHO (Fig. 6.1). Moreover, the collaboration ensures that the needs and circumstances of practice shape theory development and research. All participants (e.g., clients, therapists, managers, educationalists, students, researchers) take on the role of 'practice scholars', sharing responsibility for developing and applying MOHO. MOHO is, therefore, driven by practice concerns, and practice shapes how its theory is articulated and applied. This approach has not only ensured MOHO's usefulness in practice, but has also enhanced the profile of occupational therapists, resulting in greater client understanding and satisfaction, and more respect from managers, policy-makers and interdisciplinary colleagues for the contribution occupational therapy makes.

In 1985 the book *A Model of Human Occupation: Theory and Application* introduced an expanded theory and a wide range of clinical applications (Kielhofner 1985). Revisions of the model were completed in 1995, 2002 and 2008. The latest edition of the text was published in 2017 (Taylor 2017) For therapists who wish to apply MOHO, this text is a necessary resource.

Other published literature provides additional sources of theoretical discourse, discussions of programmatic applications, cases examples and research findings. The literature on this model is published worldwide.

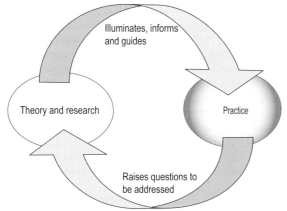

Fig. 6.1 Scholarship of Practice. (From Kielhofner G., Challenges of the New Millennium: Keynote Address, World Federation of Occupational Therapists Conference, Stockholm 2003. With permission.)

MOHO THEORY

A conceptual model of practice proposes theory to address certain phenomena with which the model is concerned (Kielhofner 2008). MOHO provides theory to explain occupation and occupational problems that arise in association with illness and disability.

Its concepts address
- the motivation for occupation
- the routine patterning of occupational performance
- the nature of skilled performance
- the influence of environment on occupation.

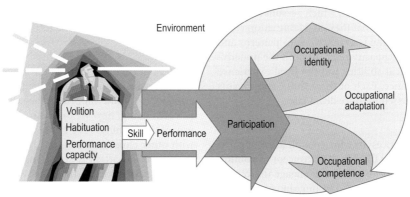

Fig. 6.2 Model of Human Occupation concepts. (From Kielhofner, G., 2008. *A Model of Human Occupation: Theory and Application,* (4th ed.). Baltimore: Lippincott Williams & Wilkins. With permission.)

The following section will address the main conceptual ideas in MOHO (Fig. 6.2), namely embracing the complexity of human occupation:
1. Components of the person
2. Environment
3. Occupational performance.

EMBRACING THE COMPLEXITY OF HUMAN OCCUPATION IN PRACTICE

MOHO recognizes that occupation (i.e., what a person does in work, play and self-care) is influenced by many factors inside and outside the person. MOHO further emphasizes that each person's inner characteristics and external environment are linked together into a dynamic whole. To embrace this complexity, MOHO theory includes a range of concepts. These concepts seek not only to offer explanations of the factors that influence occupation, but also to provide a framework for gathering data about a client's circumstances, generating an understanding of the client's occupational strengths and limitations, and selecting and implementing a course of occupational therapy.

Further, MOHO theory views therapy as a process in which people are helped to do things to shape their occupational abilities and occupational identities. MOHO provides a framework for successfully and meaningfully engaging people in occupations, which helps to maintain, restore or reorganize their occupational lives.

COMPONENTS OF THE PERSON

To explain how occupational participation is chosen, organized and performed, MOHO conceptualizes people as composed of three interconnected ideas:
• volition
• habituation
• performance capacity.

Volition refers to the process by which persons are motivated towards and choose what they do. Habituation refers to a process whereby doing is organized into patterns and routines. Performance capacity refers to both the underlying mental and physical abilities and the lived experience that shapes performance. Each of these three components of the person is discussed in more detail later.

Volition

Volition refers to the process by which people are motivated towards and choose what they do. The concept of volition asserts that all humans have a desire to engage in occupations, and that this desire is shaped by ongoing experiences as we do things. Volition consists of thoughts and feelings that occur in a cycle of anticipating possibilities for doing,

choosing what to do, experiencing what one does, and subsequent interpretation of the experience. These thoughts and feelings are concerned with three issues:
• how effective one is in acting on the world (personal causation)
• what one holds as important (values)
• what one finds enjoyable and satisfying (interests).

Personal Causation

Personal causation is reflected in our awareness of present and potential abilities (Harter 1983, Harter & Connel 1984) and our sense of how able we are to do what we want to do (Rotter 1960, Lefcourt 1981). Our own culture and social environment tell us what capacities we should have and why they matter. For example, a performer on stage, a taxi driver in a large city, a secondary school teacher and a farmer in the countryside will each be concerned about very different kinds of ability. Also, developmental level will affect the experience of personal causation. A young child typically will be concerned with developing such skills as walking and playing with toys. An older child may be mostly concerned with school performance and ability to get along with peers and perform in sports. Adolescents usually begin to think about capacity for further or higher education and entry into a line of work. Adults will focus on such things as the capacity for work performance and management of other adult responsibilities such as parenting. Older adults will often be concerned with loss of capacity associated with ageing and how to maintain abilities for personally important things.

Consequently, personal causation is never static, but rather a dynamic unfolding set of thoughts and feelings about our capacities and our efficacy in doing what we want to do. Our unique personal causation influences how we anticipate, choose, experience and interpret what we do. Consequently, the thoughts and feelings that make up personal causation are powerful motivational influences and they also guide how we experience what we do and how we look forward to the future.

Values

Choices of occupations are also influenced by our values. Values are beliefs and commitments that define what we see as good, right and important; they shape our sense of what is worth doing, how we ought to act, and what is the right way of doing things (Lee 1971). The child who plays nicely with other children because he has learned that playing in this way is important is expressing values. The worker who feels she needs to excel, the father who believes it is important to spend time with his children, and the old person who feels compelled to volunteer his services to his church are all examples of people whose values shape what they do.

When we cannot live up to our values, we may feel guilty or inadequate and we experience a lack of meaning (Bruner 1990). The worker who has a stroke and subsequently loses his job, the mother whose mental illness interferes with parenting her child, the child whose learning disability makes it difficult to do as well in school as he thinks he should, and the elderly person whose fear of falling interferes with being able to engage in meaningful occupations are all examples of persons who are unable to enact their values.

Interests

Being interested in an occupation means that one feels an attraction based on anticipation of a positive experience in doing that occupation. The experience of pleasure and/or satisfaction in doing something may come from positive feelings associated with either the exercise of capacity, intellectual or physical challenge, fellowship with others, aesthetic stimulation, or other factors. We are more likely to enjoy what we can perform with some level of proficiency when skill is involved in the performance. Csikszentmihalyi (1990) describes flow, a form of ultimate enjoyment in occupations that occurs when a person's capacities are optimally challenged. Often, this preference is manifested as a pattern of related interests such as athletic interest or cultural interests, including theatre and art. Preferring certain occupations over others influences what we are motivated to choose to do.

Illness or impairment can interfere with doing what one is interested in. For instance, a person might lose the capacity to do something he previously enjoyed, or an individual may find that engaging in an interest is no longer pleasurable because it evokes too much pain or fatigue. Persons with depression may find that they no longer enjoy doing what was previously pleasurable. Being able to engage in occupations that interest us and provide us with enjoyment and satisfaction is essential to well-being, and when illness or impairment interferes with this engagement, quality of life is reduced.

Summary

Our interests, values and personal causation affect what everyday activity we are motivated to do, what activities we choose to engage in and how we experience doing them. Illness and disability can interfere with volition in many ways. When this is the case, occupational therapists need to be able to assess and address volitional problems.

Additionally, volition is critical to the occupational therapy process. To provide therapy, occupational therapists must enable clients to engage in meaningful activity. Choosing a therapeutic activity and experiencing it as meaningful is a function of volition. Therapy cannot be meaningful unless occupational therapists attend to their client's volition.

The outcomes of therapy also depend on volition. It is not enough to improve a client's capacity. If the client leaves therapy and has no volitional motivation to use that capacity by engaging in activities of value and interest, then the client will not use what he or she has gained in therapy. Thus, therapy should always support the client's volition. Good therapy outcomes require that clients will *choose* to use their capacity, to develop new capacities, or make adjustments for their limitations because they can see these efforts as providing a life with value and satisfaction over which they can exercise reasonable control.

HABITUATION

Occupation is more than simply doing things. Every person has some kind of life pattern that is made up of everyday routines and roles. Habituation refers to the process by which people organize their occupational performance into the recurrent patterns of behaviour. These patterns integrate us into our physical and temporal world (when and where we do things) and our social and cultural world (doing things that reflect what we are expected to do by virtue of our position in society). Moreover, they allow us to carry out our daily lives efficiently and automatically. Habituated patterns of action are governed by

- habits
- roles.

HABITS

Habits involve learned ways of doing occupations that unfold automatically. The way we bathe and dress ourselves each morning, and how we drive, take a bus or ride a bike to work or school are examples of habits. We learn these habits through repeated experience. When we learn a habit, we acquire a way of appreciating and behaving in our familiar environments. So, for instance, we recognize the ring of the alarm clock as an indication that it is time to rise and bathe and dress; we know where to find the toothbrush and reach for it without thinking. We know how to turn on the shower and do it unreflectively. Because we do not have to think about these things as we go about our morning routine, our routines take less effort and concentration. Our habits always involve co-operation with our environment (Dewey 1922). When our environment changes, our habits may no longer work automatically. For instance, when we find ourselves in an unfamiliar environment such as a hotel room, we may suddenly find that we have consciously to think about and figure out how to do a routine task such as turning on the shower. As the example illustrates, when habits cannot guide our behaviour automatically, it takes more concentration and effort to complete our routines. Consequently, habits give us our bearings throughout daily life and allow us to do routine things with relative ease.

Habits also organize our underlying capacities. When we reach for the toothbrush or turn on the shower, we are using our vision, our cognition and our motor capacity. If we were to experience a loss of any of these capacities, our habits would disintegrate. For example, if the power is out and one has to feel one's way about the bathroom at night without the benefit of sight, habits go out of the window. If one has a broken arm and one's dominant hand is in a cast, simple things like turning on the shower, brushing one's teeth or putting on clothes take a lot more thinking and effort or may be impossible. When clients develop impairments, their habits become disrupted and their everyday routines take additional effort and thought or cannot be done without help. When one suddenly must use a wheelchair, the environment is changed and familiar habits no longer work. Getting into the shower and reaching to the medicine cabinet for the toothbrush are suddenly no longer habitual or possible. All the familiarity and ease of everyday life is disrupted. An important function of occupational therapy is to help clients develop new habits of everyday life to restore some of the ease and familiarity of daily life.

ROLES

People see themselves as students, workers and parents, and recognize that they should behave in certain ways to enact these roles. Much of what we do is done as a spouse, parent, worker, student and so on (Mancuso & Sarbin 1983). The presence of these and other roles helps ensure that what we do is regular (e.g., we go to school or work according to a schedule). Roles also give us a sense of identity and belatedly a sense of what we are obligated to do. When we tell someone we are a parent, a student, a worker or a member of some group, we are telling them who we are. Moreover, we know what is expected of us in those roles. Parents take care of children. Students attend lectures, study and take exams. Members of a bicycling club plan and go on bicycle trips together.

The roles that we have internalized serve as a kind of framework for looking out on the world and for engaging in occupation. When one is engaging in an occupation within a given role, it may be reflected in how one dresses, one's demeanour, the content of one's actions and so on. For instance, one would dress differently for work from when engaging in a leisure role. We do quite different things when we are in the role of student from when we are in the role of a friend.

Having an impairment can compromise one's ability to engage in meaningful life roles. If the impairment is severe, it can prevent or alter the way a person engages in all of their life roles. People with chronic disabilities often inhabit many fewer roles than those who do not have impairments. As a consequence, they have fewer opportunities to develop a sense of identity and to fill their lives with meaningful activities. To understand fully how a disability has influenced a client, the occupational therapist must understand its impact on their roles. Moreover, the aim of occupational therapy should be to support clients to enable them to engage in those roles that are most important or necessary for them.

SUMMARY

Habituation regulates the patterned, familiar and routine features of what we do. Habits and roles give regularity, character and order to what we do and how we do it. They make our everyday lives familiar and they give us a sense of who we are. Disability can invalidate established habits and roles. Having a disability may require one to develop new habits for managing everyday routines and it may interfere with being able to engage in a role or alter how one can do that role. Understanding how a disability affects any person requires that the occupational therapist pays careful attention to the client's habituation.

Moreover, it is not sufficient that a client develops skills for doing everyday routines; it is also critical that the client develops the habits to integrate these skills into effective ways of doing everyday life tasks. Similarly, having abilities does little good, if clients are not able to access and identify with roles that call upon them to use those abilities. Therapy that focuses only on augmenting capacity without considering how the client will go about organizing everyday life is incomplete. Moreover, knowing what roles and habits are part of a client's life will also provide important information to enable us to prioritize the kinds of skill development on which to focus. Clients do not simply do things; they do them to enact daily routines and discharge their roles.

PERFORMANCE CAPACITY

The capacity for performance is affected by the status of one's musculoskeletal, neurological, cardiopulmonary and other bodily systems. A number of occupational therapy frameworks provide detailed concepts for understanding performance capacity. For example, the biomechanical framework seeks to explain human movement as the function of a complex organization of muscles, connective tissue and bones (Trombly 1989), while the sensory integration framework (Ayres 1986) explains how the brain organizes sensory information for executing skilled movement. Because these frameworks already address performance capacity, MOHO does not address this aspect of performance capacity. Consequently, occupational therapists using MOHO routinely use other frameworks for understanding and addressing performance capacity.

MOHO (Kielhofner 2008) concepts offer a different but complementary way of thinking about performance capacity. This view of performance capacity builds upon phenomenological concepts from philosophy (Husserl 1962, Merleau-Ponty 1962) and focuses on the subjective experience of performing. It asks occupational therapists to pay more attention to how it feels to perform with a disability. By having a better understanding of a client's pain, fatigue, confusion or other subjective aspects of performance, therapists can be more client-centred and more helpful in assisting clients to learn or relearn skills.

Interweaving of Volition, Habituation and Performance Capacity

The things we do reflect a complex interplay of our motives, habits and roles, and performance capacity. Volition, habituation and the subjective experience of performance always operate in concert with each other. We cannot fully understand a client's occupation without considering all these contributing factors. For example, a person with low personal causation will tend to feel anxious when attempting to perform. This anxiety in turn can negatively affect performance. Another example is that if a person does not have interests and values that lead him to use his capacities, those capacities will diminish through disuse. For this reason, it is important that occupational therapists gather information about all the aspects of a client (performance capacity, values, interests, personal causation, roles and habits) in order truly to understand that client and provide the best services.

The Environment

Just as volition, habituation and performance capacity are inter-related and inter-dependent, people and their environments are also inseparable (Kielhofner 2008). Our environments offer us opportunities, resources, demands and constraints. Whether and how these environmental potentials affect us depend on our values, interests, personal causation, roles, habits and performance capacities. Because each individual is unique, any environment will have somewhat different effects on each individual within it.

The physical environment consists of natural and human-made spaces and the objects within them. Spaces can be the result of nature (e.g., a forest or a lake) or the result of human fabrication (e.g., a house, classroom or theatre). Similarly, objects may be those that occur naturally (e.g., trees and rocks) or those that have been made (e.g., books, cars and computers). The social environment consists of groups of persons, and the occupational forms or tasks that persons belonging to those groups perform. Groups allow and prescribe the kinds of things their members can do. Occupational forms or tasks refer to the things that are available to do in any social context (e.g., in a classroom the kinds of things that are typically done include writing notes, giving a lecture, answering questions, taking exams and so forth). Every context has certain occupational forms or tasks associated with it.

Any setting within which we perform is made up of spaces, objects, occupational forms/tasks and/or social groups. Typical settings in which we engage in occupational forms are the home, neighbourhood, school or workplace. The environment can be both a barrier and an enabler for disabled persons. For example, snow dampens the sound used by blind persons to help navigate without sight and may make the pavement inaccessible to the wheelchair user. Much of the built environment limits opportunities and poses constraints on those with disabilities because it often has been designed for persons without impairments. However, careful design of spaces can facilitate daily functioning of disabled persons. Similarly, while most fabricated objects in the environment are created for use by able-bodied, sighted, hearing and cognitively intact individuals, there are also a large number of objects designed to compensate for impairments. Occupational therapists are experts in providing and training clients in the use of these specialized objects.

People with a physical and mental impairment often contradict cultural values, making others uncomfortable and evoking a range of reactions. These attitudes can limit the person with disability. Moreover, disability may remove people from or alter the positions they can assume in social groups. The occupational forms available to the person with a disability may be limited or altered. Performance limitations can make doing some occupational forms impossible. Persons with disabilities often must give up or relinquish to others occupational forms that have become impossible to do. In short, the physical and social environment can have a multitude of positive or negative impacts on the disabled person, which can make all the difference in that person's life. The environment is not only a pervasive factor influencing disability. It is a critical tool for supporting positive change in the disabled person's life. A therapist may purposefully alter the physical setting to remove constraints or to facilitate function. An example of this is a ramp that replaces inaccessible steps. Therapists can remove objects that are barriers or provide objects such as assistive technology that facilitate functioning. The therapist may provide, monitor or seek to change social groups such as families or work colleagues. Finally, the therapist may provide or help a client select occupational forms to undertake, or help them modify how an occupational form is done.

UNDERSTANDING OCCUPATIONAL PERFORMANCE

Personal causation, values and interests motivate what we choose to do. Habits and roles shape our routine patterns of doing. Performance capacities and subjective experience provide the capacity for what we do. The environment provides opportunities, resources, demands and constraints for our doing. We can also examine the doing itself and what consequence it has over time. Doing can be examined at different levels:

- skills
- occupational performance
- occupational participation
- occupational identity/occupational competence
- occupational adaptation.

Skills

Within occupational performance we carry out discrete purposeful actions called skills. For example, making a cup of tea has a culturally recognizable occupational form in the United Kingdom. To do so, one engages in such purposeful actions as gathering together tea, kettle and a cup, handling these materials and objects, and sequencing the steps necessary to brew and pour the tea. These actions that make up occupational performance are referred to as skills (Fisher & Kielhofner 1995, Fisher 1999a, Forsyth et al 1998). In contrast to performance capacity (which refers to underlying ability, e.g., range of motion, strength, cognition), skill refers to the discrete actions seen *within* an occupation performance. There are three types of skills: motor skills, process skills, and communication and interaction skills.

If a person has difficulty 'reaching', an occupational therapist may conclude that the client has a limited range of motion in the shoulder joint. However, using Figure 6.2 to support theoretical clinical reasoning, we could hypothesize other reasons for the client not 'reaching'. For example, the client may not think he has the capacity to reach (personal causation); he may not see the activity as important and therefore fail to reach (values); he may not find the activity satisfying or enjoyable and therefore fail to reach (interest); it may not be part of his role responsibilities and therefore he fails to reach as he knows someone else will do this for him (roles); the environment may not

be supporting the reach; the occupational form may not be within the person's culture and so they do not know they need an object to complete the occupational form and so fail to reach; and so on. Skills can therefore be influenced by a range of personal and environmental factors. Having a theoretical framework supports clinical reasoning to understand why a client is having difficulty exhibiting skill to complete the occupational form.

Occupational Performance

When we complete an occupational form or task, we perform. Occupational forms for a lecturer may include lecturing, writing, administering and marking exams, creating courses and counselling students. Taking care of ourselves may involve performing the occupational forms of showering, dressing and grooming. Other examples of occupational performance are when persons do such tasks as walking the dog, baking a chicken, vacuuming a rug or mowing the lawn. These people are performing those occupational forms.

Occupational Participation

Participation refers to engagement in work, play, or activities of daily living that are part of one's sociocultural context and are desired and/or necessary to one's well-being. Examples of occupational participation include working in a full- or part-time job, engaging routinely in a hobby, maintaining one's home, attending school and participating in a club or other organization. This definition is consistent with the World Health Organization's view that participation is 'taking part in society along with their experiences within their life context' (World Health Organization 1999, p.19). Each area of occupational participation involves a cluster of related things that one does. For example, maintaining one's living space may include paying the rent, doing repairs and cleaning.

Occupational Identity and Occupational Competence

Our participation helps to create our identities. Occupational identity is defined as a composite sense of who one is and who one wishes to become as an occupational being, generated from one's history of occupational participation. Occupational identity includes one's sense of capacity and effectiveness for doing; what things one finds interesting and satisfying to do; who one is, as defined by one's roles and relationships; what one feels obligated to do and holds as important; a sense of the familiar routines of life; perceptions of one's environment and what it supports and expects. These are garnered *over time* and become part of one's identity. Occupational identity reflects accumulative life experiences that are organized into an understanding of who one has been and a sense of desired and possible directions for one's future.

Occupational competence is the degree to which one sustains a pattern of occupational participation that reflects identity. Competence has to do with putting your identity into action. It includes fulfilling the expectations of one's roles and one's own values and standards of performance; maintaining a routine that allows one to discharge responsibilities; participating in a range of occupations that provide a sense of ability, control, satisfaction and fulfilment; and pursuing one's values and taking action to achieve desired life outcomes.

Occupational Adaptation

Occupational adaptation is the construction of a positive occupational identity and achieving occupational competence over time in the context of the environment.

RESOURCES FOR PRACTICE

MOHO was initiated with the specific goal of *developing resources to guide and enhance occupation-focused practice.*

Practitioners have collaborated in the development of a wide range of tools for partnerships. Academic/practice partnerships were built around how the tools developed. This ensured that the tools were theoretically driven and had robust research to support them while simultaneously being flexible and useful within busy clinical workplaces.

MOHO tools are specifically built to support occupation-focused practice.

Examples are:

- a range of assessments that operationalize concepts from the model (Box 6.1 and Fig. 6.3)
- published case examples, as well as videotapes, illustrating application of the model in assessment, treatment planning and intervention (Box 6.2)
- published papers and manuals describing the implementation of programmes based on the model (Box 6.3). There is an evidence-based search engine and downloadable evidence briefs on the MOHO website (https://www.moho.uic.edu/default.aspx) making it easier for practitioners to focus on the evidence for their areas of practice.

BOX 6.1   Model of Human Occupation Assessment Tools

Overview Assessments

Most Model of Human Occupation (MOHO) assessments are available at https://www.moho.uic.edu. Assessments marked with an * are available on request from kforsyth@qmu.ac.uk

Occupational Performance History Interview (OPHI-II)

As a historical semistructured interview, the OPHI-II seeks to gather information about a patient or client's past and present occupational performance. The OPHI-II is a three-part assessment, which includes

- a semi-structured interview that explores a client's occupational life history
- rating scales that provide a measure of the client's occupational identity, occupational competence and the impact of the client's occupational behaviour settings
- a life history narrative designed to capture salient qualitative features of the occupational life history.

Occupational Circumstances Interview and Rating Scale (OCAIRS)

The OCAIRS is a semi-structured interview focused on the present and seeks to understand clients' occupational abilities on the full range of MOHO issues. It is an outcome measure. It is appropriate for clients who are

conversational and is used when time is limited, as it is shorter than the OPHI-II interview.

Occupational Self-Assessment (OSA) and the Child Occupational Self-Assessment (COSA)

The OSA is an update of the Self-Assessment of Occupational Functioning (SAOF) and is designed to capture clients' perceptions of their own occupational competence and of the impact of their environment on their occupational adaptation. As such, the OSA is designed to be a client-centred assessment, which gives voice to the client's view. Once clients have had an opportunity to assess their occupational participation and their environments, they review the items to establish priorities for change, which can be translated into therapy goals.

Model of Human Occupational Screening Tool (MOHOST) and Short Child Occupational Profile (SCOPE)

These are relatively new assessments based on MOHO. Similar in format and administration, they were developed with clinicians in response to their request for a comprehensive assessment that is quick and simple to complete. MOHOST and SCOPE may be scored by the therapist using any combination of observation, interview, information from others who know the client and chart audit.

Continued

BOX 6.1   Model of Human Occupation assessment tools—cont'd

Because of their flexibility, the two tools can be used in a wide range of settings and with a wide range of clients. Moreover, the tools can be administered in a way that is client centred.

Making It Clear (MIC)*

This is a self-report assessment that indicates occupational participation needs for entry into a prevention programme delivered by support staff with supervision of an occupational therapist. The assessment captures the person's own views of their occupational participation. It has been designed to be quick and easy to use and indicates which intervention strategies would be helpful to allow the person to engage with their community and prevent a reduction in occupational participation.

Model of Human Occupation—Exploratory Level Outcome Ratings (MOHO-ExpLOR)

This assessment is a formal observational assessment. It was designed for people with multiple and complex needs. It is sensitive enough to assess subtle changes in skills. It is used extensively with people who have moderate to severe dementia and people with significant learning disability.

ACHIEVE Assessment*

This is an assessment that is focused on the occupational participation of children. This is a self-report format for teachers and parents of children with difficulties in their occupational participation. The profile of teachers and parents can be directly compared as the items are the same across both. This allows the occupational therapist to understand how the child's occupational participation is impacted by either school or home environment.

Observational Assessments
Assessment of Communication and Interaction Skills (ACIS)

The ACIS is a formal observational tool designed to measure an individual's performance in an occupational form and/or within a social group of which the person is a part. The instrument aims to assist occupational therapists in determining a client's ability in discourse and social exchange in the course of daily occupations.

Assessment of Motor and Process Skills (AMPS)

The AMPS (Fisher 1999b) represents a fundamental and substantive reconceptualization in the development of occupational therapy functional assessments. The AMPS is a structured, observational evaluation. It is used to evaluate the quality or effectiveness of the actions of performance (motor and process skills) as they unfold over time when a person performs daily life tasks.

Volitional Questionnaire (VQ) and the Paediatric Volitional Questionnaire (PVQ)

Traditionally, it has been difficult to assess volition in clients who have communication and cognitive limitations, because of the complex language requirements of most assessments of volition. The Volitional Questionnaire is an attempt to recognize that, while such clients have difficulty formulating goals or expressing their interests and values verbally, they are often able to communicate them through actions. The client is observed in a number of occupational behaviour settings so that a picture of the person's volition and the environmental supports required to support the expression can be identified.

Self-Reports
Interest Checklist and the Paediatric Interests Profiles (PIP)

Although a number of versions of the Interest Checklist exist, the revised version appears to be the one most commonly used by occupational therapists using the (Model of Human Occupation) and will be the one referred to in this discussion. This version consists of 68 activities or areas of interest. There is a paediatric version available.

National Institutes of Health Activity Record (NIH ACTRE)

The NIH ACTRE was developed as an outcome measure for a study of patients with rheumatoid arthritis. This instrument provides a 24-hour log of a patient's activities and is an adaptation of the Occupational Questionnaire (described later). The ACTRE aims to provide details of the impact of symptoms on task performance, individual perceptions of interest, significance of daily activities, and daily habit patterns.

Occupational Questionnaire (OQ)

The OQ is a pen-and-paper, self-report instrument that asks the individual to provide a description of typical use of time and utilizes Likert-type ratings of competence, importance, and enjoyment during activities. The client completes a list of the activities they perform each half-hour on a typical weekday. After listing the activities, the client is asked to answer four questions for each activity.

BOX 6.1   Model of Human Occupation assessment tools—cont'd

Role Checklist

The Role Checklist is a self-report checklist that can be used to obtain information about the types of roles people engage in and which organize their daily lives. This checklist provides data on an individual's perception of their roles over the course of their life and also the degree of value, that is, the significance and importance that they place on those roles. The Role Checklist can be used with adolescents, adults or geriatric populations.

Vocational Assessments

Worker Role Interview (WRI)

The WRI is a semi-structured interview designed to be used as the psychosocial/environmental component of the initial rehabilitation assessment process for the injured worker. The interview is designed to have the client discuss various aspects of their life and job setting that have been associated with past work experiences. The WRI combines information from an interview with observations made during the physical and behavioural assessment procedure of a physical and/or work capacity assessment. The intent is to identify the psychosocial and environmental variables that may influence the ability of the injured worker to return to work.

Work Environment Impact Scale (WEIS)

The WEIS is a semi-structured interview designed to gather information about how individuals with disabilities experience and perceive their work settings. The focus of the interview is the impact of the work setting on a person's performance, satisfaction and well-being. An important concept underlying this scale is that workers are most productive and satisfied when there is a 'fit' or 'match' between the worker's environment and their needs and skills. Hence, the same work environment may have a different impact on different workers. It is important to remember that the WEIS does not assess the environment. Rather, it assesses how the work environment affects a given worker.

School Assessments

Occupational Therapy Psychosocial Assessment of Learning (OT PAL)

The OT PAL is an observational and descriptive assessment tool. It assesses a student's volition (ability to make choices), habituation (roles and routines) and environmental fit within the classroom setting. The observational portion consists of 21 items that address the major areas of making choices, habits/routines and roles. In addition to the observation portion, there is a preobservation form and interview guidelines. The preobservation form is designed to gather environmental information, as well as assist in determining an appropriate time to complete the observation. The semi-structured interviews of the teacher, the student and the parent(s) are designed to have the teacher, student and parent describe various psychosocial aspects of learning related to school.

The School Setting Interview (SSI)

The SSI is a semi-structured interview designed to assess student–environment fit and identify the need for accommodations for students with disabilities in the school setting. The SSI is a client-centred interview intended to assist the occupational therapist in the planning of intervention by examining the student's interaction with the physical and social environments at school. The SSI provides the occupational therapist with a picture of the child's functioning in 14 content areas. This assessment is designed to be used collaboratively with the student and is therefore intended for students who are able to communicate adequately enough to discuss their feelings.

CIRCLE Assessments*

These assessments (nursery, primary and secondary versions) measure children's occupational participation within schools. The assessments are teacher-completed and allow the teachers to analyze the child's challenges. There are complimentary intervention strategies that provide teachers with ways of supporting the child within the school.

Environmental Assessments

Residential Environmental Impact Scale (REIS)

This is a therapist-rated assessment of residential environments. It is measuring environmental impact on a group of residents rather than for any particular resident. It has been used in populations with supported accommodations, for example, people with learning difficulties or people with complex mental health challenges.

Environmental Social Participation and Inclusion (ESPI) Assessment*

This is a therapy-rated assessment of a person's environmental impact. It is often used after the MOHOST if more detailed environmental information is required. The areas covered include physical spaces/objects, enabling relationships and structure of activities. If on a home visit, both the MOHOST and the ESPI can be completed as part of the write-up of the visit.

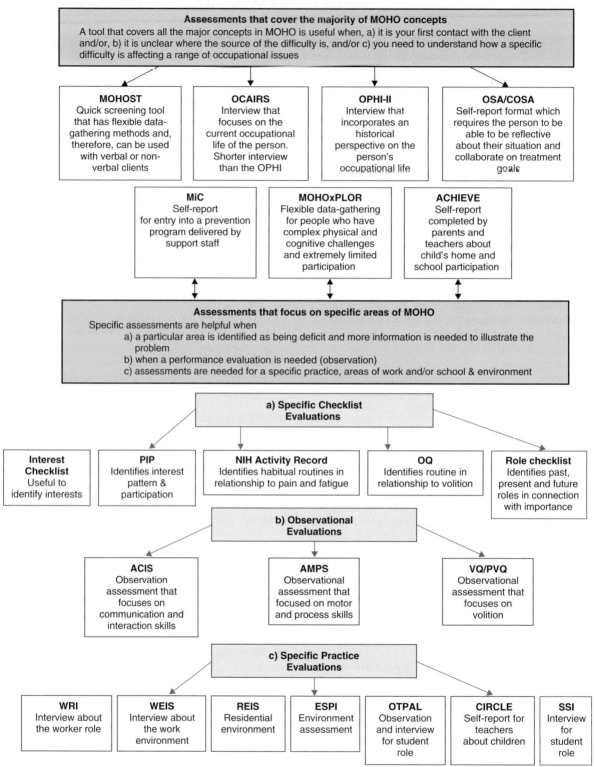

Fig. 6.3 Choosing a Model of Human Occupation Assessment. *NIH*, National Institutes of Health. (Modified from Kielhofner, G., 2008. *A Model of Human Occupation: Theory and Application*, (4th ed.). Baltimore: Lippincott Williams & Wilkins.)

BOX 6.2   Published Articles

There are a large number of published case examples, illustrating application of MOHO in assessment, treatment planning and intervention. A selection are referenced here:

Case Illustrations Through Articles

Affleck, A., Bianchi, E., Cleckley, M., et al., 1984. Stress management as a component of occupational therapy in acute care settings. *Occupational Therapy in Health Care, 1* (3), 17–41.

Baron, K.B., Littleton, M.J., 1999. The model of human occupation: A return to work case study. *Work, 12* (1), 37–46.

Barrett, L., Beer, D., Kielhofner, G., 1999. The importance of volitional narrative in treatment: An ethnographic case study in a work program. *Work, 12* (1), 79–92.

Curtin, C., 1991. Psychosocial intervention with an adolescent with diabetes using the model of human occupation. *Occupational Therapy in Mental Health, 11* (2/3), 23–36.

DePoy, E., Burke, J.P., 1992. Viewing cognition through the lens of the model of human occupation. In Katz, N., (ed.)., Cognitive rehabilitation: Models for intervention in occupational therapy. Butterworth-Heinemann, Stoneham, MA, 240–257.

Froehlich, J., 1992. Occupational therapy interventions with survivors of sexual abuse. *Occupational Therapy in Health Care, 8* (2/3), 1–25.

Gusich, R., 1984. Occupational therapy for chronic pain: A clinical application of the model of human occupation. *Occupational Therapy in Mental Health, 4* (3), 59–73.

Helfrich, C., Kielhofner, G., 1994. Volitional narratives and the meaning of occupational therapy. *American Journal of Occupational Therapy, 48,* 319–326.

Helfrich, C., Kielhofner, G., Mattingly, C., 1994. Volition as narrative: an understanding of motivation in chronic illness. *American Journal of Occupational Therapy, 42,* 311–317.

Kavanaugh, J., Fares, J., 1995. Using the model of human occupation with homeless mentally ill patients. *British Journal of Occupational Therapy, 58* (10), 419–422.

Mentrup, C., Niehaus, A., Kielhofner, G., 1999. Applying the model of human occupation in work-focused rehabilitation: A case illustration. *Work, 12* (1), 61–70.

Neville, A., 1985. The model of human occupation and depression. *Mental Health Special Interest Section Newsletter, 8,* 1–4.

Oakley, F., 1987. Clinical application of the model of human occupation in dementia of the Alzheimer's type. *Occupational Therapy in Mental Health, 7* (4), 37–50.

Pizzi, M.A., 1990. The model of human occupation and adults with HIV infection and AIDS. *American Journal of Occupational Therapy, 44,* 257–264.

Pizzi, M.A., 1990. Occupational therapy: Creating possibilities for adults with human immunodeficiency virus infection, AIDS related complex, and acquired immunodeficiency syndrome. *Occupational Therapy in Health Care, 7* (2/3/4), 125–137.

Series, C., 1992. The long-term needs of people with head injury: A role for the community occupational therapist? *British Journal of Occupational Therapy, 55* (3), 94–98.

Woodrum, S.C., 1993. A treatment approach for attention deficit hyperactivity disorder using the model of human occupation. *Developmental Disabilities Special Interest Section Newsletter, 16* (1), 1–2.

BOX 6.3   Example Manuals for Model of Human Occupation-based Programmes (Available from https://www.moho.uic.edu)

Remotivation Process
  Population: People with poor volitional status
  Author: Carmen Gloria de las Heras
Work Readiness: Day Treatment for Persons with Chronic Disabilities
  Population: Unemployed adults with chronic disabilities
  Author: Linda Olson
Work Rehabilitation in Mental Health Programs
  Population: Adults with mental illness
  Authors: Trudy Mallinson, Dorianne LaPlante, Jan Holmann-Smith

QUESTIONS AND ANSWERS

Over the past four decades, the development of this model has been accompanied by questions and critiques including the following:

- Can MOHO be used with other models of practice?
- Is MOHO client-centred?
- Is MOHO flexible enough to embrace a range of social, geographic and cultural environments?
- Why is there specific language?
- Can MOHO embrace the complexity of human occupation?
- Is MOHO applicable to lower-functioning clients?
- Is MOHO an evidence-based choice?
- Can MOHO be used when selecting adaptive equipment?

We will address each of these issues in turn.

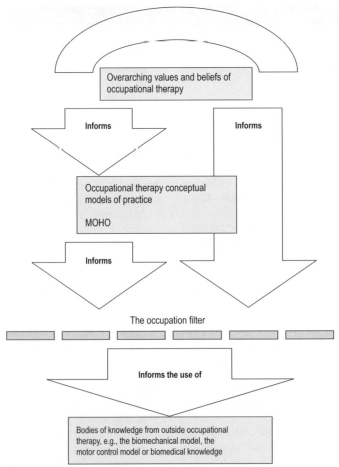

Fig. 6.4 Model of Human Occupation Integration. (From Forsyth K, McMillan I, personal communication, 2001.)

Can MOHO Be Used Together with Frames of Reference?

Yes. A common question is 'Is it MOHO or nothing?' This question involves the extent to which MOHO can be used in an integrative way with other approaches. As mentioned above, MOHO does not provide theoretical arguments to understand the capacity for performance that is supported by one's musculoskeletal, neurological, cardiopulmonary, mental or cognitive abilities such as memory and planning, and other bodily systems. A number of occupational therapy frames of reference seek to explain performance capacities that make possible occupational performance. These models provide detailed concepts for understanding some aspect of performance capacity. Consequently, occupational therapists using MOHO will also need to use other frameworks to understand and address performance capacity. A combination of frameworks can, therefore, be used to support a full understanding of the client's occupational engagement. Fig.

6.4 identifies how this can be achieved. Overarching values and beliefs of occupation therapy (e.g., occupation is important for health, it is important to consider both the mind and the body, it is important to be client-centred etc.) inform occupation-focused conceptual models of practice (e.g., MOHO). MOHO has very specific detail on how to carry out occupation-focused practice. Both the values and beliefs of occupational therapy and MOHO provide support for the concept of an 'occupation filter' (Mallinson & Forsyth personal comunication 2000). The occupation filter is a way of viewing knowledge from outside occupational therapy and bringing it into our practice in an occupation-focused way (Fig. 6.5). This allows the integration of a range of theories, yet avoids the 'cutting and pasting' of bodies of knowledge from outside occupational therapy into our practice and calling it occupational therapy when it in fact closely resembles other professionals' practice. For example, 'cutting and pasting' cognitive–behavioural therapy into occupational

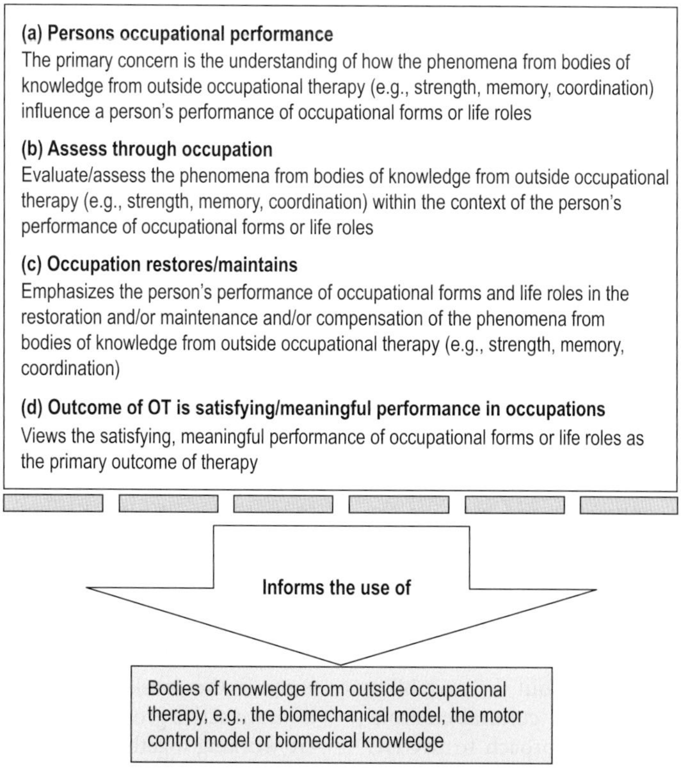

(a) **Persons occupational performance**
The primary concern is the understanding of how the phenomena from bodies of knowledge from outside occupational therapy (e.g., strength, memory, coordination) influence a person's performance of occupational forms or life roles

(b) **Assess through occupation**
Evaluate/assess the phenomena from bodies of knowledge from outside occupational therapy (e.g., strength, memory, coordination) within the context of the person's performance of occupational forms or life roles

(c) **Occupation restores/maintains**
Emphasizes the person's performance of occupational forms and life roles in the restoration and/or maintenance and/or compensation of the phenomena from bodies of knowledge from outside occupational therapy (e.g., strength, memory, coordination)

(d) **Outcome of OT is satisfying/meaningful performance in occupations**
Views the satisfying, meaningful performance of occupational forms or life roles as the primary outcome of therapy

Informs the use of

Bodies of knowledge from outside occupational therapy, e.g., the biomechanical model, the motor control model or biomedical knowledge

Fig. 6.5 Components of the Occupational Filter. (From Mallinson, T, Forsyth, K, personal communication, 2000.)

therapy without using an 'occupation-focused filter' will result in practice that looks like that of a psychologist and perpetuate role confusion within occupational therapy.

Is MOHO Client-Centred?

MOHO is recognized as a model consistent with client-centred practice (Law 1998, Sumsion 1999). MOHO concepts require therapists to have knowledge of their client's values, sense of capacity and efficacy, value, roles, habits, performance experience and personal environment. MOHO-based assessments are designed to gather information on clients and provide them with opportunities to provide their perspectives on these factors. The client's unique characteristics, in combination with the theory, guide the development of an understanding of the client's unique situation. The understanding of the client, in turn, provides the rationale for therapy. Moreover, because MOHO conceptualises the client's own doing, thinking and feeling as the central dynamic in achieving change, therapy must support the client's choice, action and experience.

MOHO is, therefore, inherently a client-centred model in two important ways. Firstly, it views each client as a unique individual whose characteristics fundamentally influence the rationale for and nature of the therapy goals and strategies. MOHO theory both focuses the therapist on the unique characteristics of the client and provides concepts that allow the therapist to appreciate the client's perspective and situation more deeply. Secondly, MOHO views what the client does, thinks and feels as the central mechanism of change (Kielhofner 2002). MOHO concepts also propose that the client's occupational engagement (i.e., what the client does, thinks and feels) is the central dynamic of therapy (Kielhofner 2002). MOHO-based intervention supports the client's doing, thinking and feeling to achieve change. MOHO-based practice, therefore, requires a client–therapist relationship in which the therapist must understand, respect and support their client's values, sense of capacity and efficacy, value, roles, habits, performance experience and personal environment.

Is MOHO Flexible Enough to Embrace a Range of Social, Geographic and Cultural Environments?

Some have questioned whether MOHO is flexible and pragmatic enough to be used in a wide range of social, geographic and cultural environments.

With respect to the social environment, the third edition of MOHO has been influenced by the disabilities studies literature (Miller & Oertel 1983, Hull 1990, Gill 1997). This literature argues that many of the problems faced by persons with disabilities can more properly be located in the environment—in everything from physical barriers to stigmatising attitudes and outright discrimination. A growing theme is that disability occurs because of a lack of fit between person and environment. This implies, of course, that change must include altering the environment. Accordingly, MOHO calls attention to the environment as both an enabler of and a barrier to occupation (Kielhofner 2002). Throughout, an effort has been made to call attention to circumstances both within the person and within the environment that contribute to a person's motivation, patterns of behaviour and occupational performance. The assessment tools that have been developed routinely contain an environmental component and examine the fit between the person and their environment. A MOHO-based assessment that is entirely focused on the environment has been developed (Moore-Corner et al 1998), and others incorporate the environment as an aspect of the assessment.

There have been questions raised about the portability of MOHO to different geographic and cultural environments. The scholarship of practice approach to MOHO development has encouraged an international community of occupational therapists to use and contribute to the development of MOHO. MOHO has, therefore, become an international conceptual practice model. MOHO has received significant attention, including criticism, elaboration, application and empirical testing, from occupational therapists throughout the world in such diverse countries as Australia, New Zealand, the Netherlands, Sweden, Denmark, Japan, Korea, Spain, Italy, Portugal, Chile and Colombia.

The theory itself incorporates a respect for each client's individuality and cultural narrative into its concepts, and many of the assessments are specifically designed to capture a client's unique cultural perspective. For example, the Occupational Performance History Interview II (OPHI-II) (Kielhofner et al 1997) elicits and considers culturally influenced values, interests and roles through the use of narrative ethnography as a predominant interviewing method. For this reason, the OPHI-II and similar assessments are particularly useful when therapists desire to gather information about the client's culturally influenced thoughts, feelings and actions. Concepts of occupational form can also be helpful in identifying how different cultures define how everyday occupations are completed. Each culture includes a wide range of occupational forms that constitute the opportunities and demands that culture will put on its members for doing everyday things. Knowing how occupational forms are culturally defined for each client (e.g., the occupational form of dressing has different social expectations based on cultural norms from culture to culture) helps occupational therapists to be sensitive to cultural differences in the ways of doing everyday activity.

Assuring that assessments are relevant and valid with persons from diverse cultural backgrounds requires ongoing development and research. Such work is being undertaken across the MOHO-based assessments. Assessments have been developed in collaboration with therapists and clients representing multiple cultures and languages. Many of the MOHO standardized assessments are now translated into different language versions. Research indicates that many of the MOHO-based assessments do not reflect cultural biases. For example, studies of the Worker Role Interview (WRI; Haglund et al 1997), the Work Environment Impact Scale (WEIS) (Kielhofner et al 1999), the OPHI-II (Kielhofner et al 2001), the Assessment of Communication and Interaction Skills (ACIS) (Forsyth et al 1997) and the Occupational Self Assessment (Kielhofner & Forsyth 2001) indicate that these assessments are valid cross-culturally. Occupational therapy in the United Kingdom is very influential in the development of MOHO theory and application. An active group of both researchers and practitioners are working together to contribute to the development of MOHO.

Why Is There Specific Language?

The words that are selected to describe therapy are very important. Complex conditions or procedures can be conveyed and immediately understood when such professional terminology is used. Occupational therapists acquire the professional languages of several disciplines. In college we learn medical language to support our communication with medical colleagues. For example, we can say 'Alzheimer disease' and immediately the multidisciplinary team members have a sense of the issues faced by the person under discussion and then can enter into specifics of how the condition has affected this particular person. The medical definition of Alzheimer disease is very long and having language to name and frame the issue supports effective communication with others who are familiar with the terms. Therefore one strength of having a unique language is that MOHO terminology can be used in consultation with others who are familiar with the model to convey complex concepts accurately and succinctly. For example, the term *volition* conveys a complex set of ideas about how people are motivated towards their occupations. When someone refers to a client having a volitional challenge, those who know the terminology can anticipate that the challenge involves the client's values, personal causation and interests, and how this manifests in the way clients anticipate, choose, experience and interpret what they do every day. In this way, MOHO terminology can succinctly convey information.

Deciding whether and how to use MOHO terminology in communication and documentation requires consideration of several factors. MOHO terms, like those of any other professional language, offer benefits and pose challenges. The major disadvantage of all professional language is that everyone needs to have a common understanding of the terms. It is, therefore, ineffective to use MOHO terms (or, indeed, any medical term) with colleagues, clients and others who will not understand what the words mean. Therefore, therapists should carefully decide when

and how they use MOHO terms in communicating to clients, lay persons and other professionals. Because practitioners, clients and settings differ greatly in terms of their knowledge and understanding of languages associated with particular theoretical models, it is ultimately the clinicians' responsibility and judgement that count in terms of translating the MOHO terms into verbal and written language that accurately conveys the intended knowledge. Two examples follow where MOHO was used to understand the client's situation. Example 1 involves a situation where the occupational therapist decided not to use MOHO terminology and example 2 describes a situation where the occupational therapist found it helpful to use the terminology.

CASE VIGNETTE 1 Occupational Therapist Decides Not to Use MOHO Terminology

The following is an example of an entry into a multidisciplinary record. It frames Sophie's occupational life using MOHO; however, specific MOHO terminology was not used because the multidisciplinary team was not familiar with MOHO language. MOHO constructs have been placed in brackets for illustration only.

'Sophie states she was previously a very active person (occupational identity). She worked behind the bar of a local pub (role) for 20 years before her retirement (role change) 5 years ago. She was very social and felt that a lot of the "regulars" at the pub were like friends (social environment). She enjoyed (interests) the social aspect of her job. Since retirement (role change) she has felt isolated (social environment). She is extremely house proud (values), always had high standards

(values) of cleaning and ran the household very efficiently (homemaker role). It was important (values) for Sophie always to present herself well. She took great care of her appearance (self-care role), liked to be "well turned out" (values) and had her hair set once a week (habit). She enjoyed spending time with her daughter and family (interest/social environment). She was particularly close to her granddaughter (role) and they had previously spent time together every Saturday out in the community (habit). She also enjoyed board games and knitting (interest). She previously volunteered at a local sheltered housing complex (role), where she made soup and meals. She was involved in church events (role) and ran charity events for the women's guild (role).'

CASE VIGNETTE 2 Occupational Therapist Decides to Use MOHO Terminology

The following is an example of using MOHO language to help understand a client called Jane. An occupational therapist may routinely document in their notes the following statement:

Statement A

'Jane lacks confidence and is overly dependent.'

Using MOHO framework and language makes the definition of the challenge Jane faces more specific:

Statement B

'Jane's personal causation is characterised by lacking a clear sense of her own capacity. As a result, she anticipates performance situations with anxiety and frequently chooses to avoid doing things for which she has adequate skills. She also habitually seeks advice and help from others, which leads to her being unnecessarily dependent on others.'

In this situation the therapist decided to use statement B because using the terminology of MOHO resulted in documentation that was more precise and detailed. Moreover, although statement A describes Jane's behaviour, it does not explain it. The MOHO framework and language in statement B offered an explanation that also provides a rationale for the following interventions:

- Advise Jane on a course of occupational therapy that will support a graded engagement in occupations to challenge her sense of capacity increasingly.
- Provide Jane with feedback around her occupational performance to enable a more accurate sense of her own capacities to engage in occupations.
- Encourage Jane to sustain occupational performance in the face of anxiety.
- Structure the environment to provide the opportunity for Jane to practice engaging in occupations with more autonomy.

Precision in language, including the use of theoretical terms, can clarify what we understand clients' occupational challenges to be and how we plan to address them.

Can MOHO Embrace the Complexity of Human Occupation?

Human occupation is complex (Creek 2003). Most people come into occupational therapy with significant impairments and major disruptions to their lives. Others struggle with declining function or recurring exacerbations of their diseases. A large proportion of clients face the task of rebuilding all or part of their lives. In short, their occupational problems tend to be complex and challenging. The strength and application of MOHO is neither simple nor formulaic. Instead, it aims to understand important multiple dimensions of each client's unique experience and bring a sophisticated understanding to bear on the life issues facing each client in practice.

In occupational therapy, a number of frameworks address aspects of occupational performance and the capacities that underlie it, but these theories tend to exist in isolation from one another. For example, occupational therapy theories that concentrate on physical performance have generally attended to the bodily components (brain and musculoskeletal system) involved in physical doing, whereas motives have been seen as part of a separate domain. By contrast, MOHO offers an approach to thinking about the capacity for occupational performance that complements existing theory. There is growing recognition of the importance of considering body and mind together in explaining phenomena (Kielhofner 1995, Trombly 1995). After all, motivation for a task can influence the extent of physical effort directed to that task (Yoder et al 1989, Riccio et al 1990), whereas physical impairments can weigh down the desire to do things (Murphy 1987, Toombs 1992). Conceptually, MOHO seeks to avoid dividing humans into separate physical and mental components, and instead embraces the complexity of human occupation. MOHO seeks to explain how occupation is motivated, patterned and performed, and implicates both body and mind in each of these major concepts. By offering explanations of such diverse phenomena, MOHO offers a broad and integrative view of human occupation. Consequently, it can be used to explain and guide practice involving a wide range of phenomena and corresponding concepts. Moreover, as stated above, therapists often use MOHO in combination with other conceptual models of practice or with theories borrowed from other disciplines or professions.

Is MOHO Applicable to Lower-Functioning Clients?

Some have questioned the relevance of MOHO in addressing issues of motivation in children and in lower-functioning clients. This perception is perplexing because those clients who are least able to self-describe and self-advocate most deserve careful assessment of their volition. This can be achieved through careful observation of the client's volitionally relevant actions. The Volitional Questionnaire (VQ) (de las Heras et al 2001), the Pediatric Volitional Questionnaire (PVQ; Geist et al 2001) and the Model of Human Occupation Screening Tool (MOHOST) (Parkinson et al 2001) work well with such clients. A therapist can, therefore, readily gain insight into the volition of children or lower-functioning clients. Additionally, therapists can make good use of unstructured means of assessment for such clients (Kielhofner 2002) that allow for complete flexibility within the assessment process.

Is MOHO an Evidence-Based Choice?

Yes. Since MOHO was first published in the early 1980s it has built up an evidence base. The majority of these studies were completed in the last decade, indicating an accelerating growth in research on MOHO, and it is now the most internationally researched and occupation-focused conceptual model of practice. MOHO provides theoretical evidence for its practice theory and it provides research evidence for its tools for practice.

Theoretical Evidence for Practice

Such research examines whether the concepts of MOHO theory are supported by evidence. It also involves asking whether the theory can account for and predict the kinds of client change it seeks to explain. Therefore, theoretical evidence on MOHO has included the following types of study:

- construct validity studies that seek to verify MOHO concepts
- correlative studies that examine the accuracy of relationships between constructs proposed in MOHO theory
- studies comparing groups on concepts from MOHO theory to test whether they explain group differences
- prospective studies that examine the potential of MOHO concepts and propositions to predict future behaviour or states
- qualitative studies that explore MOHO concepts and propositions in depth.

This kind of theoretical evidence for practice yields findings that may lead one to have confidence in the theory and/or to eliminate, change or expand a concept and/or proposition.

Evidence for Technology for Practice Application

In addition to offering a practice-based theory to embrace the complexity of therapy, conceptual models of practice like MOHO additionally generated a technology for

application (e.g., assessments and intervention strategies) for use in practice. Examples of this kind of research are
- psychometric studies leading to the development of outcome measures
- studies of how MOHO concepts influence therapeutic reasoning and practice
- studies that examine what happens in therapy
- outcomes studies that identify the effectiveness of occupational therapy services
- predictive studies that identify whether certain occupational outcomes can be predicted by the occupational therapist.

This kind of research provides practical tools for therapists to use within their practice and evidence to argue for additional occupational therapy resources. Although we can distinguish theoretical and application research within the MOHO research base, it is important to recognize that many MOHO-based studies incorporate both theoretical and application research aims, addressed simultaneously. This is reflective of a 'scholarship of practice' approach to building evidence for the field, whereby research for theory and application are simultaneously achieved. For example, some studies that primarily sought to examine the dependability of an assessment tool have identified new concepts that were later incorporated into the theory (Mallinson et al 1998).

Can MOHO Be Used When Selecting Adaptive Equipment?

Yes. Social service colleagues have asked the question, 'How would I apply MOHO to a client who is having difficulty bathing?' A biomechanical way of framing this challenge may be to state that the person is having difficulty 'physically getting in and out of the bath'. A MOHO way of framing the challenge is to state that the person is having 'difficulty engaging in the bathing activity'. MOHO, therefore, supports therapists in embracing the complexity of bathing rather than reducing it to only an issue of moving the client's body into/out of the bath. MOHO would support the therapist in asking the following questions:
- Does the person feel confident doing this activity?
- Have they had difficult past experiences doing this activity? (personal causation)
- Do they find this activity enjoyable/satisfying? (interest)
- How important is this activity for them?
- How important is it that they complete the activity alone?
- What meaning will adaptive equipment have for the person? (values)
- Can they physically do the activity? (motor skills)
- Do they have enough concentration—sequencing and so on—to complete the activity? (process skills)

- Do they have the full responsibility for doing the activity? (role)
- Does someone help them? (social environment)
- Where do they bathe?
- Where do they undress?
- Do they have any equipment to help them?
- Can they describe the environment when the bath is full—slippy, with lots of steam and so on? (physical environment)
- Do they have a routine when doing this activity?
- What time of day do they bathe? (habits)
- Are they satisfied with their morning/evening routine and when bathing happens?
- How does the time of day affect their abilities to bathe? (habits)

MOHO can, therefore, provide a framework for understanding the life within which occupational therapy is entering and whether adaptive equipment is appropriate. It also provides an understanding of the meaning attached to the equipment and how it might be adapted into the routine of the client. A lack of attention to these details may mean that the equipment is hidden away because of the client not wanting to be seen as 'disabled', or the equipment being removed because it was not adopted into the client's habitual routine.

Can You Use MOHO as an Activity Analysis Structure?

Yes. The analysis of occupations and their use within therapy are among the unique skills of the occupational therapist (Hagedorn 2000). There are many structures that provide a framework for analyzing activity. Recently, however, there has been some discussion that advocates using theories as a framework for activity analysis (Crepeau 2003, Toglia 2003).

> *Practitioners analyse activities from the perspective of practice theories to understand problems in performance and intervention strategies.*
>
> Crepeau 2003, p.191

MOHO provides an evidence-based practice theory that supports a therapist in *analyzing* a person's occupational life. Practice-based theories have the added advantage of providing an understanding of how different elements of analysis relate to each other and provide an insight into the change process (Creek 2009). MOHO has an established evidence base to support how different theoretical constructs relate to each other (e.g., Lederer et al 1985, Barris et al 1986, Ebb et al 1989, Davies Hallet et al 1994, Peterson et al 1999, American Occupational Therapy Association 2002) and has a theory of how therapeutically supported change happens (Kielhofner 2002). It could, therefore, be argued that using evidence-based theory (e.g., MOHO) to analyze activities has several advantages over traditional activity analysis frameworks. MOHO-driven activity analysis simultaneously

- provides an analysis of the person's occupational life
- examines how the different aspects of this analysis relate to each other
- looks at how this analysis relates to the changes that potentially can be made to support the client's re-engagement in everyday life.

This view has been supported by the inclusion of motor and process skills (Fisher & Kielhofner 1995, Kielhofner 2002), along with communication and interactions skills (Forsyth et al 1998) in the occupational therapy practice framework (Butts & Nelson 2007). As described in a previous section, MOHO would need to be used with other frameworks (e.g., biomechanical, motor control, sensory integration, etc.) to support a complete activity analysis that included analyzing performance capacities.

CASE VIGNETTE 3

This case illustrates the use of the MOHO framework to understand the occupational participation of a client called Sophie Bronson. The occupational therapy report shown was developed from observations of Sophie within her home environment, and from face-to-face discussion with Sophie and Sophie's husband, in addition to telephone contact with Sophie's daughter. The therapist decided not to use MOHO terminology in the report because of the multidisciplinary audience.

Sophie: Occupational Therapy Report[a]
Name: Sophie Bronson
Address: 12 Church Street, Edinburgh
Date of Birth: 12.03.30
GP: Dr Watson
Consultant: Dr Wallace
Data sources:
14 March 2005 Home visit with Sophie and her husband present
15 March 2005 Telephone contact with Sophie's daughter
Date of report: 16 March 2008

Referral and Reason for Assessment
The referral was received from Sophie's GP, Dr Watson, on 24 February 2005. The referral stated that Sophie was now reporting 'difficulties with coping and mobility'. It also stated that Sophie has been diagnosed as having early dementia and has a previous medical history of osteoarthritis and congestive heart failure. The reason for the assessment, therefore, was to look at Sophie's engagement with everyday activity and make recommendations to support Sophie in feeling as if she can 'cope and manage her mobility' issues and with other potential unidentified difficulties engaging in activity.

Sources of Information for Report
This report is a compilation of information gathered on a home visit (Sophie, her husband and her occupational therapist present) and a telephone contact with Sophie's daughter.

History of Activity
Information from Sophie
She was previously a very active person. She worked behind the bar of a local pub for 20 years before her retirement. She was very social and felt that a lot of the 'regulars' at the pub were like friends. She enjoyed the social aspect of her job. Since retirement she has felt isolated. She is extremely house-proud, always had high standards of cleaning and ran the household very efficiently. It was important for Sophie always to present herself smartly. She took great care of her appearance, liked to be 'well turned out' and had her hair set once a week. She enjoyed spending time with her daughter and family. She was particularly close to her granddaughter and they had previously spent time together every Saturday out in the community. She also enjoyed board games and knitting. She previously volunteered at a local sheltered housing complex, where she made soup and meals. She was involved in church events and ran charity events for the women's guild.

Information from Sophie's Husband and Daughter
They both confirmed the above information from Sophie and so it could be concluded that Sophie is an accurate historian. They stated that Sophie's activity levels reduced when she retired 5 years ago. There has been a gradual deterioration in activity levels over a 12-month period. She has been sitting in her chair all day doing very little since her recent hospital admission 6 months ago.

Current Mental/Physical Health
A. Current Mental Health
On the visit, Sophie was observed to be responsive and cooperative; she reported that her mood has been low for 6 months and that she no longer took any interest in activities that were once meaningful. Sophie identified the source of her low mood as including

- her inability to mobilise out of doors
- her recent hospital admission (6 months ago)
- a flood incident in the flat above.

CASE VIGNETTE 3—CONT'D

She states that she is not coping with any activities that were previously meaningful to her and she is frustrated by this.

Sophie's daughter feels that her mother's current low mood is caused by social isolation since retiring and to having reduced mobility ascending/descending stairs because of her painful and swollen feet. Sophie's social isolation has worsened recently because she is not taking as much care of her physical appearance and now would not want anyone to see her in an unkempt state.

B. Current Physical Health

Sophie needs a Zimmer frame to mobilise around her environment. She was observed to mobilise in her flat independently and safely using this frame. She has not gone outside for the past 12 months because of her inability to ascend/descend stairs. She was observed to have swollen feet, with hyper-extended big toes. The podiatrist and physiotherapist are involved, which has improved the situation; however, Sophie still reports pain. She wears glasses, although states she is able to read without them. She reports deteriorated eyesight since a cataract operation. She states that she has hearing aids, which she was not wearing during the visit. She was observed to be answering questions appropriately and followed the conversations; therefore, she could hear people talking.

Current Engagement in Activity

A. Physical Environment

Sophie was observed to live in a two-bedroomed first-floor flat. External access is by two steps (no rails) into the building, a 100-yard paved corridor, then 16 steps broken halfway with a landing (with rail right side ascending). The physical condition of the flat was well maintained; it is centrally heated and connected by a telephone.

B. Social Environment

Sophie states that she has had a home carer for the last 3 months who attends three times per day, 7 days a week. Sophie says she has not been enjoying the company of her granddaughter recently and feels guilty about this.

Sophie lives with her husband and he states that he is in good health. He says he is frustrated by his wife's lack of engagement in activities and her perception that he is not completing tasks to her standards.

Sophie's daughter states that she and her husband live close by. They both work full-time but Sophie's daughter visits every evening to support her parents. She has two teenage children, a son and a daughter, who now only visit sporadically.

Sophie has asked friends not to visit any longer. She states that she does not want them to see her unkempt.

C. Daily Routine

Sophie's husband states that she rises at 9 AM when the home care assistant attends. She goes through her morning routine then has breakfast at 9.30 AM. She sits in her lounge chair watching TV all day and evening. The home care assistant attends at 1 PM to carry out domestic tasks. She then attends at 10 PM to support Sophie with her night routine. Sophie states that she is not happy with this routine but cannot 'be bothered to do anything'.

D. Roles

i. Self-care

Sophie's self-care routine takes place entirely within her bedroom. Because of a lack of confidence in her balance, Sophie does not

- strip-wash at the bathroom sink
- use the shower
- use the perch stool.

Sophie states that to wash herself she has an established routine and sits on the bedside commode. The care assistant arranges needed objects to support this lack of mobility and provides verbal encouragement (to support Sophie's lack of confidence). Sophie and her daughter both state that she then has the skills to dress herself independently on the commode. Grooming herself is very important to Sophie; she says that she is currently unable to set her hair and can no longer get out of her flat to access the hairdresser. Sophie was observed on the visit to

- independently transfer on/off a 40-cm high commode using a Zimmer frame with a safe technique
- independently transfer on/off a 40-cm high toilet, using a 5-cm raised toilet seat and right wall grab rail, with a safe technique.

Bed transfer was not observed. Sophie did not want to attempt shower transfer, as she is not currently using the shower and is comfortable with her current arrangement of strip-washing at the bedside.

ii. Productivity

- *Cooking.* The kitchen was observed to have a gas cooker with overhead grill, microwave, electric kettle, continuous surfaces, and a table and chairs. Although Sophie stated that she previously enjoyed cooking for the sheltered housing volunteer position, her husband now does all the cooking and makes the hot drinks at home. She states that she has 'no interest' in cooking

Continued

CASE VIGNETTE 3—CONT'D

now, although does occasionally help prepare meals with her husband. She feels she cannot do the cooking now and feels she will not be able to do this independently. They have a diet of toast in the morning, banana and bread for lunch and a cooked meal in the evening. Sophie states that she does not eat the vegetables because her husband does not prepare them well enough. Sophie's husband feels that Sophie still has the skill, supportive environment and previous habits to cook but she is not motivated to do so. He is frustrated by his wife's lack of engagement with cooking.

- *Task on visit: making a hot drink.* Sophie stated that she would not be able to manage to complete the activity. She did, however, manage to make the hot drink independently with the following skill level:
  - *Motor skills.* She was unsteady at times and slow, but managed physically without intervention. She demonstrated some stiffness and reduction in strength. She appeared to lack energy and sat at regular intervals during the activity.
  - *Process skills.* Sophie managed to use knowledge, plan and organise the activity. She did, however, have challenges problem solving.

Sophie did not view this as an achievement because it was not completed to her standard.

- *Laundry/cleaning and shopping.* These activities are completed by the home carer and Sophie's husband. They are happy to continue to support; however, Sophie feels these activities are not completed to 'her standards'.
- *Volunteer job.* Sophie has not been involved with her volunteer job for 3 years. She states she misses the social contact and the feeling of 'being useful'.

iii. Leisure

Sophie could identify interests that she engaged in the past. She specifically identified the social aspect of these interests as being enjoyable and satisfying.

Sophie now appears to have reduced leisure opportunities. She could identify specific TV programmes that she enjoys watching. She now receives a weekly visit at home from the church. She could not identify anything else that she does that brings her enjoyment.

Sophie's daughter is particularly concerned that Sophie is not engaging with previous leisure activities. Her daughter states she feels that this is the key for supporting her mother to 're-engage in life'.

E. Goals

Sophie was unable to identify any goals for the future. Sophie feels very pessimistic about her ability to return to a meaningful life. She states she feels 'hopeless' about the future.

F. Readiness for Change

Sophie's current situation is not supportive of her mental or physical health. The combination of high performance standards and less skill means that Sophie lacks motivation to engage in doing activities that were meaningful to her in the past and she cannot identify any goals, develop plans and follow them through. Although socially isolated by not being able to ascend/descend external stairs, Sophie stated that she is not prepared to consider moving to alternative accommodation on the ground floor. The couple have been buying their council flat and moving would be 'too large an upheaval'. Sophie now has carer support and has developed strong habits and dependence on this support. Although Sophie is unhappy with her circumstances, she is not ready to change independently and, therefore, requires further extended occupational therapy input.

Occupational Therapy Perspective (Fig. 6.6)

Sophie gives the impression of a person who has given up on life. She has previously been an active woman but has had a reduction in activity in the past 5 years since retiring; this has further reduced in the past 12 months and was accelerated within the last 6 months following a hospital admission. This situation was brought about primarily by a difficult transition from working to retirement, physical limitations and pain when mobilising. This has been compounded by the identification of the start of a dementia process.

Motivation for Activity

Currently Sophie lacks motivation to engage in previously held meaningful activity. Specifically, she has difficulty appraising her own abilities, leading to her being dependent on others. She does not expect success in the future, which leads to fear of failing and not meeting her high standards. She cannot identify any activities that bring her enjoyment and is unable to set goals for the future. These characteristics create a situation where Sophie does not make choices to do activity, apart from basic self-care.

CASE VIGNETTE 3—CONT'D

Pattern of Activity

Sophie has had substantial role loss over the last 5 years, which has led to an empty routine, a poor sense of belonging and avoidance of previously held responsibility. She demonstrates an unwillingness to agree to changes in her current routines and ways of doing activities, even though these habits do not support her preferred lifestyle.

Skill for Activity

Sophie has adequate communication and interaction skills but is now having challenges maintaining relationships. She has physical difficulties with balance, stiffness, strength and energy. She has adequate processing skills but has difficulty with problem-solving.

Environment

Sophie's physical environment is problematic because her flat is accessed by stairs and she cannot ascend/descend them. This will not be easily resolved. Her social environment is very supportive; however, carers are not supporting the development of Sophie's ability to engage in daily activities.

Overall Recommendation

Sophie's current situation is not supportive of her mental or physical health. Although Sophie wants to change her circumstances, she is not ready to change independently and therefore requires further extended occupational therapy input.
NAME: Kirsty Forsyth
GRADE: Senior I
LOCATION: Edinburgh Community Rehabilitation Team
cc: GP, PT.

[a]The Model of Human Occupation Screening Tool (MOHOST) was used to complete this assessment, from: Parkinson, S., Forsyth, K., Kielhofner, G., 2002. A User's Manual for the Model of Human Occupation Screening Tool (MOHOST), Version 1.0, Research Version. MOHO Clearinghouse, University of Illinois at Chicago.

Client: Sophie Bronson				**Assessor:** K. Forsyth	
Age: 70	**Date of birth:** 01/02/34			**Designation:** Senior IOT	
Sex:	Male:	Female:		Signature:	
Status:	Inpatient:	Outpatient;		Date of assessment: 16/03/05	
Ethnicity: White:		Black:	Asian:	Treatment setting: Home	
Disabling condition:		Dementia			

4	Strength	Supports occupational participation
3	Difficulty	Minor interference with or risk to occupational participation
2	Weakness	Major interference with occupational participation
1	Problems	Prevents occupational participation

ANALYSIS OF STRENGTHS AND LIMITATIONS

Sophie is currently having difficulty engaging in meaningful daily activity and appears to have given up on life. This situation is not supportive of her physical or mental health. Although Sophie is dissatisfied with her present circumstances she is not ready to independently change, and therefore requires further extended occupational therapy. See ratings below.

Fig. 6.6 The Model of Human Occupation Screening Tool (MOHOST). (Copyright Parkinson, S., Forsyth, K., Kielhofner, G., 2005. The Model of Human Occupation Tool (MOHOST), version 2.0. Reproduced with the permission of Parkinson, Forsyth and Kielhofner.)

SUMMARY OF RATINGS

Motivation of occupation				Pattern of occupation				Communication and interaction skills				Process skills				Motor skills				Environment			
Appraisal of abilities	Expectation of success	Interest	Commitment	Routine	Adaptability	Responsibility	Roles	Non-verbal skills	Conversation	Vocal expression	Relationships	Knowledge	Planning	Organization	Problem-solving	Posture and mobility	Coordination	Strength and effort	Energy	Physical space	Physical resources	Social groups	Occupational demands
4	4	4	4	4	4	4	4	(4)	(4)	(4)	4	(4)	(4)	(4)	4	4	4	4	4	4	4	(4)	4
3	3	3	3	3	3	3	3	3	3	3	3	3	3	3	3	3	(3)	(3)	3	3	3	3	(3)
(2)	2	(2)	2	2	2	(2)	2	2	2	2	(2)	2	2	2	(2)	(2)	2	2	(2)	2	2	2	2
1	(1)	1	(1)	(1)	(1)	1	(1)	1	1	1	1	1	1	1	1	1	1	1	1	(1)	(1)	1	1

MOTIVATION FOR OCCUPATION		
Appraisal of ability	4	Realistic, recognizes strengths, aware of limitations, shows pride in assets
Understanding of strengths and limitations	3	Reasonable tendency to over/underestimate own abilities, recognizes some limitations
Self-awareness and realism	(2)	Over/underestimates own abilities leading to inappropriate occupations
Belief in skill	1	Does not reflect on skills, fails to realistically estimate or lacks pride in own abilities
		Comments : ....
Expectation of success	4	Anticipates success and seeks challenges, confident about overcoming obstacles
Optimism	3	Has some hope for success, adequate self-belief but has some doubts, may need encouraging
Self-efficacy	2	Requires support to sustain confidence about overcoming obstacles or overly confident
Sense of control	(1)	Pessimistic, feels hopeless or highly overconfident, gives up in the face of obstacles
Hope		*Comments* : ....
Interest	4	Keen, curious, lively, tries new occupations, expresses pleasure, perseveres, appears content
Expressed enjoyment	3	Has adequate interests that guide choices, has some opportunities to pursue interests
Satisfaction	(2)	Difficulty identifying interests, interest is short-lived, ambivalent about choice of occupations
Curiosity	1	Easily bored, unable to identify interests, apathetic, lacks curiosity even with support
Participation		*Comments* : ....
Commitment	4	Clear preferences and sense of what is important, motivated to work towards occupational goals
Values and standards	3	Mostly able to make choices, may need encouragement to set and work towards goals
Goals and projects	2	Difficulties identifying what is important or setting and working towards goals, inconsistent
Choices and preferences	(1)	Cannot set goals, impulsive, chaotic, goals are unattainable or based on antisocial values
Sense of purpose		*Comments* : ....

Fig. 6.6, cont'd

PATTERN OF OCCUPATION		
Routine	4	Able to arrange a balanced routine that supports responsibilities and goals (steady)
Balance	3	Generally able to maintain an organized and productive daily schedule
Structure	2	Difficulty organizing routines to meet occupational responsibilities without support
Productivity	(1)	Chaotic or empty routine, unable to support responsibilities and goals (erratic/imbalanced)
Activity		Comments : ....
Adaptability	4	Anticipates change, alters actions or routine to meet demand (flexible/accommodating)
Anticipation	3	Generally able to modify behaviour, may need time to adjust, hesitant
Flexibility	2	Difficulty adapting to change, reluctant, passive or habitually overreacts
Response to change	(1)	Rigid, unable to adapt routines or tolerate change
Frustration tolerance		Comments : ....
Responsibility	4	Willingly takes on responsibilities and meets expectations (reliable/dependable)
Awareness	3	Accepts responsibility for most personal actions, can generally utilize constructive feedback
Handling expectation		
Fulfilling obligations	(2)	Difficulty recognizing responsibilities, avoids extra responsibilities or feels over-responsible
Acceptance	1	Unable to recognize responsibilities, denies responsibilities or responds inappropriately
		Comments : ....
Roles	4	Has a sense of identity that comes from roles, is committed to their roles and fits in well
Involvement	3	Generally meets obligations of several roles or maintains one major productive role
Belonging	2	Limited involvement in roles or has difficulty meeting role demands due to overload/conflict
Response to demand	(1)	Poor sense of belonging, has negligible role demands, does not identify with any role
Role variety		Comments : ....

COMMUNICATION AND INTERACTION SKILLS		
Non-verbal skills	(4)	Appropriate (possibly spontaneous) body language, given culture and circumstances
Physicality	3	Demonstrates questionable ability to display or control appropriate body language
Eye contact	2	Difficulty controlling/displaying appropriate body language (delayed/limited/disinhibited)
Gestures		
Orientation	1	Unable to display appropriate body language (absent/incongruent/unsafe/violent)
		Comments : ....
Conversation	(4)	Appropriately initiates, discloses and sustains conversation (clear/direct/open)
Disclosing	3	Demonstrates questionable ability to effectively exchange information
Initiating and sustaining	2	Difficulty initiating, disclosing or sustaining conversation (hesitant/abrupt/limited/irrelevant)
Speech content		
Language	1	Uncommunicative, disjointed, bizarre or inappropriate disclosure of information
		Comments : ....
Vocal expression	(4)	Assertive, articulate, uses appropriate tone, volume and pace
Intonation	3	Demonstrates questionable ability in vocal expression
Articulation	2	Difficulty with expressing self (unclear/pressured speech/monotone)
Volume	1	Unable to express self (incomprehensible/too quiet or loud/too fast)
Pace		Comments : ....

Fig. 6.6, cont'd

Relationships	4	Sociable, supportive, aware of others, sustains engagement, friendly, relates well to others
Cooperation	3	Demonstrates questionable social skills
Collaboration	(2)	Difficulty with cooperation or makes few positive relationships
Rapport	1	Unable to cooperate with others or make positive relationships
Respect		*Comments :* ....

PROCESS SKILLS

Knowledge	(4)	Seeks and retains relevant information, selects tools appropriately, shows understanding
Seeking and retaining information	3	Demonstrates questionable ability to seek and retain information and use tools
	2	Difficulty selecting and using tools, difficulty in asking for help (forgetful/unaware/confused)
Use of knowledge, including use of objects	1	Unable to complete occupation, disoriented or lacking knowledge or ability to use tools
Understanding, orientation		*Comments :* ....
Planning	(4)	Plans ahead, sustains concentration, starts and completes occupation at appropriate times
Thinking through from beginning to end	3	Demonstrates questionable ability to plan for and during occupations
Timing	2	Difficulty planning, fluctuating concentration or distractible, difficulty initiating and completing
Concentration	1	Unable to plan ahead, unable to concentrate, unable to initiate or complete occupations
		Comments : ....
Organization	(4)	Efficiently searches for, gathers and restores tools/objects needed in occupation (neat)
Arranging space and objects	3	Demonstrates questionable ability to search, gather and restore needed tools/objects
Neatness	2	Difficulty searching for, gathering and restoring tools/objects, appears disorganized/untidy
Preparation	1	Unable to search for, gather and restore tools and objects (chaotic)
		Comments : ....
Problem-solving	4	Shows good judgement, anticipates difficulties and generates workable solutions (rational)
Judgement	3	Demonstrates questionable ability to make decisions based on difficulties that arise
Adaptation	(2)	Difficulty anticipating and adapting to difficulties that arise, seeks reassurance
Decision-making	1	Unable to anticipate and adapt to difficulties that arise and makes inappropriate decisions
Responsiveness		*Comments :* ....

MOTOR SKILLS

Posture and mobility	4	Stable, upright, independent, flexible, good range of movement (possibly agile)
Stability walking	3	Demonstrates questionable ability to maintain posture and mobility in occupation
Alignment reaching	(2)	Unsteady at times, slow or manages with difficulty
Positioning bending	1	Extremely unstable, unable to reach and bend or unable to walk
Balance transfers		*Comments :* ....
Coordination	4	Coordinates body parts with each other, uses smooth fluid movements (possibly dextrous)
Manipulation	(3)	Some awkwardness or stiffness
Ease of movement	2	Difficulty coordinating movements (clumsy/tremulous/awkward/stiff)
Fluidity	1	Unable to coordinate, manipulate and use fluid movements
Fine motor skills		*Comments :* ....

Fig. 6.6, cont'd

Strength and effort	4	Grasps, moves and transports objects securely with adequate force/speed (possibly strong)
Grip lifting	(3)	Demonstrates questionable ability in strength and effort
Handling, transporting	2	Has difficulty with grasping, moving, transporting objects with adequate force and speed
Moving, calibrating	1	Unable to grasp, move, transport objects with appropriate force and speed (weak/frail)
		Comments : ....
Energy	4	Maintains appropriate energy levels, able to maintain tempo throughout occupation
Endurance	3	Demonstrates questionable energy (whether low or high)
Pace	(2)	Difficulty maintaining energy (tires easily/evidence of fatigue/distractible/restless)
Attention	1	Unable to maintain energy, lacks focus, lethargic, inactive or highly overactive
Stamina		Comments : ....

ENVIRONMENT		
Physical space	4	Affords a range of opportunities, supports and stimulates valued occupations
Home and neighbourhood	3	OT questions whether the physical space adequately supports valued occupations
Work and/or leisure facilities	2	Affords a limited range of opportunities and curtails performance of valued occupations
Privacy and accessibility	(1)	Restricts opportunities and prevents performance of valued occupations
Stimulation and comfort		Comments : ....
Physical resources	4	Allow occupational goals to be achieved safely, easily and independently
Finance	3	Have questionable impact on ability to achieve occupational goals
Equipment and tools	2	Restrict ability to achieve occupational goals safely, easily and independently
Possessions and transport	(1)	Have major impact on ability to achieve occupational goals, lead to high risks
Safety and independence		Comments : ....
Social groups	(4)	Offer practical support, values and attitudes support optimal functioning
Family dynamics	3	OT questions the support of social groups due to under- or over-involvement
Friends and social support	2	Offer reduced support, or detracts from functioning, supported in some groups but not others
Work climate	1	Do not support functioning due to lack of interest or inappropriate involvement
Expectations and involvement		Comments : ....
Occupational demands	4	Match well with abilities, interests, energy and time available
Social and leisure activities	(3)	OT questions whether the demands are consistent with abilities, interest, energy or time
Daily living tasks	2	Some inconsistencies with abilities and interest, or energy and time available
Work and/or domestic responsibilities	1	Inconsistent with abilities and motivation, under or overdemanding
		Comments : ....

Fig. 6.6, cont'd

SUMMARY

MOHO provides a way for occupational therapists to embrace the complexity of human occupation within their practice. It provides an understanding of the choice, order and performance of occupation within people's lives. It also provides assessment and intervention techniques to support the integration of MOHO theory into practice. MOHO is built for and with an international community of occupational therapists, with the ultimate goal of fully embracing the unique occupational characteristics of our clients and supporting them in their re-engagement with meaningful self-care, productivity and leisure.

✴ REFLECTIVE LEARNING

Think of a recent occupational therapy client you have been involved with (either as a student on placement or as a qualified occupational therapist) and ask yourself the following questions:

- What is the person's occupational identity? (Prompt: what roles do they identify with? Father, brother, sibling, worker?)
- What is the person's occupational competence? (Prompt: what skills does the person feel they have to meet role responsibilities? Is this accurate appraisal?)
- What are the positive occupational issues for the person? (Prompt: think about engagement in self-care, work and/or leisure and personal causation, values, interests, habits, role, performance capacity, skills or environment? Or a combination of these?)
- Why is the person unable to engage in occupations or having challenges engaging in them? (Prompt: think about challenges engagement in self-care, work and/or leisure and personal causation, values, interests, habits, role, performance capacity, skills or environment? Or a combination of these?)
- Write a summary statement using the answers to the above questions to capture the main occupational issues for the client.

REFERENCES

American Occupational Therapy Association. (2002). Occupational therapy practice framework: Domain and process. *American Journal of Occupational Therapy*, 56, 609–639.

Ayres, A. J. (1986). *Developmental dyspraxia and adult onset apraxia*. Torrance, CA: Sensory Integration International.

Butts, D. S., & Nelson, D. L. (2007). Agreement between Occupational Therapy Practice Framework classifications and occupational therapists' classifications. *American Journal of Occupational Therapy*, 61(5), 603–604.

Barris, R., Kielhofner, G., Burch, R. M., Gelinas, I., Klement, M., & Schultz, B. (1986). Occupational function and dysfunction in three groups of adolescents. *Occupational Therapy Journal of Research*, 6, 301–307.

Bruner, J. (1990). *Acts of meaning*. Cambridge, MA: Harvard University Press.

Creek, J. (2002). The knowledge base of occupational therapy. In J. Creek (Ed.), *Occupational therapy and mental health*. Edinburgh: Churchill Livingstone.

Creek, J. (2003). *Occupational therapy defined as a complex intervention*. London: College of Occupational Therapists.

Creek, J. (2009). Occupational therapy defined as a complex intervention: A 5-year review. *British Journal of Occupational Therapy*, 72(3), 105–115.

Crepeau, E. (2003). Activity analysis: A way of thinking about occupational performance. In E. B. Crepeau, B. Schell, & E. Cohn (Eds.), *Willard and Spackman's occupational therapy*. Philadelphia: Lippincott Williams & Wilkins.

Csikszentmihalyi, M. (1990). *Flow: The psychology of optimal experience*. New York: Harper & Row.

Davies Hallet, J., Zasler, N., Maurer, P., & Cash, S. (1994). Role change after traumatic brain injury in adults. *American Journal of Occupational Therapy*, 48, 241–246.

de las Heras, C. G., Geist, R., Kielhofner, G., et al. (2001). *The Volitional Questionnaire (VQ) (Version 4.1). Model of Human Occupation Clearinghouse*. Chicago: Department of Occupational Therapy, College of Applied Health Sciences, University of Illinois at Chicago.

Dewey, J. (1922). *Human nature and conduct*. New York: Henry Holt.

Ebb, E. W., Coster, W., & Duncombe, L. (1989). Comparison of normal and psychosocially dysfunctional male adolescents. *Occupational Therapy in Mental Health*, 9, 53–74.

Fisher, A., & Kielhofner, G. (1995). Skill in occupational performance. In G. Kielhofner (Ed.), *A model of human occupation: theory and application* (2nd ed.). Baltimore: Williams & Wilkins.

Fisher, A. G. (1999a). Uniting practice and theory in an occupational framework. *American Journal of Occupational Therapy*, 532(7), 509–520.

Fisher, A. G. (1999b). *Assessment of motor and process skills* (3rd ed.). Ft. Collins, CO: Three Star Press.

Forsyth, K., Salamy, M., Simon, S., et al. (1997). *Assessment of communication and interaction skills*. Chicago: University of Illinois, Model of Human Occupation Clearinghouse.

Forsyth, K., Salamy, M., Simon, S., et al. (1998). *A user's guide to the Assessment of Communication and Interaction Skills (ACIS). Chicago: Model of Human Occupation Clearinghouse*. Chicago: Department of Occupational Therapy, College of Applied Health Sciences, University of Illinois at Chicago.

Geist, R., Kielhofner, G., Basu, S., et al. (2001). *The Pediatric Volitional Questionnaire (PVQ) (Version 1.1). Model of Human Occupation Clearinghouse*. Chicago: Department of Occupational Therapy, College of Applied Health Sciences, University of Illinois at Chicago.

Gill, C. J. (1997). Four types of integration in disability identity development. *Journal of Vocational Rehabilitation*, 9, 39–46.

Hagedorn, R. (2000). *Tools for practice in occupational therapy.* Edinburgh: Churchill Livingstone.

Haglund, L., Karlsson, G., Kielhofner, G., & Lei, J. S. (1997). Validity of the Swedish version of the Worker Role Interview. *Scandinavian Journal of Occupational Therapy, 4*(1–4), 23–29.

Haglund, L., Ekbladh, E., Thorell, L., & Hallberg, I. R. (2000). Practice models in Swedish psychiatric occupational therapy. *Scandinavian Journal of Occupational Therapy, 7*(3), 107–113.

Harter, S. (1983). The development of the self-system. In M. Hetherington (Ed.), *Handbook of child psychology: Social and personality development* (vol. 4). New York: John Wiley.

Harter, S., & Connel, J. P. (1984). A model of relationships among children's academic achievement and self perceptions of competence, control, and motivation. In J. Nicholls (Ed.), *The development of achievement motivation.* Greenwich, CT: JAI.

Hull, J. M. (1990). *Touching the rock: An experience of blindness.* New York: Vintage.

Husserl, E. (1962). *Ideas: General introduction to pure phenomenology.* London: Collier (W.R.B. Gibson, Trans.).

Kielhofner, G. (1980a). A model of human occupation, part three. Benign and vicious cycles. *American Journal of Occupational Therapy, 34,* 731–737.

Kielhofner, G. (1980b). A model of human occupation, part two. Ontogenesis from the perspective of temporal adaptation. *American Journal of Occupational Therapy, 34,* 657–663.

Kielhofner, G. (1985). *A model of human occupation: Theory and application.* Baltimore: Williams & Wilkins.

Kielhofner, G. (1995). *A model of human occupation: Theory and application* (2nd ed.). Baltimore: Williams & Wilkins.

Kielhofner, G. (1997). *Conceptual foundations of occupational therapy.* Philadelphia: FA Davis.

Kielhofner, G. (2002). *A model of human occupation: Theory and application* (3rd ed.). Baltimore: Williams & Wilkins.

Kielhofner, G. (2008). *A model of human occupation: Theory and application* (4th ed.). Baltimore: Lippincott Williams & Wilkins.

Kielhofner, G., & Burke, J. P. (1977). Occupational therapy after 60 years: An account of changing identity and knowledge. *American Journal of Occupational Therapy, 31,* 675–689.

Kielhofner, G., & Burke, J. (1980). A model of human occupation, part one. Conceptual framework and content. *American Journal of Occupational Therapy, 34,* 572–581.

Kielhofner, G., & Forsyth, K. (2001). Development of a client self-report for treatment planning and documenting therapy outcomes. *Scandinavian Journal of Occupational Therapy, 8*(3), 131–139.

Kielhofner, G., Burke, J., & Heard, I. C. (1980). A model of human occupation, part four. Assessment and intervention. *American Journal of Occupational Therapy, 34,* 777–788.

Kielhofner, G., Mallinson, T., Crawford, C., Nowak, M., & Rigby, M. (1997). *A user's guide to the occupational performance history interview-II (OPHI-II) (version 2.0). Model of Human Occupation Clearinghouse.* Chicago: Department of Occupational Therapy, College of Applied Health Sciences, University of Illinois at Chicago.

Kielhofner, G., Lai, J. S., Olson, L., Haglund, L., Ekbadh, E., & Hedlund, M. (1999). Psychometric properties of the work environment impact scale: A cross-cultural study. *Work, 12*(1), 71–77.

Kielhofner, G., Mallinson, T., Forsyth, K., & Lai, J. S. (2001). Psychometric properties of the second version of the Occupational Performance History Interview (OPHI-II). *American Journal of Occupational Therapy, 55,* 260–267.

Law, M. (1998). *Client-centred occupational therapy.* Thorofare, NJ: Slack.

Law, M., & McColl, M. A. (1989). Knowledge and use of theory among occupational therapists: A Canadian survey. *Canadian Journal of Occupational Therapy, 56*(4), 198–204.

Lederer, J., Kielhofner, G., & Watts, J. (1985). Values, personal causation and skills of delinquents and non delinquents. *Occupational Therapy in Mental Health, 5,* 59–77.

Lee, D. (1971). Culture and the experience of value. In A. H. Maslow (Ed.), *Neural knowledge in human values.* Chicago: Henry Regnery.

Lee, S., Kielhofner, G., & Taylor, R. (2009). Choice, knowledge, and utilization of a practice theory: A national study of occupational therapists who use the Model of Human Occupation. *Occupational Therapy in Health Care, 23*(1), 60–71.

Lefcourt, H. M. (1981). Assessment and methods. *Research with the locus of control construct* (Vol. 1). New York: Academic Press.

Mallinson, T., Mahaffey, L., & Kielhofner, G. (1998). The Occupational Performance History Interview: Evidence for three underlying constructs of occupational adaptation. *Canadian Journal of Occupational Therapy, 65*(4), 219–228.

Mancuso, J., & Sarbin, T. (1983). The self-narrative in the enactment of roles. In T. R. Sarbin, & K. E. Scheibe (Eds.), *Studies in social identity.* New York: Praeger.

Merleau-Ponty, M. (1962). *Phenomenology of perception.* London: Routledge & Kegan Paul. [Translated by C. Smith from the French original version, Phénoménologie de la perception.].

Miller, J. F., & Oertel, C. B. (1983). Powerlessness in the elderly: Preventing hopelessness. In J. F. Miller (Ed.), *Coping with chronic illness: Overcoming powerlessness.* Philadelphia: FA Davis.

Moore-Corner, R., Kielhofner, G., & Olsen, L. (1998). *Work Environment Impact Scale (WEIS) (Version 2). Model of Human Occupational Clearinghouse.* Chicago: Department of Occupational Therapy, College of Applied Health Sciences, University of Illinois at Chicago.

Murphy, R. (1987). *The body silent.* New York: Henry Holt.

National Board for Certification in Occupational Therapy. (2004). A practice analysis study of entry-level occupational therapist registered and certified occupational therapy assistant practice. *OTJR, Occupation, Participation and Health, 24*(supplement 1) S3–S31.

Parkinson, S., Forsyth, K., & Kielhofner, G. (2001). *The Model of Human Occupation Screening tool (MOHOST), version 1.0. Model of Human Occupation Clearinghouse.* Chicago: Department of Occupational Therapy, College of Applied Health Sciences, University of Illinois at Chicago.

Peterson, E., Howland, J., Kielhofner, G., et al. (1999). Falls self-efficacy and occupational adaptation among elders. *Physical & Occupational Therapy in Geriatrics, 16*, 1–16.

Reilly, M. (1962). Occupational therapy can be one of the great ideas of 20th century medicine. *American Journal of Occupational Therapy, 16*, 1–9.

Riccio, C. M., Nelson, D. L., & Bush, M. A. (1990). Adding purpose to the repetitive exercises of elderly women. *American Journal of Occupational Therapy, 44*, 714–719.

Rotter, J. B. (1960). Generalized expectancies for internal versus external control of reinforcement. *Psychological Monographs: General Applications, 80*, 1–28.

Shannon, P. (1970). The work-play model: A basis for occupational therapy programming. *American Journal of Occupational Therapy, 24*, 215–218.

Sumsion, T. (1999). *Client-centred practice in occupational therapy: A guide to implementation*. Edinburgh: Churchill Livingstone.

Taylor, R. R. (2017). *Kielhofner's research in occupational therapy: Methods of inquiry for enhancing practice*. Philadelphia: FA Davis.

Taylor, R., Braveman, B., & Forsyth, K. (2002). Occupational science and the scholarship of practice: Implications for practitioners. *New Zealand Journal of Occupational Therapy, 49*, 37–40.

Taylor, R. R., Lee, S. W., Kielhofner, G., & Ketkar, M. (2009). Therapeutic use of self: A nationwide survey of practitioners' attitudes and experiences. *American Journal of Occupational Therapy, 63*, 198–207.

Toglia, J. P. (2003). The multicontext treatment approach. In E. B. Crepeau, B. Schell, & E. Cohn (Eds.), *Willard and Spackman's occupational therapy*. Philadelphia: Lippincott Williams & Wilkins.

Toombs, K. (1992). *The meaning of illness: A phenomenological account of the different perspectives of physician and patient*. Boston: Kluwer Academic.

Trombly, C. A. (1989). *Occupational therapy for physical dysfunction*. Baltimore: Williams & Wilkins.

Trombly, C. (1995). Occupation: Purposefulness and meaningfulness as therapeutic mechanisms. *American Journal of Occupational Therapy, 49*, 960–972.

World Health Organization. (1999). *ICIDH-2: International Classification of Functioning and Disability. Beta-2 draft, full version*. Geneva: WHO.

Yoder, R., Nelson, D., & Smith, D. (1989). Added-purpose versus rote exercise in female nursing home residents. *The American Journal of Occupational Therapy, 43*(9), 581–586.

7

Canadian Model of Occupational Performance and Engagement (CMOP-E): A Tool to Support Occupation-Centred Practice

Helene J. Polatajko, Jane A. Davis

◎ HIGHLIGHTS

- Two perspectives that have dominated practice are discussed: occupation as means and occupation as ends.
- These perspectives serve to frame the form of our practice.
- Practice is described as occupation-centred, with the ultimate objective to enable occupational performance and occupational engagement.
- The CMOP-E can be used as a tool to give form to occupation-centred practice through a way of organizing information about our clients.
- The CMOP-E grid can be used to organize occupation-centred practice information and to support professional reasoning.

Occupational therapy practice is complex and multifaceted, hence our difficulties with explaining what we do. We can as readily be seen crafting a splint, as redesigning a home, or advocating for workplace accommodations, teaching one-handed dressing, carrying out a kitchen assessment, running a craft group, enabling community integration, or, or, or … the list is endless. How does one make sense of such diversity; how do we, as a profession, make sense of such diversity? At the risk of being accused of gross oversimplification, the answer is occupation. Underlying each of the examples listed, indeed all occupational therapy practice, is the intent to improve occupational outcomes. In some instances the intended occupational outcome is immediately apparent (e.g., teaching one-handed dressing, advocating for workplace accommodations) while in others less so (e.g., creating a splint, running a craft group). The degree to which the intended occupational outcome is apparent in what we do reflects our perspectives on the role of occupation in practice. Historically, two perspectives have dominated practice: occupation as means and occupation as

ends. In this chapter, we discuss these perspectives and how they serve to frame the form of practice. We suggest that the particular form practice assumes is determined by the particular perspective we adopt; we argue for an occupation-centred perspective on practice. We introduce the Canadian Model of Occupational Performance and Engagement (CMOP-E), describe it and discuss how it can be used as a tool to give form to occupation-centred practice. We start the chapter with a discussion of the means/end duality and we end with a case vignette demonstrating the use of the CMOP-E.

A DUALITY OF PERSPECTIVES: MEANS AND ENDS

Two dominant perspectives have guided, and continue to guide, the approaches to practice seen in occupational therapy. These perspectives, most commonly captured by the phrase *means* versus *ends*, stand in contrast to each other. The *means* perspective, generally associated with the term *therapeutic use of activity*, is entrenched in the medical model and is focused on 'curing' or 'fixing' underlying deficits. In this perspective, occupation is typically referred to as activity rather than occupation and is viewed as our primary therapeutic agent (Fisher 2013). When adopting this perspective, occupational therapists operate on the premise that activity has curative/therapeutic value and use a variety of activities—chosen for their potential to address underlying deficits or to build capacity in the components that underlie function—to effect change. Running a craft group designed to improve attention span and organizational skills is consistent with this perspective. The *ends* perspective is entrenched in the occupational model and is focused on enabling occupation. In this perspective, occupation is viewed as the primary goal of the occupational therapy intervention (Fisher 2013). When adopting this perspective, occupational therapists operate on the premise that there are numerous ways to enable occupation, and they use a variety of techniques, such as redesigning a home, or advocating for workplace accommodations or teaching one-handed dressing.

Occupation at Our Core: Means and Ends

The terms *means* and *ends* have been used in our literature not only to evoke these two dominant practice perspectives, but also to signal the nature of the profession. On the one hand, it is argued that our profession is named occupational therapy to convey the *means* by which we do our work (i.e., through occupation, also known as activity). On the other hand, it is argued that our profession is named occupational therapy to convey the *ends* towards which we focus our work (i.e., occupation; Polatajko et al 2013). In the case of the former, the therapeutic use of activity was not necessarily aimed at enabling a client's occupation. Similarly, in the case of the latter, the use of occupation (also known as activity) was not necessarily seen as the active agent.

Since the late 20th century, it has been considered that occupation has a central role in occupational therapy. As articulated in the Canadian guidelines for occupational therapy practice (see Townsend & Polatajko 2013), it is now considered that the primary domain of concern of occupational therapy is occupation. This focus on occupation, given prominence near the end of the 20th century by such important scholars as Elizabeth Yerxa (1998), is an intentional departure from the focus on impairment that dominated our practice for much of the 1900s. Our former focus on impairment was well suited to the medical arena in which much of our practice was situated for significant parts of the 20th century. Much of our work then, and much of our literature, discussed theories that linked the use of activity to impairment reduction and was focused on demonstrating how activity, carefully chosen for its therapeutic value, could reduce impairment or, more positively, build capacity in the components underlying functioning (Polatajko 2001). In most instances, the therapeutic use of activity was viewed as promoting health but was divorced from any concern for occupational change (Polatajko 2001). For some, inherent in the quest for impairment reduction, or capacity-building, or health promotion, was the implicit quest for improved occupation. Nonetheless, this quest was rarely articulated and even more rarely addressed in our research. That is to say, the early research literature on intervention outcomes rarely included occupational measures. Indeed, there has been a dearth of occupational measures for much of our history, with most only introduced near the end of the 20th century.

By naming occupation as our primary domain of concern, we have also named enabling occupation as the primary objective of our profession; in other words, it is now broadly accepted that our name should convey the *ends* towards which our therapy is directed. Recently terms such as *occupation-centred*, *occupation-based* and *occupation-focused* have been introduced into our literature as practice descriptors to highlight the centrality of occupation to our profession and the various roles (*means and ends*) it plays in occupational therapy. Unfortunately, as Fisher (2013) has noted, there is insufficient clarity around the use of these terms in our literature; at times they are used to distinguish the various forms of practice seen in occupational therapy, while at times used as synonyms. Arguing that they are distinct and capture differing forms of occupational therapy practice, Fisher provided an in-depth discussion of the terms, their distinguishing features and how those features play out in practice. In this chapter, building on Fisher's work, we use these three terms to make explicit the various roles occupation takes in present day occupational therapy practice. As these three terms do not capture the full scope of the various forms of occupational therapy that are practiced, we include two additional terms, *activity-based* and *technique-based*: all are defined later.

Clarifying Terms: Occupation-Centred, Occupation-Focused and Occupation-Based

The definitions of the terms *occupation-centred*, *occupation-focused* and *occupation-based* used in this chapter are essentially those offered by Fisher (2013), with some additional qualifiers. To improve clarity, we have aligned the terms with the two dualities that support occupational therapy practices (i.e., we discuss each in relation to content [*means*] and intended outcome [*ends*]). As noted above, historically, the *means* portion of the means/ends duality referred to the focus of practice on impairment—be it impairment reduction or capacity-building in the components that underlie function—through the use of activity, generally captured by the phrase *therapeutic use of activity*. (Note. The phrase *therapeutic use of occupation* is rarely found in our literature and we suggest it should not be used, nor should the term *therapeutic occupation*; we will not use either in this chapter.) Indeed, in the interest of clarity, from here forward we will use the term *therapeutic activity* to refer to some form of client doing that is used during therapy, that is not necessarily part of the client's actual occupational repertoire but is chosen by the therapist for its perceived therapeutic potential to address the client's needs. Further, for the remainder of this chapter, also for the sake of clarity, we will use the term *activity* to refer to any form of doing that is not part of a client's established or desired occupational repertoire; we reserve the term *occupation* to refer to a client's actual or desired real-world doing.

Occupation-Centred. Occupation-centred pertains to the practice of the profession as a whole. The term indicates that occupation is at the core of our practice and requires, as stated by Fisher (2013), 'that we adopt an occupational lens *(Yerxa 1998, Wicks 2012)*, base our reasoning on the core theoretical tenets of the profession, and explicitly link what we do to that core *(Hooper 2006)*, (See Chapter 13, Fig 13.1) Those tenets pertain to our understanding of people as occupational beings, the impact of occupational challenges on their lives, and the power of occupation as a therapeutic change agent' (Fisher 2013, p.164; italics denotes changes to the original text).

By definition, any practice that is embedded in occupation is occupation-centred. It follows that intervention perspectives that are not embedded in occupation as either *means* or *ends,* that use change agents, including therapeutic activity, for the primary purpose of curing or fixing (i.e., practice embedded in the medical model), are not occupation-centred. Such perspectives are best captured by the term *impairment-centred* and are outside of the scope of this chapter.

Occupation-Focused. Occupation-focused interventions are those where the intended outcome is occupational change, but the occupations of interest are not directly addressed during the intervention. Occupation-focused interventions can use any manner of change agent to promote the desired occupational change (such as wheelchair-fitting, advocating for workplace accommodations, installing grab bars, modifying occupations or making environmental adaptations). Frequent among these are the therapeutic activity or some other technique.

Activity-Based. Interventions are those that use activities, chosen for their perceived potential to reduce or prevent impairment, or to promote change in the components that underlie function (e.g., weaving, cone stacking, macramé, navigating an obstacle course, scootering down a ramp). Activity-based intervention is to be distinguished from occupation-based. In activity-based interventions, the activities used are neither the clients' actual occupations nor the clients' occupational goals, and it cannot be assumed that the activities used will result in goal achievement; indeed, the majority of intervention evidence points to the superiority of task-specific approaches (Polatajko 2017) over activity-based interventions. In activity-based interventions the immediate concern is impairment reduction, impairment prevention or a change in the components that underlie function. If the primary intended outcome is change in the client's

real-world occupation(s), activity-based intervention is considered to be a particular class of occupation-focused interventions and, by extension, is occupation-centred. If the primary intended outcome is impairment reduction, impairment prevention or a change in the components underlying function for its own sake, they are not a form of occupation-centred practice; rather they are a form of impairment-centred practice.

Technique-Based. Interventions are those that use neither activity nor occupation during the intervention, rather they use some other agent of change, some technique that will effect change. There are a large variety of techniques available to therapists that do not directly involve the client in their occupations or in therapeutic activity, such as positioning, using inhibitive casting, fitting a wheelchair, prescribing compression garments, teaching handling techniques, fabricating and applying splints, adapting equipment or environments, designing or prescribing assistive devices, running relaxation groups or advocating policy change. If the primary intended outcome of the technique-based intervention is change in the client's real-world occupation(s), then the intervention is also considered a particular class of occupation-focused intervention and, by extension, is occupation-centred. If the primary intended outcome is impairment reduction, impairment prevention or a change in the components underlying function for its own sake, they also are not a form of occupation-centred practice, rather they are a form of impairment-centred practice.

Whether the intervention is activity-based, technique-based or some other form of enablement, (e.g., client education, advocacy, policy change, etc.), if the intent outcome is occupational change then the intervention aligns with an ends perspective. Occupation-focused interventions are, by definition, occupation-centred.

Occupation-based interventions are those that directly address the occupations that are the intended outcome during intervention; they use the clients' real-world occupation(s) or occupational goal(s) as the content of the intervention and have the client's real-world occupational goals as the intended outcome. In occupation-based interventions, the occupations of interest are specifically addressed during the intervention. This term aligns with both occupation as means and as ends and is, by definition, occupation; thus the term *occupation-based* is sufficient to convey that an intervention is occupation-focused.

SPECIFYING OCCUPATION: CONCEPTS FROM THE CMOP-E

Setting enabling occupation as the core mission of occupation-centred practice requires specifying the occupation of interest. During much of our history, enabling occupation has meant enabling the expression of human occupation, the act of purposeful doing. This meaning has often been captured by the term *occupational behaviour*. As first discussed by Reilly in 1969 (as cited in Kielhofner 2009), occupational behaviour can take many forms. Indeed, the occupational therapy literature is replete with terms intended to capture occupational forms of interest (e.g., *occupational behaviour, occupational deprivation, occupational disruption, occupational engagement, occupational identity, occupational performance;* see Townsend & Polatajko 2013 for more occupational terms and their definitions). A number of these terms are associated with particular models; for example, the Human Occupations Model (Reed & Sanderson 1980) is focused on occupational adaptation while the Model of Human Occupation (MOHO; Kielhofner 2008) is concerned not only with occupational adaptation but also with occupational competence, identity and participation. The Canadian Model of Occupational Performance and Engagement (CMOP-E; Polatajko et al 2013), the focus of this chapter, specifies performance and engagement as the aspects of occupation of interest. Accordingly, using the CMOP-E to specify the form of occupation of interest, occupation-centred practice is focused on improving occupational performance and occupational engagement. Next we describe the CMOP-E in detail and discuss how it can be used as a tool in occupation-centred practice to guide and support both occupation-focused and occupation-based interventions. First we start with definitions of occupational performance and occupational engagement.

Occupational Performance

The concept of occupational performance is one of the longest standing and most commonly used occupational terms in the profession's lexicon. Occupational performance refers to the 'observable aspects of [purposeful] doing or how an occupation is carried out' (Davis 2017, p.153). It is the 'result of a dynamic, interwoven relationship between persons, environment, and occupation over a person's lifespan; the ability to choose, organize, and satisfactorily perform meaningful occupations that are culturally defined and age appropriate for looking after oneself, enjoying life, and contributing to the social and economic fabric of a community' (Canadian Association of Occupational Therapists [CAOT], 2002, p.34).

Occupational performance captures what an individual *can* do or, when naming it as the intended outcome of therapy, what a person has the capacity, skills and knowledge to do. As portrayed in many of our occupational models (e.g., CMOP-E), occupational performance is the result of the interaction of person, occupation and environment, and it has physical, cognitive and affective components. Occupational performance, by itself, is a neutral, nonevaluative concept. Nevertheless, it is often qualified with descriptors such as weak|strong, poor|excellent and novice|expert or quantified with some form of rating scale as with the Canadian Occupational Performance Measure (COPM; Law et al 2019). Occupational performance indicates that an occupation is carried out, but not how, or how well it is carried out; the latter two understandings require the addition of other concepts such as performance analysis or occupational competence, respectively.

Occupational Engagement

The concept of occupational engagement has also been in our literature for some time. However, it has long been poorly described and defined and is often used interchangeably with a number of other terms such as *performance, participation* and *involvement*. The literature that describes occupational engagement often does so in terms of cognitive/affective dimensions and argues that the 'doing' of an occupation is not enough to conclude engagement and, in fact, may not be required for engagement (Xavier et al 2012). This perspective suggests that engagement is essentially an experiential phenomenon, involving subjective 'involvement' in the doing of the occupation. Accordingly, occupational engagement is defined as the presence of a cognitive and/or affective connection to an occupation (Xavier et al 2012).

Whereas occupational performance is directly observable occupational behaviour, occupational engagement can only be inferred through observation or self-report. It is a subjective, experiential phenomenon, drawing attention to the internal and personal reactions that result from involvement in occupation. Occupational engagement does not require physicality, although it can be a part of it, and thus allows for occupational behaviour where performance is not possible, as with individuals with severe performance limitations. Like performance, engagement is, by itself, a neutral, nonevaluative concept. However, it can be discussed along a continuum from disengagement to full engagement (Sutton et al 2012), where neither end is either necessarily desirable or undesirable. As Sutton and colleagues explain, disengagement may be an essential nature of being for some people who need to disengage so that they can be fully engaged at other times. Further, according to Egan et al (2010), more intense or frequent occupational engagement may not always be supportive of health, and people may pull back from more intense engagement for various reasons.

The CMOP-E and Its Development

The CMOP-E (Polatajko et al 2013) is a conceptual model that identifies the key elements of occupational performance and engagement—person, occupation and environment—and related concepts. The CMOP-E sits at the centre of occupational therapy practice in Canada and is broadly used around the world. It is the most recent iteration of the models of occupation that have guided Canadian practice for decades.

The first iteration of the CMOP-E, referred to as the 'occupational performance model' (OPM) was based on the 'Human Occupations Model' introduced by Reed and Sanderson (1980). The OPM, depicted in a simple black and white line drawing of three concentric circles, identifies three core elements of human occupation: individual, environment and occupation, each having a number of subcomponents. The inner circle, representing the individual, shows four performance components—the physical, mental, socio-cultural and spiritual. The middle circle, representing occupation, identifies three groupings of occupation—self-care, productivity and leisure. The outer circle, representing the environment, indicates three types of the environments that are of relevance to human occupation—physical, social and cultural.

A second iteration was published in 1997 in the 6th Canadian practice guidelines. Now named the *Canadian Model of Occupational Performance* (CMOP; CAOT 2002), this iteration depicted the same three elements of occupational performance central to the OPM but sported a new three-dimensional image and re-organized/re-named some of the components and introduced some new language. The CMOP image, designed to appear more dynamic than the previous version, was intended to portray the interactive nature of the three elements of occupational performance. At the centre of the graphic is a large triangle, representing person (rather than individual as it had been named in the earlier version), with four components: three—physical, affective, cognitive—located at the points of the triangle and the fourth—spirituality—located in a small circle at the centre of the triangle. The triangle sits atop two successively larger concentric circles representing occupation and environment, respectively. The smaller circle, occupation, as in the previous iteration, has three groupings—self-care, productivity and leisure. The larger circle, environment, has four types of environments—physical, institutional, social and cultural. The graphic shows the triangle (person) extending across both circles (occupation and environment), not sitting within both, as it had done in the previous iteration. This change is intended to indicate that the person interacts with both the environment and the occupation, and it is this 'dynamic, interwoven relationship' of all three elements that constitutes occupational performance (CAOT 2002).

The most recent iteration, the model in current use, the CMOP-E, was introduced in 2007 with the publication of the 8th Canadian practice guidelines *Enabling Occupation II: Advancing an Occupational Therapy Vision for Health, Well-Being, & Justice Through Occupation* (Townsend & Polatajko 2013). The CMOP-E comprises two images: on the left is the CMOP image, as first published in 1997; on the right is a transverse slice of that image (see Fig. 7.1). The CMOP-E expands on the previous iteration in two important ways: moving beyond performance and delimiting our domain of concern.

Moving Beyond Performance. A major contribution of the CMOP-E is to expand the specification of occupation beyond performance to include occupational engagement. This expansion was deemed necessary as it was felt that a focus on performance alone was too limiting, did not capture the full scope of our practice and, de facto, excluded many of the clients whom occupational therapists serve. Performance of an occupation often may not be our clients' goal or within their capabilities. For example, in his book *Still Me*, Christopher Reeve (1998) writes about being a sailor, an occupation of great importance to him. Well aware that because of the severity of his spinal cord injury he could not actively sail his boat again (i.e., perform the act of sailing), he endeavoured, successfully, to sail on his boat (i.e., engage in sailing). Clearly, enabling Christopher Reeve to re-engage in sailing, postinjury, was an attainable occupational outcome, whereas performing the physical act of sailing was not—the two are very different forms of occupation, requiring different approaches to intervention.

The addition of engagement to our conceptual model substantially broadens the breadth of our core purpose to not only enable individuals to *do* occupation, but also to *be* engaged in that doing. The concept of occupational engagement also broadens the scope of occupational therapy practice to help characterize people's social participation in occupation regardless of their capacity to perform an occupation.

Delimiting Our Domain of Concern. A transverse view of the CMOP graphic was included in the CMOP-E graphic to depict the primacy of occupation (Polatajko et al 2013) and its role in delimiting our concern with person and environment. With the addition of the transverse view, occupation is visually identified as the primary domain

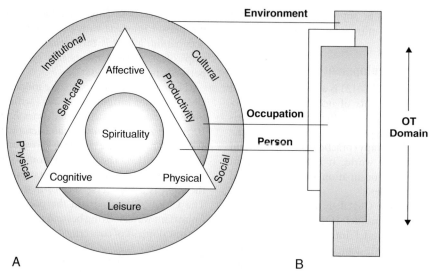

Fig. 7.1 The CMOP-E: Specifying our domain of concern. **A** was referred to as the CMOP in Enabling occupa-tion (1997, 2002) and CMOP-E in Enabling oED:ccupation II (2007, 2013). **B** is the trans-sectional view of the CMOP-E. (Copyright by CAOT Publications ACE. Reprinted with permission: Polatajko, H.J., Townsend, E.A., Craik, J., 2013. Canadian Model of Occupational Performance and Engagement (CMOP-E). In: Townsend, E.A., Polatajko, H.J. *Enabling Occupation II: Advancing an Occupational Therapy Vision of Health, Well-Being, & Justice Through Occupation*. Ottawa, ON: CAOT Publications ACE, 23.)

of concern of occupational therapy (Polatajko et al 2013). Positioning occupation atop person and environment is intended to convey that our interest in person and environment is delimited by occupation; that is, our concern with aspects of the person and the environment is limited to the interaction between person, occupation and environment that results in occupational performance and engagement. The transverse section, which in part depicts occupation atop person and environment alone, is also intended to convey that our concern can extend to situations where occupation and person interaction alone are considered, as may happen when conducting a job demands analysis. Similarly, our concern can extend to situations where occupation and environment interaction alone are considered, as in the analysis of the effect of policy on occupational engagement.

The Key Elements of the CMOP-E

The CMOP-E identifies the key elements that interact to effect occupational performance and occupational engage-ment—person, occupation and environment. Each appears with its related concepts.

Person. In the CMOP-E, person refers to all humans regardless of age, sex, gender, race, ethnicity, ability or nationality. The CMOP-E identifies four aspects of the

person: three person components—cognitive, affective and physical—which appear at the corners of the triangle in the graphic, and spirituality—which appears at the centre of the triangle.

Cognitive. The cognitive component of the person comprises aspects such as memory, orientation, concentration, intellect, insight, judgement and general knowledge. It covers how we think and remember and what we know.

Affective. The affective component of the person involves aspects that describe emotions, mood, affect, volition, body image, coping skills, and reaction and adaptation to illness or injury.

Physical. The physical component of the person pertains to aspects of movement, strength, co-ordination, balance, endurance, sensation, pain, appearance, and physical illness and/or injury of body systems and/or structures.

Spirituality. In the centre of the person triangle sits a small circle depicting spirituality. Although some might argue that spirituality is a component of the person, its location is intended to indicate that spirituality is at the core of occupational performance and engagement, relevant to all aspects of the model. Spirituality, or the 'essence of the self' (CAOT 2002, p.43), is viewed as infused through the person, occupation and environment, in that not only are people regarded as spiritual beings, but occupations and environments are viewed as containing spiritual elements that are experienced by people (CAOT 2002). Spirituality is 'a pervasive life force, manifestation of a higher self, source of will and self-determination, and a sense of meaning, purpose and connectedness that people experience within the context of their environment' (CAOT 2002, p.182).

Occupation

Occupation refers to all manner of doing. Occupations are 'groups of activities and tasks of everyday life, named, organized, and given value and meaning by individuals and a culture. Occupation is everything people do to occupy themselves, including looking after themselves (self-care), enjoying life (leisure), and contributing to the social and economic fabric of their communities (productivity)' (CAOT 2002, p.34). The three groupings of occupation named in this definition are depicted in the model within the occupation circle. These groupings have been a part of the model since its inception in 1983 and are acknowledged as groupings based on purpose. As the above definition indicates, it is recognized that the purpose ascribed to any particular occupation, that is, how any particular occupation is understood and named is defined, and hence decided, by the individual and culture.

Self-Care. Occupations designated as self-care are those that serve any aspect of personal care such as grooming, dressing, bathing, feeding and toileting. Some people may include such activities as exercise, meditation and sleep under self-care, whereas others may view these aspects as leisure. As noted earlier, how any particular occupation is understood and named is defined, and hence decided, by the individual and culture. In practice, the occupational therapy client would determine what particular group of activities compose their self-care.

Leisure. The leisure category is meant to capture occupations that are performed or engaged in for their own sake such as hobbies, games, collecting, sports and recreation. Leisure occupations often fill free time, fulfil cultural, creative or social interests, and can include such things as participating in clubs, joining groups, enjoying nature, going to a party or attending theatre. Leisure occupations may bring joy, relaxation, rest or rejuvenation. An ongoing debate in occupational therapy remains with respect to the categorization of the play of children. In the CMOP-E, play would generally fall under leisure, even though some argue that 'play is the work of children'. The notion that 'play is the "work" of children' has long been argued, whereas others assert that children play and children work, and the nature of children's play and work differs.

Productivity. Occupations classified as productivity are those that provide remuneration, such as paid employment, as well as occupations that contribute to others, the community or society, such as volunteering, homemaking and schooling.

Environment. The environment refers to the surroundings or conditions in which a person lives or operates. The CMOP-E identifies four aspects of the environment—physical, social, cultural and institutional.

Physical environment. The physical environment encompasses all built and natural aspects of the environment from the micro, such as the type of doorknobs, to the macro, such as cities, oceans and mountains. It includes everything from indoor features of a house or building to outdoor features of both built and naturally occurring spaces. The environment also includes nontangible aspects such as air quality, noise and atmosphere.

Social environment. The social environment comprises the people in the environment, known, unknown, family, friends, acquaintances, strangers, individuals, groups and so on. It includes our relationships with them, the networks we can leverage when requiring assistance and the general availability of assistance to support living. Social environments can vary depending on the institutional environments as described subsequently.

Cultural environment. The cultural environment comprises the set of values, conventions or social practices under which we operate. It includes the customary beliefs, social forms and material traits of the societies that surround us. It extends from the micro, such as personal or family rituals, to the macro, such as expectations and attitudes of the broader culture. The extent to which a person 'takes up' a culture will shape their behaviours, rituals and practices.

Institutional environment. The institutional environment comprises the significant practices, relationships or organizations in a society or culture or an established organization or corporation (such as a bank or university), especially of a public character. It refers to structural and systemic elements composing the broad-level social environment. The institutional environment is viewed as not only comprising governmental and organizational structures, policies and practices, but also often hidden or under-considered social determinants of health such as income, education, unemployment, aboriginal status, race, gender and disability, as well as stigmatizing, fear-mongering and bullying systemic practices.

Using the CMOP-E

Forming the starting point for the Canadian occupational therapy practice guidelines, the CMOP-E can be used to facilitate the identification of occupational performance and/or occupational engagement issues and the setting of occupational goals, to support our professional reasoning in generating explanatory hypotheses and intervention options, and to organize client information.

Identifying Occupational Issues—Setting Goals.

Using the CMOP-E to guide occupation-centred practice suggests that occupational therapy should focus on enabling occupational performance and/or engagement or, more specifically, the performance of and/or engagement in self-care, productivity and leisure. Accordingly, an important step, generally the first step, in the occupational therapy process would be to identify the occupational performance and/or occupational engagement issues (OPI/Es) that clients are experiencing and set their occupational goals (OGs).

The CMOP-E supports two approaches to establishing goals in occupational therapy: a direct, client-centred approach and an indirect, analysis-centred approach. Either is consistent with occupation-focused practice, but only the former is consistent with occupation-based practice.

Client-Centred Goal-Setting. This is based on the premise that our clients are the experts in their own occupation and are in the best position to identify their own specific OGs. This approach is derived from client-centred practice, a collaborative approach in which therapists work in partnership with clients, demonstrating respect, involving them in decision-making and otherwise recognizing their experience and knowledge (CAOT 2002). This approach can be undertaken in an informal manner by using the areas of occupation as a basis for discussion with our clients. There are also formal tools to guide this process. One example is the COPM (Law et al 2019), designed specifically to be used in conjunction with the Canadian model. Another is the Occupational Performance History Interview (OPHI-II; Kielhofner et al 2004), designed as a goal-setting measure to accompany the MOHO. Client-centred goal-setting often results in quite specific OGs (e.g., Christopher Reeve's sailing goal), lending itself well to occupation-focused practice, in general, and occupation-based practice, in particular. Indeed, research has shown that client-centred goal-setting leads to occupation-based practice (Colquhoun et al 2012, Hunt et al 2015).

Analysis-Centred Goal-Setting. This is derived through a professional reasoning process, often rooted in the medical model. In analysis-centred goal-setting, the therapist uses the information she/he has about the client, often including medical diagnosis and health status, to determine client needs and identify intervention goals. The CMOP-E can be used to guide this process and move it beyond the medical model. The components of person, occupation and environment can each be explored for their contribution to the OPI/Es. This approach to goal-setting can lead to person change goals of impairment reduction, capacity-building or skill acquisition; occupation change goals such as occupational adaptation or modification; or environment change goals such as physical, social or institutional environmental adaptations or modifications. This approach to goal-setting is typically seen in impairment-centred practice but can also be of use in occupation-centred practice if the analysis is related to occupational performance or engagement goals.

Supporting Our Professional Reasoning. Another important step in the occupational therapy process is to generate explanatory hypotheses and intervention options related to the OPI/Es or OGs. This step is accomplished through a process of professional reasoning that is driven by an understanding of the client's OPI/Es or OGs, relevant theories and the body of evidence. The CMOP-E points to the elements that should be considered.

Theories

In occupational therapy, including in this text, theories are often discussed in the context of frame of reference: 'a structure for identifying relevant information from one or more theories and customising that information to develop a theoretical base for use by occupational therapists to guide evaluation and interventions, and overall application to practice' (Hinojosa et al 2010, p.6). In this chapter we focus on theories because these support understanding of the various aspects of the CMOP-E and their relationships. There are formal and informal theories. In occupational therapy practice both are used, often in combination. Formal theories are well articulated (often published); comprise key concepts, definitions and postulates; explain a phenomenon; offer predictions; and have a body of evidence to support them. Informal theories are those that are generated from experience, from repeated observations of a phenomenon; they are not formally tested and do not have clear body of evidence to support them, and are often combined in practice. There are numerous theories available, both in occupational therapy literature and beyond, that align with the CMOP-E. Indeed, the CMOP-E can be used to identify theories of interest (e.g., theories of motivation that may underlie engagement, biomechanical theories that may underlie performance; for an overview of these see Polatajko and Davis 2005, and the frames of reference chapters within this text). The particular theory chosen depends on the aspect of the CMOP-E of relevance to the client's OPI/Es or OGs.

Body of Evidence

Using the CMOP-E to identify the body of evidence relevant to occupation-centred practice suggests that the research must address occupational performance or engagement specifically. If the research examines an intervention, to be relevant it must demonstrate an effect on occupational performance or occupational engagement. This effect is most clearly demonstrated by using outcome measures that specifically address occupation, such as the COPM, School Function Assessment (Coster et al 1998), Pediatric Activity Card Sort (Mandich et al 2004) and the Assessment of Motor Process Skills (Fisher & Bray Jones 2014).

Organizing Client Information

The CMOP-E grid ('the grid' see Fig. 7.2) is a two-dimensional matrix designed to support professional reasoning and organize client information. The grid uses the elements of the CMOP-E down the left vertical side to structure the professional reasoning process. The top row is used to list the OPI/Es of interest. The resultant cells provide a place to enter and organize the relevant information: the specifics of the OPI/Es in relation to person, occupation and environmental factors. The grid is completed by considering each aspect of the CMOP-E for each OPI/E. Filling in the grid ensures all aspects are fully considered, and the client information is organized.

The CMOP-E grid is a two-dimensional chart that facilitates the organization of information about a client and their occupations and environments that underlie their agreed upon OPI/Es. Many different types of information—observational, scientific, diagnostic, narrative and interactive—can be gathered and included in the grid, to be considered in the occupational therapist's reasoning. Having this information recorded explicitly can ensure that the decisions made are well reasoned; lead to the identification of sound possible targets for change in relation to person, occupation and/or environment to support occupation-centred interventions; and can be articulated clearly to the client.

CASE VIGNETTE

Sylvia is a 45-year-old unemployed single mother of a 10-year-old son, Ryan. She worked for 12 years as a librarian at the local library, and when her son started kindergarten 5 years ago she volunteered reading to the children in her son's class. Sylvia and her son live together in a two-bedroomed home that she owns, which has been in

CMOP-E elements and concepts		OPI/E #1	OPI/E #2	OPI/E #3	OPI/E #
OCCUPATION	Self-care				
	Productivity				
	Leisure				
PERSON	Spirituality				
	Cognitive				
	Affective				
	Physical				
ENVIRONMENT	Physical				
	Social				
	Cultural				
	Institutional				

Fig. 7.2 The CMOP-E grid is a two-dimensional chart that facilitates the organization of information about a client, their occupations and environments that underlie their agreed upon occupational performance and occupational engagement issues.

her family for three generations. Three years ago, Sylvia was diagnosed with bipolar disorder and after a short admission to an inpatient mental health hospital she was referred to outpatient services through the local community health services. Sylvia was referred to occupational therapy following her initial appointment with her community-based psychiatrist and social worker.

Data Gathering and Assessment

Using the CMOP-E grid, the occupational therapist organized what Sylvia was telling her about herself, her past and current occupational repertoire, and her environments. This structure afforded the occupational therapist an organized approach to understanding how things were going for Sylvia, from an occupational perspective. The therapist asked Sylvia about each of the occupational areas. The assessment and re-assessment process used by the therapist was an informal one. The COPM (Law et al 2019) could be used to formalize this process and collect objective, numeric pre- and post intervention data.

In the area of her self-care, Sylvia identified issues with basic activities of daily living such as getting up in the morning to see her son off to school, having a shower regularly and staying out of bed after her son leaves the house. With her instrumental activities of daily living, Sylvia identified issues with budgeting her money to ensure she is paying the bills on time and allocating enough money to pay for groceries.

Sylvia's occupational issues in productivity were returning to competitive part-time work as a librarian, cooking for herself and her son, and completing household chores such as vacuuming and cleaning the bathroom and kitchen. She also identified that she would like to be able to volunteer again at her son's school.

Sylvia identified issues with her leisure pursuits in relation to participating in quiet recreation, such as flower arrangement; active recreation, such as swimming; and socializing with her family and peers. Specifically, Sylvia reported that being involved in social situations is 'hard for me and can be very stressful'.

Next, the therapist asked Sylvia to choose the issues she would like to address in intervention. Sylvia indicated that she wanted to work on performing household chores, socializing with family and peers, finding part-time work, showering daily and money management. The therapist and Sylvia then discussed an intervention plan and agreed on how to proceed.

Intervention Plan

Self-Care. To address showering, Sylvia identified that showering daily may be too difficult, but agreed that showering 3 days a week would be achievable. The occupational therapist and Sylvia prepared a monthly schedule to refer to and prompt her on the day she is required to complete her shower.

Interventions to address money management focused on helping Sylvia to budget her monthly income and prioritize her expenses. A weekly table was used for her to record her spending. This information was gathered each month and then discussed with the occupational therapist to identify when and where unnecessary spending was taking place. At the end of each month, Sylvia and the occupational therapist discussed what bills required payment and money was allocated to ensure the bills were paid. Sylvia had also allocated a specific amount of money in her budget for grocery shopping. To manage this budget, she was encouraged to prepare grocery lists in advance of her shopping by reviewing weekly flyers for specials and exploring the possibility of using coupons.

Productivity. To address obtaining competitive part-time employment, although Sylvia wanted to return to the library, she and the occupational therapist explored other possible jobs that may be of interest to her. Sylvia also identified that she would update her curriculum vitae (résumé).

In addressing household chores, Sylvia agreed that having cues such as a schedule identifying exactly what to clean on a specific day would enable her to be motivated to pursue the tasks. The use of the schedule enabled Sylvia to complete small achievable cleaning tasks.

Leisure. To address leisure, Sylvia was encouraged to attend the outpatient centre and participate in groups that promote socialization and support as well as participation in meaningful occupations. She agreed to attend a support-based group that addressed current issues and their effect on one's mental health, and a task-based group that promoted socialization with peers through completion of a meaningful activity. Her ultimate goal was to re-engage in flower arranging.

Re-Assessment

The occupational therapist checked in with Sylvia weekly at first and then biweekly for the first 6 months. At that point the therapist and Sylvia reviewed the progress being made towards meeting her OGs. Sylvia indicated that she had made improvements in showering daily, money management, budgeting and household chores. At the time Sylvia also indicated that returning to work as a part-time librarian was no longer important to her, and she decided not to pursue this goal at this time.

Conclusion

A client's occupational performance and engagement issues and goals are constantly being adjusted and changed as a result of intervention, and her or his perception of the importance of addressing the originally identified occupational performance and/or engagement issues may have changed. At the 6-month reassessment some original occupational issues were no longer relevant, new occupational issues were identified, and some original issues were still problems for Sylvia. As a result of new occupational performance issues that arose and issues that still remained, Sylvia and the therapist decided to continue intervention to address the original issues that still needed attention and the newly identified occupational performance and engagement issues.

SUMMARY

In this chapter, we have discussed two perspectives that have dominated practice: occupation as means and occupation as ends. We argue that these perspectives serve to frame the form of our practice, or what our practice looks like. We further argue that practice must be occupation-centred and offer the CMOP-E as a tool to give form to that practice. We introduce the CMOP-E and describe how it can be used support practice intent on improving occupational performance and occupational engagement. Through the vignette about Sylvia, we have demonstrated how the CMOP-E can be used to identify occupational performance and engagement issues and support intervention planning.

ACKNOWLEDGEMENT

Thelma Sumsion, Lesley Tischler-Draper and Sheila Heinicke, who authored the previous version of this chapter, are acknowledged for their work on the case vignette in their chapter; it served as the basis for the case vignette presented in this edition of the chapter.

✳ REFLECTIVE LEARNING

- What is the difference between occupation as means and occupation as ends?
- What is the core domain of concern for occupational therapy and the objective of occupation-centred practice?
- How do occupation-centred, occupation-focused and occupation-based practice relate to each other?
- What are the key elements of the CMOP-E?
- How can the CMOP-E be used to support client-centred, occupation-centred practice?

REFERENCES

Canadian Association of Occupational Therapists. (2002). *Enabling occupation: An occupational therapy perspective* (2nd ed.). Ottawa: CAOT Publications ACE.

Colquhoun, H., Letts, L. J., Law, M. C., MacDermid, J. C., & Missiuna, C. A. (2012). Administration of the Canadian occupational performance measure: Effect on practice. *Canadian Journal of Occupational Therapy, 79*(2), 120–129.

Coster, W., Deeney, T., Haltiwanger, J., & Haley, S. (1998). *School function assessment.* London: Pearson.

Davis, J. A. (2017). The Canadian model of occupational performance and engagement (CMOP-E). In M. Curtin, M. E. Egan, & J. Adams (Eds.), *Occupational therapy for people experiencing illness, injury or impairment: Promoting occupation and participation* (7th ed.) (pp. 148–168). London: Elsevier.

Egan, M. Y., Kubina, L. A., Lidstone, R. I., Macdougall, G. H., & Raudoy, A. E. (2010). A critical reflection on occupational therapy within one assertive community treatment team. *Canadian Journal of Occupational Therapy, 77*, 70–79.

Fisher, A. G. (2013). Occupation-centred, occupation-based, occupation-focused: Same, same or different? *Scandinavian Journal of Occupational Therapy, 20*, 162–173.

Fisher, A. G., & Bray Jones, K. (2014). User manual (8th ed.). *Assessment of motor and process skills* (vol. 2). Fort Collins, CO: Three Star Press.

Hinojosa, J., Kramer, P., Luebben, A.J., 2010. Structure of the frame of reference. In P. Kramer, P., Hinojosa, J. (Eds.), *Frames of reference for pediatric occupational therapy,* 3rd ed. Lippincott Williams & Wilkins, Baltimore, MD, 3–22.

Hooper, B. (2006). Beyond active learning: A case study of teaching practices in an occupation-centered curriculum. *American Journal of Occupational Therapy, 60*, 551–562.

Hunt, A. W., Le Dorze, G., Trentham, B., Polatajko, H. J., & Dawson, D. R. (2015). Elucidating a goal-setting continuum in brain injury rehabilitation. *Qualitative Health Research, 25*, 1044–1055.

Kielhofner, G. (Ed.). (2008). *Model of human occupation: Theory and application* (4th ed.) Baltimore, MD: Lippincott Williams & Wilkins.

Kielhofner, G. (2009). *Conceptual foundations of occupational therapy practice* (4th ed.). Philadelphia, PA: FA Davis.

Kielhofner, G., Mallinson, T., Crawford, C., et al. (2004). *Occupational performance history interview II (OPHI-II) version 2.1.* Chicago, IL: University of Illinois at Chicago.

Law, M., Baptiste, S., Carswell, A., McColl, M. A., Polatajko, H., & Pollock, N. (2019). *Canadian occupational performance measure* revised (5th ed.). Hamilton, ON: COPM.

Mandich, A., Polatajko, H., Miller, L., & Baum, C. (2004). *The paediatric activity card sort.* Ottawa: CAOT Publications ACE.

Polatajko, H. J. (2001). National perspective: The evolution of our occupational perspective: The journey from diversion through therapeutic use to enablement. *Canadian Journal of Occupational Therapy, 68*, 203–207.

Polatajko, H. J. (2017). History of the CO-OP approach. In D. Dawson, S. McEwen, & H. J. Polatajko (Eds.), *Cognitive orientation to daily occupational performance in occupational therapy (Chapter 1).* Bethesda, MD: AOTA.

Polatajko, H. J., & Davis, J. A. (2005). Methods of inquiry: The study of occupation. In C. Christiansen, C. Baum, & J. Bass-Haugen (Eds.), *Occupational therapy: Performance, participation, and well-being* (3rd ed.) (pp. 188–208). Thorofare, NJ: Slack.

Polatajko, H. J., Davis, J., Stewart, D., et al. (2013). Specifying the domain of concern: occupation as core. In E. A. Townsend, & H. J. Polatajko (Eds.), *Enabling occupation II: Advancing an occupational therapy vision for health, well-being, and justice through occupation* (2nd ed.) (pp. 13–36). Ottawa, ON: CAOT Publications ACE.

Polatajko, H. J., Townsend, E. A., & Craik, J. (2013). The Canadian model of occupational performance and engagement (CMOP-E). In E. A. Townsend, & H. J. Polatajko (Eds.), *Enabling occupation II: Advancing an occupational therapy vision for health, well-being, and justice through occupation* (2nd ed.) (p. 23). Ottawa, ON: CAOT Publications ACE.

Reed, K. L., & Sanderson, S. R. (1980). *Concepts of occupational therapy*. Baltimore, MD: Williams & Wilkins.

Reeve, C. (1998). *Still me*. New York, NY: Random House.

Sutton, D. J., Hocking, C. S., & Smythe, L. A. (2012). A phenomenological study of occupational engagement in recovery from mental illness. *Canadian Journal of Occupational Therapy, 79*, 142–150.

Townsend, E. A., & Polatajko, H. J. (2013). *Enabling occupation II: Advancing an occupational therapy vision for health, well-being, & justice through occupation* (2nd ed.). Ottawa, ON: CAOT Publications ACE.

Wicks, A. (2012). *Identifying occupational needs in the community, Umeå, Sweden*. Seminar presented at Umeå University, Department of Occupational Therapy, Umeå, Sweden, May 29, 2012.

Xavier, S., Ferreira, J., Davis, J., & Polatajko, H. (2012). Beyond performance: Clarifying the construct of occupational engagement. Paper presentation at the Canadian association of occupational therapists conference. *Quebec City, QC* June 6, 2012.

Yerxa, E. J. (1998). Occupation: The keystone of a curriculum for a self-defined profession. *American Journal of Occupational Therapy, 52*, 365–372.

8

The Person-Environment-Occupation-Performance Model

Carolyn M. Baum, Julie D. Bass, Charles H. Christiansen

◎ HIGHLIGHTS

The Person-Environment-Occupation-Performance (PEOP) model

- provides an occupational lens on everyday living, social participation, health and well-being
- uses a systems perspective and applies to individuals, organizations and populations
- is top down and client centred because it focuses first on the narratives and unique life situations of clients
- organizes current knowledge of person and environmental factors in evaluation and interventions
- serves as a guide to an occupational therapy process that begins with an occupational profile and emphasizes evaluations and interventions that lead to improved outcomes in performance, participation and well-being

OVERVIEW

This chapter summarizes the history and evolution of the Person-Environment-Occupation-Performance (PEOP) model, a model for practice first conceived during the mid-1980s in the United States. As a guide to occupational therapy intervention, the PEOP model can be considered a transactive systems model. The model focuses on the client and relevant person factors and environmental influences on the performance of everyday occupations. It can be applied to individuals, groups (or organizations) and populations. The PEOP model has characteristics that are similar to other social ecological models in that it identifies three relevant domains of knowledge for occupational therapy practice, all of which interact to support the occupational performance of individuals, groups or populations: (1) the person, group or population factors (previously identified as intrinsic factors); (2) the environmental factors that include the situation and context, and relevant cultural,

physical, social, policy and technological environments (previously identified as the extrinsic factors); and (3) the occupations of importance to the client's well-being (activities, tasks and roles). The PEOP model is transactive in that it views everyday occupations as being affected by, and affecting, the person factors and environment factors. The PEOP model is client-centred in that it values and requires the active involvement of clients in determining intervention goals. It is different from other models as it makes the person, environment and occupation factors explicit and applies them to occupational performance or 'doing' of occupations at the person, organizational and population level. The model provides an 'occupational lens' that considers knowledge unique to occupational therapy and from other disciplines, to build upon capabilities/enablers and address constraints/barriers in person factors and environmental factors, to support occupational performance, participation and well-being.

ORIGINS AND AIMS OF THE PEOP MODEL

In 1985, work was initiated on what was to become the PEOP model, which was first published in 1991 (Christiansen & Baum, 1991). At the time, there was a growing awareness that it was necessary to re-organize the knowledge that was being used by occupational therapists in a manner that would identify, clarify and emphasize the unique contribution of occupational therapy to the health and well-being of individuals, groups and populations. We knew that occupational therapy could provide practical and relevant interventions that enabled people to preserve or improve the quality of their lives. Yet, at that time, the most influential textbooks in the field organized content using a biomedical approach that resembled diagnosis- and pathology-focused models of practice. Influenced by writers from medicine who were calling for more complete health-oriented approaches (e.g., Engel 1977), as well as occupational therapy scholars who emphasized ideas central to the profession's founding (e.g., Shannon 1977), we set about re-framing the organizing structure for knowledge relevant to occupational therapy theory and practice. We proposed an intuitive model that would organize the knowledge relevant to performing the activities, tasks and roles necessary for everyday living and facilitate thinking in ways that would guide assessment, planning and the delivery of interventions. Our goal was to have a model that would be relevant regardless of the settings in which occupational therapists worked and the characteristics of individuals served, including ages, life stages or diagnoses. We also felt that such a model would encourage a more balanced approach to care that would encourage therapists to plan interventions with a focus on the life situations of their clients. This focus would require that therapists understand the person-related and environment-related resources and barriers to performance of the particular occupations necessary to live satisfying lives.

The PEOP model is now in its fourth iteration (Baum et al 2015). During the 33-year period since its inception, the knowledge and evidence generated from occupational therapy science, neuroscience, environmental science and other biological and social sciences have enabled us to refine and extend our original ideas and to provide a scientific basis for the constructs we believe are central to understanding the occupational performance of humans, whether as individuals or members of social groups. Throughout this process of elaboration, we have been influenced by many emerging ideas and innovations in healthcare, disability, social policy, technology, rehabilitation and public health. Although some terminology has changed, definitions have been revised and new concepts have been added, the basic philosophical orientation of the model and its central features have remained consistent. Thus we believe the PEOP model is not only conceptually sound, but parsimonious in its ability to organize a knowledge base of information useful for practice.

Collaboration

Because occupational therapy is based on a co-operative approach towards care (Meyer 1922), the PEOP model was designed to facilitate the development of a collaborative intervention plan with the client and with other professionals. Use of the term *client* is meant to apply whether the intervention is directly with a patient in a healthcare setting, a well child with special needs, an adult living in the community, a family, a group or organization, or an entire population. Clients can also be other professionals with whom an occupational therapy practitioner consults. Each of these clients may seek the knowledge and skills of the occupational therapist to address issues that influence

occupational performance or the ability of people to participate fully in their lives. Occupational therapists use a unique body of knowledge and skillset that bridge the world of the client to the world of healthcare (Engelhardt 1983). A core assumption is that people cannot truly be well if they cannot participate in and influence their life situations.

Occupational Performance

The concepts of person-environment-occupation are evident in many models of occupational therapy. In the PEOP model, we have also emphasized occupational performance, as this concept connects the individual to roles and to the socio-cultural environment (Reed & Sanderson 1999, p.93). We define occupational performance as the 'doing of meaningful activities, tasks and roles through complex interactions between the person and environment' (Baum et al 2015, p.52). We contend that when people are able to engage in life tasks that provide purpose and meaning within their social spheres, they can see themselves and be seen by others as full participants in the community.

A Systems Perspective

The PEOP model is a systems model, recognizing that the interaction of the person, environment and occupational elements are dynamic and reciprocal, and that the client must be central to the care-planning and intervention process. Only the client (whether person, family, organization or community) is able to determine the outcomes that are most important and necessary.

Client-Centred

The PEOP model provides a bridge from the biomedical model to a socio-cultural model of health. That is, it recognizes impairments that limit performance and participation but also views a person in context, including a consideration of the abilities and strengths that a person can use to enable performance. It also considers the environmental characteristics that provide supports or create barriers, whether those include places, other people, policies or technologies. Ultimately, the comprehensive assessment of a person, what that person needs and wants to do, and the context of the home and community environment, collectively determine the best interventions in a given situation. These interventions are selected because they enable the person to perform valued roles, activities and tasks that are central to living, whether these pertain to management of self and others, work or community engagement. A central theme of the PEOP model is that ultimately the client determines the performance goals towards which therapy is targeted.

DESCRIPTION OF THE PEOP MODEL

Figure 8.1 provides a graphic representation of the PEOP model. This representation is intended to convey that occupational performance is determined not only by the nature of the activity, task or role to be performed, but also by person and environmental characteristics. Performance and participation always occur in context, and ultimately determine well-being and quality of life. For a given situation or context, the applicability or importance of specific person and environmental factors will vary. The model presupposes that a complete assessment to plan intervention will include a consideration of each of the factors as well as a narrative that reflects an occupational history, perceptions, needs and goals, and attitudes and motivations.

The Narrative

The PEOP model visually represents the constructs that must come together to support both the occupational therapy practitioner and the client in developing interventions or programmes that help achieve goals related to performance, participation and well-being. Success in this process depends on the practitioner's skills in obtaining the narrative or story of the client; these skills include forming a relationship with the client, asking the right questions, and being able to access the knowledge to understand the issues and options presented by the client's occupational performance issues and goals. The PEOP model proceeds with 'a top down approach', in that it first considers the narrative of the person, organization or population, and then evaluates personal and environmental capacities/enablers and constraints/barriers. The model requires the occupational therapist to use the context obtained through the narrative to address the personal performance capabilities/constraints and the environmental performance enabler/barriers that are central to the occupational performance of the individual, organization or populations.

Person Factors

Person factors in the PEOP model that are central to occupational performance include physiological characteristics such as strength, endurance, flexibility, activity levels, stress, sleep, nutrition and health; cognitive dimensions including organization, reasoning, attention, awareness, executive function and memory—all necessary for task performance; sensory/perceptual characteristics including somatosensory, olfactory, gustatory, visual, auditory, proprioceptive and tactile; motor factors, including motor control, motor planning (praxis), motor learning and postural control; psychological factors including emotional state (affect), self-concept, self-esteem, sense of identity, self-efficacy and theory of mind (social awareness); and spiritual dimensions, which include beliefs and practices that influence personal meaning.

Environmental Factors

Environmental factors in the PEOP model that are central to occupational performance include cultural factors, social determinants of health, social support and social capital, education and policies, physical and natural

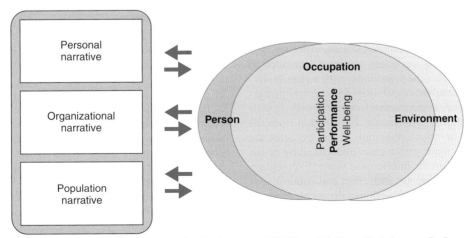

Fig. 8.1 The Person-Environment-Occupation-Performance (PEOP) model. (From Christiansen, C., Baum, C., Bass, J. (Eds.), 2015. *Occupational therapy: performance, participation, and well-being,* (4th ed.). Therefare, NJ: Slack, Inc. Reprinted with permission from SLACK incorporated.)

environments and assistive technology. Social determinants include social support (emotional support, practical or instrumental support and informational support) and social capital (interpersonal relationships [groups], social receptivity, laws and policies). The cultural environment includes values, beliefs, customs and use of time. The physical and natural environment includes physical properties, tools, geography, terrain, climate and air quality; assistive technology includes personal technology and design.

Although assistive technology is currently classified as an environmental factor in the PEOP model, it is important to note advances in digital technology are influencing both the person and the environment. Occupational therapists have long used technologies, ranging from simple tools to sophisticated mobility and environmental control devices to enable clients to pursue occupations of self-care, work, play and leisure. In the digital age, assistive technologies have now advanced to the level where they can enable individuals to control environments through cortical commands or even simulate environments to enable imagined participation in virtual worlds. Thus, digital technology has evolved to influence time use and the nature of experience throughout a person's round of daily work, rest, play/leisure and sleep, as well as immersion in temporary virtual worlds. With these considerations in mind, we see digital technology as transcending person and environment to influence quality of life and the experience of living.

THE PEOP OCCUPATIONAL THERAPY PROCESS

The PEOP Occupational Therapy Process was developed from the PEOP model and is used as a guide to create a complete occupational profile of the client, which includes a narrative about the client's perception of needs or problems and roles, interests, responsibilities and values. The assessment and evaluation phase of care is grounded in evidence and provides the practitioner with a clear understanding of both enablers/capabilities and constraints/barriers in person and environmental factors that may support or limit occupational performance. Information from the narrative and assessment/evaluation phases prepares the client and practitioner with a clear understanding of the likely outcomes from the intervention phase. Intervention is a collaborative endeavour, with effort and commitment contributed through the partnership of the client, the practitioner and significant others.

In the PEOP model, the client-centred elements change depending on whether the client is a person, an organization or a population. In each application of the PEOP Occupational Therapy Process (Fig. 8.2), evidence underpins the practitioner's decisions of the assessments to include and the interventions to employ. All professionals are held to a standard—the expectation of competent practice using methods that have been objectively shown to be effective. Evidence thus becomes a filter through which clinical decisions about the type of evaluation or assessment and the interventions that will support the client in achieving goals will be made.

The Narrative Phase
Occupational Profile

The narrative phase of the PEOP Occupational Therapy Process includes obtaining an occupational profile and history, identifying client goals and determining the match between client goals and occupational therapy scope of practice. In gathering the occupational profile and history, the practitioner tries to understand the client's "story", so that therapy makes sense in the life context of the person. An occupational profile and history include a description of leisure interests and social activities, and provides a clear understanding of the client's responsibilities for work, self and home management tasks. Another key element is the person's perception of what has happened or the current situation. People vary in the level of knowledge or understanding they have of their medical or health conditions. Thus, it is important to know what the person thinks has happened, whether they think it is serious and what they know about their likely course of treatment. It is also important to learn the impact of the current situation on their life. This information is particularly important, as occupational therapists employ self-management approaches to help people understand their conditions and employ strategies to achieve what they want and need to do.

The Client's Goals

It is important to view goals in a temporal progression. Considering longer-term goals first enables the therapist and client to determine the intermediate steps necessary to attain them. These intermediate steps can then be considered as shorter-term goals. It is imperative to consider goals in the context of the client's narrative and occupational history. By knowing the person's interests, skills, values, roles, traditions, habits and routines it is possible to help the client identify goals that are meaningful. Current standards of practice expect that therapists carefully avoid cultural stereotypes that can lead to improper assumptions in goal-setting. Therapists should also be sensitive to the lived experiences of clients in marginalized groups. Through attention to the particular narrative of a given client and collaboration during planning, the therapist and client may identify short- and long-term goals that are practical, achievable, appropriate and valued.

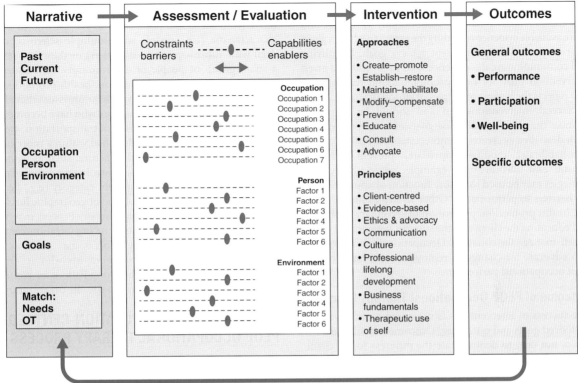

Fig. 8.2 The PEOP Occupational Therapy Process. (From Christiansen, C., Baum, C., Bass, J. (Eds.), 2015. *Occupational therapy: performance, participation, and well-being,* (4th ed.). Therefare, NJ: Slack, Inc. Reprinted with permission from SLACK incorporated.)

Match Between the Client's Needs and Occupational Therapy

The final step in the narrative phase of the PEOP Occupational Therapy Process is to determine the match between the client's goals and the occupational therapy approach. Not all goals will be appropriate for occupational therapy interventions. If there is not a match, the occupational therapist should make an appropriate referral to another professional or to other resources to address the client's goals. When there is a match the practitioner begins the second phase of the PEOP Occupational Therapy Process to determine the capabilities/enablers and barriers/constraints of person factors and environment factors that will need to be addressed to support occupational performance.

Assessment/Evaluation

Assessments are used to examine the client's occupations, person factors and environment factors along a continuum scale from constraint/barriers to capabilities/enablers. Assessments are chosen that will allow the therapist to

understand the person's capabilities and limitations in the performance of activities, tasks or occupations that are central to fulfilling valued roles or expectations. The outcome of the entire evaluation is a summary of the client's current status on multiple occupation, person and environment factors. In Figure 8.2, a continuum scale is used to represent the complex connections across different factors and summarize the client's overall current status. A marker on each continuum scale represents the therapist's evaluation of the client's current status on a specific factor along the continuum. A marker closer to the constraints/barriers end of the scale indicates a potential problem area while a marker closer to capabilities/enablers suggests a strength that may be used.

Interventions

With the information from the narrative and the practitioner's assessment and evaluation of constraints/barriers and capabilities/enablers, a client-centred intervention plan is constructed. Practitioners use their skills to help the client understand what is possible, and the issues involved in helping to achieve identified goals. The client has the right and the practitioner has the responsibility to review and share available evidence regarding the extent to which a given intervention will help the client achieve goals. Identifying and communicating the evidence used to formulate a given intervention plan not only promotes sound reasoning, it also reflects the highest principles of ethical practice.

Several interventions can and should be employed to meet the client's goals. The goals of intervention have been described as create-promote, establish-restore, main tain-habilitate, modify-compensate, prevent, educate, consult and advocate. For example, some intervention strategies may be used to restore function or compensation for barriers to performance. Other strategies may emphasize health promotion, prevention of secondary problems, and educating the client and the support network to be able to self-manage the situation. Occupational therapists may also advocate for change to remove societal barriers that limit occupational performance.

Outcome of PEOP Occupational Therapy Process

The success of interventions is measured by achievement of desired goals and outcomes. Outcomes should be measured, not only to demonstrate the progress to the client, but also to demonstrate the effectiveness of the occupational therapy interventions to the referral source, to the service provider/commissioner/payer and to the public. The effectiveness of occupational therapy must be public to shape policies of institutions and payment sources.

The entire PEOP Occupational Therapy Process leads to achieving the goals related to occupational performance, participation and well-being as identified by the client. These goals may relate to pursuit of personal interests, participation in daily life activities and performance of roles and responsibilities. Because some individuals have chronic conditions or developmental disabilities that require ongoing self-management strategies, the outcomes of the PEOP Occupational Therapy Process may focus on the needs and goals at a particular point in time. Part of the outcome may include the plans for additional services from occupational therapy, particularly if an occupational performance issue later emerges that would benefit from or require occupational therapy expertise.

APPLICATION OF THE PEOP OCCUPATIONAL THERAPY PROCESS TO POPULATIONS AND ORGANIZATIONS

The process described above focused on situations in which the occupational therapist is working with individuals or small groups of people such as families. However, an emerging area of practice for occupational therapy addresses the occupational issues of populations and organizations. Population-based care may theoretically range from the global population to groups who fit some characteristic (e.g., people with multiple sclerosis, children with autism-spectrum disorders) or they may reflect a small group of people or a community with issues of societal concern around prevention, health promotion or wellness (e.g., mid-life women with family issues that affect their work for a company, or seniors who have become isolated in a neighbourhood because of transportation issues). Sometimes, these issues are identified within a more obvious or defined organizational structure, such as within a community group or business, or involving a group of people within a designated government category (e.g., people over 65 within a designated political or geographic jurisdiction). The PEOP Occupational Therapy Process may vary in these situations. A population or organization-centred PEOP Occupational Therapy Process may serve as the starting point for occupational therapists who are interested in improving the health of populations or communities in general or working within specific organizations.

CASE VIGNETTE 1: POPULATION-CENTRED PEOP OCCUPATIONAL THERAPY PROCESS

An occupational therapist who has worked with older people in long-term care settings for several years wants to continue to work with older people but would like to work in the community with well elders to enable them to remain at home and improve their quality of life. The therapist may not have a clear understanding of the well-elder population because current work focuses on elders who have health conditions and diminished abilities in the long-term care setting. How does the therapist begin? Does one already have the background and knowledge that will enable success in this new practice arena? Is one ready to begin immediately to promote these services to organizations that work with this population or in these communities? In this situation, a population-centred PEOP Occupational Therapy Process may better prepare the therapist to understand the general characteristics and issues of the older population, the community where clients live, and most importantly to plan interventions that will meet the needs and goals of specific organizations.

The Narrative

A general description of the population or community will help the therapist define the population/community (e.g., age, gender, ethnicity, income, education, employment, religion, geographic area), obtain statistics of interest (e.g., risk factors) and identify characteristics that are associated with people who are part of this community (e.g., knowledge, attitudes, beliefs, habits, preferences, sensitivities). The narrative may support some of the therapist's assumptions and dispel myths that may be commonly held. The narrative phase also requires an examination of the critical issues for this community (e.g., barriers, policy, supports, services, motivators for change) as identified by local, national and international agencies and organizations, census information and even reports from the popular press. In a sense, the therapist is conducting an environmental/informational scan to learn more about the prioritized areas of concern for a population/community, the incidence/prevalence of the issues and the major stakeholders (e.g., transportation has been identified as a major issue for seniors living in communities). For each critical issue, the therapist uses strong critical thinking skills coupled with knowledge of factors that support or limit occupational performance, to determine whether there are occupational implications. For example, transportation issues may limit engagement in all occupations that are typically done outside the home—shopping, financial matters, socialization and so on. Identification of other areas of concern may help in preparing for the assessment/evaluation phase. Examples might include traffic, air quality, noise, the condition of pavements and parks, public lighting or issues related to accessibility and safety. These factors may intersect with goals that related to specific interventions—for example, transportation to and from shopping or recreational areas, or the safe access and use of such facilities.

The final step in the narrative is to determine the match between the community's goals and the occupational therapy approach. If there is not a match, the occupational therapist should make an appropriate referral to another professional or to other resources. When a match is identified, the practitioner should begin the second phase of the PEOP Occupational Therapy Process to determine the population's capabilities/enablers and barriers/constraints that will need to be overcome.

Assessment/Evaluation

Clinical reasoning supports the occupational therapist in applying knowledge of the person, environmental and occupational factors to the activities and tasks that are central to the older adult community. At the community level, assessment and evaluation may focus on environmental factors. For example, inadequate public transportation to support the community independence of older adults and poor or confusing signage at the senior centre may limit occupational performance participation. However, there may also be community problems that affect person factors. Examples would be air quality, water quality, limited access to fresh food and housing without lead paint.

Intervention

A client-centred intervention plan is developed from the narrative of the community and the practitioner's assessment of the person and environmental factors that serve as capabilities/enablers and barriers/constraints. When the intervention or programme entails broad population/community initiatives and responsibilities (e.g., public health, labour and legislative), one may work with others to implement these strategies as part of an overall plan. When the intervention plan involves partnerships with organizations and agencies, these overall population-based strategies may serve as the foundation for an organization-centred PEOP Occupational Therapy Process.

Outcome

The population-centred Occupational Therapy Process leads to achieving the goals identified by the older adult community that are related to occupational performance, participation and well-being. These outcomes may support the growing population of older adults as well as persons living with chronic diseases and disabling conditions to enable full participation in the community.

CASE VIGNETTE 2: ORGANIZATION-CENTRED PEOP OCCUPATIONAL THERAPY PROCESS

Case vignette 1 described an occupational therapist who used a population-centred PEOP Occupational Therapy Process for a new practice with well elders to enable them to remain at home and improve their quality of life. A senior (elderly daycare) centre has recently invited the occupational therapist to help the organization improve their programmes and services, especially for older adults with chronic conditions. An organization-centred PEOP Occupational Therapy Process begins with a narrative of the types of clients served by the organization. This step in the process enables the occupational therapist to approach the organization with a level of credibility that will open doors of opportunity. After developing expertise with regard to a specific population, an occupational therapist may not need to perform this step in an explicit manner. Rather, the knowledge base of the professional includes this foundational information. Less experienced practitioners, however, may need to begin gaining an understanding of the population served by the organization as a preliminary step and prior to any discussions with a specific organization.

The Narrative

Once there is an understanding of the population served by the organization, its needs, its resources and its goals, the next step in an organization PEOP Occupational Therapy Process is to fully describe the organization. An understanding of the organization's mission, history, focus, values, activities, funding, clients and stakeholders is essential for assessing their need and potential for occupational therapy services. This senior (elderly daycare) centre describes its mission as providing 'physical, social and intellectual opportunities to support individuals' journey to ageing successfully'. Information, like the mission, may be obtained in publications about the organization. Other information may be acquired through initial conversations with a contact person in the organization or its members. The occupational therapist then begins to explore the organization's areas of concern and unmet needs for the clients they serve. Many of these concerns may be expressed in terms of general issues. For example, the senior centre may be concerned about members with visual impairments, recent immigrants who do not speak the primary language of the community or the mental health of some older adult groups. This same organization may also be concerned about older adults who have diminished cognitive capacity that affects their skills in using the centre's website as well as meeting the needs of members who are still working or serving as caregivers for family members. In the narrative phase, the occupational therapist also uses critical reasoning skills to identify and communicate the occupational issues that may be influencing the general areas of concern for the organization.

The goals of the organization and its stakeholders are considered next in the process, especially as related to occupational areas of concern. The practitioner also asks for information that will allow him or her to determine the organization's commitment and ability to achieve these goals. The final step in the narrative is to evaluate the match between the organization's goals and the occupational therapy services one can provide. The therapist will use all the information gathered about the organization, and discussions with people in the organization to decide whether to continue the process. At this point, the therapist's personal investment in the organization has been limited. However, if one continues the process, the therapist and the organization may make a considerable commitment of personnel and resources for assessment/evaluation and interventions.

Assessment/Evaluation

The occupational therapist selects appropriate tools to understand the factors that are enabling as well as constraining the occupational performance of the organization. At the organization level, many of the primary factors will be environmental. Examples might be inadequate staff training to foster full participation of older adults with disabilities in the centre's programmes, limited environmental modifications for older adults with physical impairments or insufficient health education programmes for older adults who have low literacy levels.

Intervention

In this phase, the therapist develops an organization-centred intervention plan to help the organization achieve its general and occupational goals. The therapist may want to consider the initial population-centred PEOP Occupational Therapy Process to identify the aspects of this plan that are appropriate for the organization and the current evidence that is available. It also may be important to pilot any interventions, especially if this represents a new of area of occupational therapy practice. Pilot studies are a way to establish relationships with organizational clients and demonstrate initial outcomes that can pave the way for additional work and funding. The organization will use the time to evaluate a therapist's capacity to help them achieve their goals. Implementation of the occupational therapy intervention plan may include any of the strategies identified in the person-centred or population-centred PEOP Occupational Therapy Process. However, promotion/prevention and education/consultation strategies are probably most common and effective when the target of an intervention involves an organization and its stakeholders.

Outcome

Therapists' success with this organization can only be verified and documented if an evaluation of the effectiveness of the interventions is conducted based on attainment of identified goals. This step is important in helping therapists solidify their relationship with the organization. Additionally, it serves as a useful step in preparing therapists to work with other related organizations. Disseminating the outcomes of interventions to the broader community is also essential for expanding practice into new arenas. The entire process leads to achieving the occupational performance goals identified by the organization with the possibility that such outcomes extend benefits to other clients they serve.

SUMMARY

The PEOP model and PEOP Occupational Therapy Process emphasize the transactions between the narrative of persons, populations or organizations and the person and environment factors to support occupational performance, participation and well-being. Occupational therapists have a widespread reputation for 'doing good work'. Although this work seems to employ 'common sense' strategies, there is a systematic and complex thought process and multiple sources of knowledge required to make specific recommendations. By using the PEOP Occupational Therapy Process, the practitioner is provided appropriate language to use in reports and recommendations that will communicate the complexity of the process and the care that has gone into the resulting plan. In the end, we are confident that the PEOP Occupational Therapy Process provides a means for applying the PEOP model so that individuals, communities and organizations can accomplish goals related to improved well-being and quality of life despite the presence of conditions that may limit or restrict occupational performance.

REFLECTIVE LEARNING

1. What do the authors mean by the term the *occupational therapy lens*?
2. How is the PEOP model similar to and different from the Model of Human Occupation (MOHO; Chapter 6), the Canadian Model of Occupational Performance and Engagement (CMOP-E; Chapter 7) or the Occupational Therapy Intervention Process Model (OTIPM; Chapter 9)?
3. Reflect on the narrative of a person you know or have observed in a clinical setting. How did the narrative influence the occupational therapy goals, assessment/evaluation, intervention and outcomes?
4. As healthcare focuses more on health promotion and prevention, how does the PEOP model and PEOP Occupational Therapy Process help practitioners contribute programmes and services to these efforts?
5. How could occupational therapists use a population-centred and organization-centred PEOP approach to contribute to a school's goal to reduce bullying of students with special needs?
6. Rapid advances in digital technologies, such as assessments and interventions using virtual environments or interactions with clients in distant locations, are changing the face of healthcare. What are some implications of these technologies that may require adjustments in the application of the PEOP model in such situations?

REFERENCES

Baum, C., Christiansen, C., & Bass, J. (2015). Person-Environment-Occupation-Performance (PEOP) model. In C. Christiansen, C. Baum, & J. Bass (Eds.), *Occupational therapy: Performance, participation and well-being* (4th ed.). Thorofare, NJ: Slack, Inc.

Christiansen, C., & Baum, M. C. (1991). *Occupational therapy: Overcoming human performance deficits*. Thorofare, NJ: Slack, Inc.

Engel, G. E. (1977). The need for a new medical model. *Science, 196*, 129–136.

Engelhardt, H. T., Jr. (1983). Occupational therapists as technologists and custodians of meaning. In G. W. Kielhofner (Ed.), *Health through occupation: Theory and practice in occupational therapy* (pp. 139–145). Philadelphia: FA Davis.

Meyer, A. (1922). The philosophy of occupational therapy. *Archives of Occupational Therapy, 1*(1), 1–10.

Putnam, R. (1995). Bowling alone: America's declining social capital. *Journal of Democracy, 6*(1), 65–78.

Reed, K., & Sanderson, S. (1999). *Concepts of occupational therapy*. Philadelphia, PA: Lippincott Williams and Wilkins.

Shannon, P. D. (1977). The derailment of occupational therapy. *American Journal of Occupational Therapy, 31*, 229–234.

9

The Occupational Therapy Intervention Process Model

Lou Ann Griswold

OVERVIEW

The Occupational Therapy Intervention Process Model (OTIPM) is unique among models of practice because it combines a process model, a conceptual model of occupation and legitimate intervention models. Together, these models provide occupational therapists with an overarching occupation-centred and true top-down reasoning model for planning and implementing authentic occupational therapy services.

The OTIPM is primarily a process model that guides the step-by-step process from initial evaluation through to re-evaluation and ascertaining outcomes. During this process, the occupational therapist links to a conceptual model, the Transactional Model of Occupation. This model, based on a transactional perspective on occupation and introduced in occupational science by Aldrich (2008) and Dickie et al (2006), is unique in that occupation is viewed as a transactional whole, where three elements of occupation (occupational performance, occupational experience and participation) and various elements of the situational context (i.e., client elements, environmental elements, sociocultural elements, geopolitical elements, temporal elements and task elements) all mutually interact to influence each other. Finally, the OTIPM is intimately linked with four intervention models: adaptive occupation, occupation-focused educational and training programmes, acquisitional occupation and restorative occupation, all of which are associated with principles that guide the provision of services that are occupation-based and/or occupation-focused. This chapter presents how the OTIPM is applied in practice. A case example highlights how the occupational therapist uses the OTIPM to plan and implement evaluations and interventions that reflect the unique focus of our profession—occupation.

HIGHLIGHTS

- The OTIPM provides a true top-down and client-centred model for occupational therapy practice.
- The OTIPM is primarily a process model, guiding occupational therapy practice that is occupation-based and occupation-focused.
- The OTIPM provides clear instructions on implementing occupation-based performance analyses that support clear documentation, goal writing and intervention planning, focused on occupation.
- Occupation includes three interwoven elements: occupational performance (the doing); occupational experience (how the person experiences occupational performance); and participation (doing combined with the personal value the client places on the occupation).
- Occupation occurs within a situational context—elements that influence occupation, are influenced by the occupation, and influence one another.
- The interweaving of the occupational elements and situational elements provides the basis for a conceptual model that is linked to the OTIPM for understanding the complexity of occupation.
- The OTIPM also provides intervention models and four continua for critically evaluating the evaluation and intervention methods used in practice.
- The OTIPM emboldens authentic occupational therapy practice, the identity of each occupational therapist, and the unique focus of the profession of occupational therapy.

INTRODUCTION

Anne G. Fisher introduced the Occupational Therapy Intervention Process Model (OTIPM) in her Eleanor Clarke Slagle Lecture at the American Occupational Therapy

Conference in 1998 (Fisher 1998). She has expanded the OTIPM and how it is graphically presented over the years (Fisher 2009, Fisher 2013, Fisher & Jones 2017), based on evolution of her own thinking as she practiced, conducted research, critically evaluated the literature, talked with colleagues and provided education throughout the world. Most recently, Fisher and Marterella (2019) provided an extensive revision of the OTIPM, including the intimately linked intervention models and the Transactional Model of Occupation, in their text *Powerful Practice: A Model for Authentic Occupational Therapy*.

Various models of occupational therapy practice offer practitioners different perspectives to guide professional reasoning. As the name implies, the OTIPM provides a clear *process model* in which occupation is central to guiding professional reasoning. As Fisher and Marterella (2019) indicated, the OTIPM gives practitioners a detailed occupation-centred model to delineate a process for evaluation and intervention that is client-centred, occupation-based and occupation-focused. Fisher and Marterella defined each of these highlighted terms that support occupational therapists' reasoning to reflect the occupation-centred perspective that is unique to the profession. The Transactional Model of Occupation that is intimately linked to the OTIPM provides a conceptualization of occupation, describing occupation as a complex transactional whole where the elements of occupations and the elements of situational contexts mutually influence one another. Thus, the OTIPM also includes a conceptual model. Finally, the OTIPM includes a variety of intervention models that emphasize occupation-based and occupation-focused intervention methods. Understanding and applying the OTIPM in practice supports occupational therapists' identities as they provide occupational therapy services with clients alongside their colleagues from other professions. When occupational therapists apply the OTIPM when working with clients, the clients, clients' family members and other professionals recognize and appreciate the unique contribution of occupational therapy.

Definitions of Key Concepts for Occupational Therapy

Understanding the theoretical underpinnings for any model of practice is essential. Embracing the concepts of the OTIPM allows occupational therapists to demonstrate the values of the profession. Fisher and Marterella (2019) specified that when occupational therapists are client-centred, they collaborate with clients to understand their perspective regarding their occupational needs, choices, desires, strengths and concerns, and their desired occupational outcomes and priorities. When practising in a client-centred manner, occupational therapists make decisions collaboratively with clients throughout the occupational therapy process. Fisher and Marterella specified that decisions that are based solely on the client's perspective or on that of the occupational therapist are both unilateral and missing the collaboration between the two. Fisher (2009) and Fisher and Marterella recognized that 'clients' may be an individual person referred to occupational therapy; a *client group* (i.e., a group of more than one person referred to occupational therapy); or a *client constellation*, when an individual has been referred to occupational therapy but others are impacted by the individual's concerns. For example, a parent or teacher may also be experiencing difficulty in parenting or teaching the child. According to Fisher and Marterella, a client may also be an *organization*, a *community* or a *population*. For example, a company may want an occupational therapist to help address safety concerns in a work environment. Another example might be a population of university students for whom an occupational therapist introduces strategies to support time management and reduction of stress as part of a university-led programme for all first-year students. Regardless of who is the client, the occupational therapist will want to understand the perspectives of those considered to be the client regarding their occupational strengths, concerns and desired outcomes.

Occupation-centred indicates occupational therapists' perspective, our way of thinking about people, specifically what people do, and how we can support their doing—supporting their occupations. Occupation-based practice and occupation-focused practice result from occupation-centred thinking. Occupation-based refers to occupational therapists' method of evaluation or intervention, in which the client engages in real, desired occupations for evaluation and/or intervention, for example, observing a person get dressed or prepare a meal, or observing a group of co-workers interacting to collaborate on a project at work. In these examples, the client is engaged in real occupation (e.g., getting dressed, preparing a meal, interacting with co-workers), making the occupation the 'base' of the evaluation or intervention (Fisher 2013, Fisher & Marterella 2019).

Occupation-focused refers to the 'immediate (versus future) focus of an evaluation or purpose of an intervention' on occupation (Fisher & Marterella 2019, p.76), for example, focusing on the quality of a person's occupational performance when dressing, preparing a meal or interacting with co-workers. The immediate focus is on occupation. In contrast, nonoccupation-focused evaluation or intervention methods are focused proximally on situational factors (e.g., body functions such as range of motion or memory, task demands such as complexity of the meal being prepared, or elements of the social environment such as the number of co-workers or the presence of a manager in the room). When occupational therapists change their focus to any of these situational factors, they have lost the 'immediate' or 'proximal' focus on occupation. Even though they might think that occupational performance is the result of the factors evaluated, or that providing interventions that are proximally focused on these situational factors will result in improved occupation, they are making the occupation 'distal' or putting it in the future of their thinking. In these situations, the occupation is not the proximal focus.

When we use the term *occupation*, occupational therapists may assume we have a shared understanding of the term. However, various authors have defined 'occupation' in different ways. Fisher and Marterella (2019) conceptualized occupation as having three interwoven elements: *occupational performance*, the doing of the occupation; *occupational experience*, how the person experiences the doing; and *participation*, a combination of doing and the value the client places on the occupation. Occupational performance refers to 'doing'—what the client does. Occupational therapists evaluate the quality of 'doing' by observing task performances and analysing the quality of the performances. Occupational therapists also ask about the clients' occupational experiences (e.g., level of satisfaction with their performances). Finally, when the clients are doing something and experiencing personal value in what they are doing, they are participating. All three occupational elements are interwoven. For example, an occupational therapist may watch a client as he washes the dishes and evaluate the quality of the observed actions as he washes, rinses and stacks the dishes (occupational performance). The client may report that he washed dishes without any difficulty and that he is satisfied (occupational experiences) but also report that washing the dishes is something he does out of obligation—it is 'just a task that needs to be done'. When doing (washing the dishes) is associated with an experience of personal value, participation occurs. Fisher and Marterella consider occupational engagement and participation to be synonyms.

Fisher and Marterella (2019) further explained that in the OTIPM, occupation is not produced by people, nor separate from the client or the situational context within which it occurs. Rather occupation occurs in response to situational contexts and likewise influences those contexts, making occupation and the situational context an intertwined transactional whole.

THE OTIPM AS A PROCESS MODEL

The OTIPM, as a process model, is illustrated by a graphic design, shown in Fig. 9.1. (A colour version of this same graphic design is available on the Powerful Practice website:

www.powerfulpractice.com.) The OTIPM is divided into three primary phases: evaluation and goal setting, intervention, and re-evaluation. Each is represented by one or more ribbons in Fig. 9.1. Within the graphic design of the OTIPM, Fisher and Marterella (2019) have provided arrows to guide occupational therapists when using the model. The arrows near the top of the figure going between the ribbons indicate the order of progression from one ribbon to the next and between the phases. The downward arrows in some of the ribbons indicate that occupational therapists work through each step, one at a time, before proceeding to the next step. When there are no arrows between the vertical boxes, the steps can be performed in any order or simultaneously. The dark arrow that extends below the re-evaluation phase ribbon indicates that the occupational therapist can circle back and re-enter the process at any phase as needed to modify occupational therapy services. The horizontal band across the top of the graphic design acknowledges the ongoing collaboration between the occupational therapist and client throughout the evaluation, intervention and re-evaluation process. Finally, the band across the bottom of the figure indicates that the occupational therapist can decide to continue or terminate occupational therapy services at any point in the process.

The left to right and top to bottom stepwise progression supports true occupation-centred and top-down reasoning. When using a true top-down approach, the occupational therapist gathers information to understand the client's strengths and concerns, and the situational contexts of the client's occupations. Based on what the client indicates are concerns, and what tasks the client prioritizes, the occupational therapist then observes the client perform these tasks and evaluates the quality of the client's occupational performance. After collaborating with the client to set goals, the occupational therapist and client will consider how various situational elements (e.g., environmental, sociocultural, client) within the Transactional Model of Occupation might be influencing occupational performance, occupational experience and participation. Only then, and only if absolutely needed, does the occupational therapist administer tests of the client's body functions, environmental factors or other situational factors. Thus, the true top-down approach helps ensure the occupational therapist remains focused on occupation.

Gather Initial Information

Looking more closely at the ribbons in each phase of the OTIPM (Fig. 9.1), we begin with the ribbon titled *Gather Initial Information*. During this phase, the occupational therapist gathers information about the client to learn about his or her occupations and the situational contexts of the occupations. The occupational therapist gathers

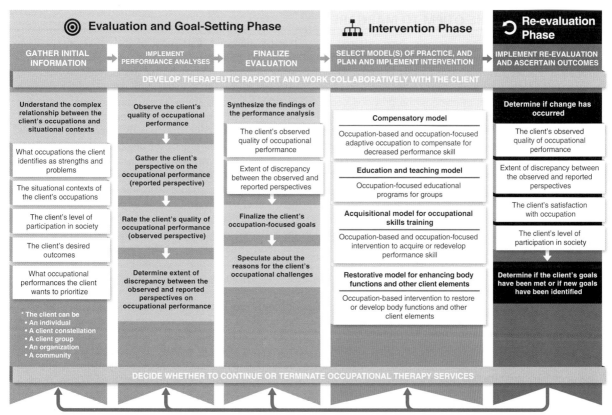

Fig. 9.1 Graphic representation of the Occupational Therapy Intervention Process Model (OTIPM). From: www.powerfulpractice.com with permission.

information from multiple sources: the person who was referred to occupational therapy, others who know the person well, the client's chart or other professionals on the team. If the client is a group, organization or population, the occupational therapist would gather information from members of the group, organization or population, as well as others who know the members well. It is important to gather adequate information to fully understand the transactional whole in which occupations and situational contexts influence one another.

The information can be gathered in any order, but the occupational therapist wants to learn about what occupations the client indicates are strengths and problems, the situational contexts of the occupations, the client's overall level of participation, the client's desired outcomes and their occupational priorities. The occupational therapist keeps the focus on occupation and specific tasks brought up by the client. The occupational therapist asks about the client's performance of tasks (e.g., what tasks are easy and what tasks are challenging), how the client is experiencing the occupations (e.g., how the client feels when

doing a given task—if the client is satisfied, whether the client enjoys the occupation) and the client's level of participation in an occupation (e.g., the personal value the client places on doing—engaging in occupation). The occupational therapist will discuss occupations related to self-care, household tasks such as cooking or cleaning, providing care for others, work, leisure or socializing with others in different situational contexts. During the interview, questions should flow as a conversation, with the goal of understanding the relationship between the client's occupations and their situational contexts.

The client's occupational concerns and priorities will guide the occupational therapist and client to collaboratively identify specific tasks or social interactions to consider for evaluation (e.g., making a pot of coffee, interacting with co-workers to make decisions). The specific tasks or social exchanges selected by the client will be those the occupational therapist observes. Thoroughly gathering information from the client to identify tasks that are valued and challenging supports client-centred and occupation-focused practice, reflecting true top-down reasoning.

APPLICATION OF THE OTIPM TO MARGARET

Margaret, a woman in her late 80s, was referred to Jarod, an occupational therapist. Jarod works in community-based practice, allowing him to visit clients in their homes. Jarod frames his professional reasoning using the OTIPM. He believes that in doing so he provides occupation-based, occupation-focused and client-centred therapy services. Because of Jarod's work setting, he sees patients with a variety of diagnoses and needs. Using a model that encourages him to maintain his occupation-centred perspective is critical for his practice. Using the OTIPM keeps Jarod focused on occupation, maintaining his professional identity.

When Margaret saw her physician for her annual physical, Margaret's ongoing memory problems were evident, but the physician observed that she seemed guarded in reporting any difficulties. The physician referred Margaret to community-based occupational therapy for evaluation and intervention to support her ability to continue living in her own home.

Gathering Initial Information from Margaret

Jarod visited Margaret in her home. Her adult daughter, Christine, was present and added information during their initial meeting. Jarod learned that Margaret lives with her husband in a two-storey house where they have lived for nearly 40 years. Margaret and her husband are both in their late 80s and Margaret firmly stated that they intend to live in their house 'for the rest of their lives'. Christine wants to support her parents' wishes and make sure that is possible. She explained that her parents currently share most household tasks of cooking and daily cleaning tasks: 'they seem to compensate for the other one's weaknesses'. Christine lives too far to drive to her parents more than once a month and therefore is limited in participating in their daily care.

Margaret said she had been a librarian in the town library for 35 years and her husband had taught in the private school in town. As a result of their longevity in the community and their past jobs, Margaret said they have many friends. Different friends drop by the house two or three evenings a week, often bringing food to contribute to a shared dinner. Margaret said she appreciates that she does not have to cook every night, although admitted that her husband does most of the cooking now. Margaret says she volunteers at her church one morning a week, folding the bulletins for the Sunday service. She also volunteers at a local food pantry and attends a monthly book club at the library. Margaret stated that her community activities are very important to her because they offer social connections with others and she feels she is 'making a difference' by being able to contribute to community organizations.

Christine said that several of the women from the food pantry have shared with her their concern about her mother's memory. Christine is not worried about her mother's ability to continue with volunteering, because the tasks are relatively easy and repetitive, and she is glad her mother can be with other people. However, Christine is concerned that her mother's memory is starting to limit her ability to be safe at home. She has noticed that her mother has had 'issues' cooking that raise safety concerns. For example, she sometimes puts a pot on a hot burner and then 'forgets' she put it there. Christine is grateful that her dad does most of the cooking. However, she knows that her mother still participates in cooking tasks. She is less concerned about housework because her parents have someone clean their house once a week. Nevertheless, Margaret worries about the hair her cats leave on the carpet in the living room, so she still vacuums at least once a week, between cleanings.

Jarod asked Margaret what types of activities she does or would like to continue doing around the house. Margaret said that she often makes sandwiches for lunch, and frequently makes a salad as part of dinner. She again mentioned that she vacuums the living room mid-week. She said the tasks are important to do and she enjoys doing them. She also reported that she does these tasks 'just fine'. Christine's facial expression let Jarod know that these tasks may be a bit challenging for Margaret. Jarod, therefore, suggested to Margaret that he watch her do a couple of the tasks that she needs to do and enjoys doing. He said that after observing her do the tasks, he might be able to give her suggestions on how to make the tasks go 'even better'. Margaret agrees, and she decided to make a salad and vacuum the living room.

Implement Performance Analyses

The next ribbon in the evaluation phase builds on the initial information gathering process as the occupational therapist implements a *performance analysis* following the clearly delineated steps shown in Fig. 9.1 (Fisher & Marterella 2019). The occupational therapist first observes the client perform relevant tasks, or engage in relevant social exchanges, ones the client prioritized as problems and would like to address in occupational therapy. The client performs real tasks or social exchanges in ecologically relevant situations, supporting occupation-based evaluation. The occupational therapist may choose to gather the client's perspective on the task performance just after each task observation. The occupational therapist then uses notes taken during the observations and rates the client's quality of performance by considering (1) the overall quality of the performance and (2) the effectiveness of performance skills, the observable, goal-direction actions that together comprise a performed task. Implementing a performance analysis and evaluating the quality of occupational performance highlights the expertise of occupational therapists.

When rating the overall quality of performance of a task involving tangible objects, the occupational therapist uses the *Occupational Therapy—Quality of Performance: Motor and Process Skills Rating Form*. (The rating forms are available on the Powerful Practice website: www.powerfulpractice.com.) A performance analysis using the OTIPM begins by rating the client's overall level of effort, efficiency, safety and frequency of assistance for tasks involving tangible objects or rating the overall quality of social interaction for tasks involving interacting with others. The same general criteria are used to rate all five criteria: no problem, minimal problem, moderate problem or substantial problem (Fisher & Marterella 2019).

Rating the effectiveness of specific performance skills provides a sensitive analysis of the client's quality of performance. The OTIPM includes three groups of performance skills: motor skills, process skills and social interaction skills. A list of all skills and their definitions is in Table 9.1. Each performance skill refers to an observable, goal-directed action, which may be thought of as an individual link in a chain of actions that together comprise a task performance or a social interaction. When conducting a performance analysis, the occupational therapist considers the quality of each skill observed throughout the client's performance of the task or the social exchange. Fisher and Marterella

---

TABLE 9.1A   Performance Skills: Motor Skills

Within the context of performing a chosen and ecologically relevant task, observable task actions related to effectively moving self and tangible task objects

Effectively Positioning the Body
- **Stabilizes**—moves through task environment and interacts with task objects without momentary propping or loss of balance
- **Align**—interacts with task objects without evidence of persistent propping or persistent leaning
- **Positions**—positions oneself an effective distance from task objects and without evidence of awkward arm or body positions

Effectively Obtaining and Holding Objects
- **Reaches**—effectively extends the arm, and when appropriate, bends the trunk, to effectively get or place task objects that are out of reach
- **Bends**—flexes or rotates the trunk as appropriate when sitting down or when bending to grasp or place task objects that are out of one's reach
- **Grips**—effectively pinches or grasps task objects such that the objects do not slip (e.g., from between one's fingers, from between the teeth, from between one's hand and a supporting surface)
- **Manipulates**—uses dexterous finger movements, without evidence of fumbling, when manipulating task objects (e.g., manipulating buttons when buttoning)
- **Co-ordinates**—uses two or more body parts together to manipulate and hold task objects without evidence of fumbling task objects or task objects slipping from one's grasp

Effectively Moving Self and Objects
- **Moves**—effectively pushes or pulls task objects along a supporting surface, pulls to open or pushes to close doors and drawers, or pushes on wheels to propel a wheelchair
- **Lifts**—effectively raises or lifts task objects without evidence of increased physical effort
- **Walks**—during the task performance, ambulates on level surfaces without shuffling the feet, becoming unstable, propping or using assistive devices
- **Transports**—carries task objects from one place to another while walking or moving in a wheelchair
- **Calibrates**—uses movements of appropriate force, speed or extent when interacting with task objects (e.g., not crushing task objects; pushing a door with enough force that it closes but does not bang)
- **Flows**—uses smooth and fluid arm and wrist movements when interacting with task objects

Effectively Sustaining Performance
- **Endures**—persists and completes the task without obvious evidence of physical fatigue, pausing to rest, or stopping to catch one's breath
- **Paces**—maintains a consistent and effective rate or tempo of performance throughout the entire task performance

TABLE 9.1B   Performance Skills: Process Skills

Within the context of performing a chosen and ecologically relevant task, observable task actions related to effectively selecting, interacting with and using tangible task objects, and carrying out individual actions and steps in a timely manner . Paces is both a motor skills and a process skill. it should only be evaluated once, based on the person's overall rate or tempo of staff performance.

Effectively Sustaining Performance (Continued)
- **Paces**—maintains a consistent and effective rate or tempo of performance throughout the entire task performance
- **Attends**—does not look away from what he or she is doing, interrupting the ongoing task progression
- **Heeds**—carries out and completes the task originally agreed upon or specified by another person

Effectively Applying Knowledge
- **Chooses**—selects necessary and appropriate type and number of task objects for the task, including the task objects that one was directed to use (e.g., by a teacher) or that were specified by the person
- **Uses**—applies task objects as they are intended (e.g., using a pencil sharpener to sharpen a pencil, but not to sharpen a crayon) and in a hygienic fashion
- **Handles**—supports or stabilizes task objects in an appropriate manner, protecting them from damage, slipping, moving or falling
- **Inquires**—(1) seeks needed verbal or written information by asking questions or reading directions or labels, and (2) does not ask for information in situations where one was fully oriented to the task and environment and had immediate prior awareness of the answer

Effectively Organizing Timing
- **Initiates**—starts or begins the next task action or task step without any hesitation
- **Continues**—performs single actions or steps without any interruptions such that once an action or task step is initiated, one continues without pauses or delays until the action or step is completed
- **Sequences**—performs steps in an effective or logical order and with an absence of (1) randomness or lack of logic in the ordering and/or (2) inappropriate repetition of steps
- **Terminates**—brings to completion single actions or single steps without inappropriate persistence or premature cessation

Effectively Organizing Space and Objects
- **Searches/locates**—looks for and locates task objects in a logical manner
- **Gathers**—collects related task objects into the same workspace and re-gathers task objects that have spilled, fallen or been misplaced
- **Organizes**—logically positions or spatially arranges task objects in an orderly fashion within a single workspace, and between multiple appropriate workspaces, such that the workspace is not too spread out or too crowded
- **Restores**—puts away task objects in appropriate places and ensures that the immediate workspace is restored to its original condition
- **Navigates**—moves the arm, body or wheelchair without bumping into obstacles when moving in the task environment or interacting with task objects

Effectively Adapting Performance
- **Notices/responds**—responds appropriately to (1) nonverbal task-related cues (e.g., heat, movement), (2) the spatial arrangement and alignment of task objects to one another and (3) cupboard doors or drawers that have been left open during the task performance
- **Adjusts**—effectively (1) goes to a new workspace, (2) moves task objects out of the current workspace and (3) adjusts knobs, dials, switches or water taps to overcome problems with ongoing task performance
- **Accommodates**—prevents ineffective performance of all other motor and process skills and asks for assistance only when appropriate or needed
- **Benefits**—prevents ineffective performance of all other motor and process skills from recurring or persisting

(2019) provide definition, detailed examples of diminished skill and rating criteria for each skill based on the degree of disruption the skill has on the task performance or social interaction. The rating criteria are as follows:
- Competent No disruption in the task performance or social interaction
- Minimally diminished skill Mild disruption
- Moderately diminished skill Modest disruption
- Markedly diminished skill Severe disruption

Motor skills refer to skills observed when moving oneself or task objects during a task performance. When doing a performance analysis, the occupational therapist

TABLE 9.1C Performance Skills: Social Interaction Skills

Observable actions related to effectively communicating and interacting with others within the context of engaging in daily life task performances that involve social interaction

Initiating and Terminating Social Interaction
- **Approaches/starts**—approaches or initiates interaction with the social partner in a manner that is socially appropriate
- **Concludes/disengages**—effectively terminates the conversation or social interaction, brings to closure the topic under discussion and disengages or says goodbye

Producing Social Interaction
- **Produces speech**—produces spoken, signed, or augmentative (i.e., computer-generated) messages that are audible and clearly articulated
- **Gesticulates**—uses socially appropriate gestures to communicate or support a message
- **Speaks fluently**—speaks in a fluent and continuous manner, with an even pace (not too fast, not too slow) and without pauses or delays during the message being sent

Physically Supporting Social Interaction
- **Turns towards**—actively positions or turns the body and the face towards the social partner or the person who is speaking
- **Looks**—makes eye contact with the social partner
- **Places self**—positions oneself at an appropriate distance from the social partner during the social interaction
- **Touches**—responds to and uses touch or bodily contact with the social partner in a manner that is socially appropriate
- **Regulates**—does not demonstrate irrelevant, repetitive or impulsive behaviours that are not part of social interaction

Shaping Content of Social Interaction
- **Questions**—requests relevant facts and information and asks questions that support the intended purpose of the social interaction
- **Replies**—keeps conversation going by replying appropriately to suggestions, opinions, questions and comments
- **Discloses**—reveals opinions, feelings, and private information about oneself or others in a manner that is socially appropriate
- **Expresses emotions**—displays affect and emotions in a way that is socially appropriate
- **Disagrees**—expresses differences of opinion in a socially appropriate manner
- **Thanks**—uses appropriate words and gestures to acknowledge receipt of services, gifts or compliments

Maintaining Flow of Social Interaction
- **Transitions**—handles transitions in the conversation or changes the topic without disrupting the ongoing conversation
- **Times response**—replies to social messages without delay or hesitation and without interrupting the social partner
- **Times duration**—speaks for a reasonable length of time given the complexity of the message sent
- **Takes turns**—takes one's turn and gives the social partner the freedom to take his or her turn

Verbally Supporting Social Interaction
- **Matches language**—uses a tone of voice, dialect and level of language that is socially appropriate and matched to the social partner's abilities and level of understanding
- **Clarifies**—responds to gestures or verbal messages from the social partner signalling that the social partner does not comprehend or understand a message, and ensures that the social partner is 'following' the conversation
- **Acknowledges/encourages**—acknowledges receipt of messages, encourages the social partner to continue interaction, and encourages all social partners to participate in the social interaction
- **Empathizes**—expresses a supportive attitude towards the social partner by agreeing with, empathizing with or expressing understanding of the social partner's feelings and experiences

Adapting Social Interaction
- **Heeds**—uses goal-directed social interactions focused towards carrying out and completing the intended purpose of the social interaction
- **Accommodates**—prevents ineffective or socially inappropriate social interaction
- **Benefits**—prevents problems with ineffective or socially inappropriate social interaction from recurring or persisting

considers the degree of physical effort or clumsiness the person demonstrated during the observed task performance.

Process skills refer to the skills observed as a person uses time, space and tools and materials. The occupational therapist considers how efficiently a person carries out steps and actions (e.g., without hesitations or pauses), locating, choosing, spatially arranging and using tools and materials for the task, and modifying performance to address any problems that occur.

Social interaction skills refer to the skills observed as a client interacts with others during a social interaction in any situation. The occupational therapist considers the quality of initiating and terminating a social interaction, producing social interaction, physically and verbally supporting a social interaction, shaping the content of a social interaction, maintaining the flow of the interaction and adapting when a problem in interaction arises.

It is important to stress that performance skills are small units of observable occupation, *not* underlying body functions. For example, the occupational therapist can observe how skilfully a person walks over to the kitchen cupboard, reaches up, grasps a glass and gathers the glass to the counter. The occupational therapist can also observe him choose milk, the beverage he said he would choose, and pour a glass of milk, stopping pouring once the glass is full, but before milk spills over the rim of the glass (terminates). In contrast, the occupational therapist cannot observe strength or range of motion, nor can the occupational therapist observe memory. What the occupational therapist observes is that the person skilfully reached up for the glass and chose the type of beverage he said he would choose.

The 16 motor skills, 20 process skills and 27 social interaction skills in the OTIPM are considered universal performance skills. They are universal in that the motor and process skills are observed in virtually any daily life task performance in which a client interacts with tangible objects (Fisher & Marterella 2019). The task performances may be related to personal or domestic activities of daily living, work, schoolwork tasks, play or leisure. Likewise, the social interaction skills are observed in nearly any social exchange, in all types of occupation in which clients interact with others. The three groups of performance skills have been operationally defined in the standardized assessments: *Assessment of Motor and Process Skills* (AMPS; Fisher & Jones 2012, 2014), *School Version of the Assessment of Motor and Process Skills* (School AMPS; Fisher et al 2007) and the *Evaluation of Social Interaction* (ESI; Fisher & Griswold 2018), supporting their validity.

The occupational therapist may conduct a nonstandardized performance analysis (see Fisher & Griswold 2019, Fisher & Marterella 2019) or use a standardized assessment such as the AMPS (Fisher & Jones 2012, 2014), the School AMPS (Fisher et al 2007) or the ESI (Fisher & Griswold 2018). Using standardized performance analysis allows occupational therapists to provide criterion-referenced and norm-referenced interpretation of the results. The standardized results can be particularly helpful in making decisions regarding eligibility for occupational therapy services, guiding planning intervention and making decisions for discharge planning. Standardized assessment results also allow for objectively measuring progress over time, supporting the effectiveness of occupational therapy services. To ensure valid and reliable administration and scoring of the standardized performance analyses, the AMPS, School AMPS and ESI each require training and certification. Gathering the person's perspective on task performance after completing a task or social exchange can also be done in a nonstandardized manner or in a standardized manner using the *Assessment of Compared Qualities – Occupational Performance* (ACQ-OP; Fisher et al 2017) or the *Assessment of Compared Qualities – Social Interaction* (ACQ-SI; Fisher et al 2017), companion assessment tools to the AMPS and ESI, respectively.

PERFORMANCE ANALYSIS FOR MARGARET

Jarod observed Margaret make a fruit salad for two persons and vacuum the living room, the two tasks that Margaret had prioritized for occupational therapy. We will focus on the task of making a fruit salad. Margaret made the salad in her kitchen. She said she would put an apple, a banana, a pear and an orange in the salad. Jarod wanted to ensure that Margaret had everything she needed to complete the task, so he had her show him where all needed tools and materials were stored. Jarod told Margaret to make the fruit salad in the way she usually would and that he would stand back to watch and take notes. After Margaret made her fruit salad, Jarod asked her how she thought she did when making the fruit salad and if she had any concerns. He also asked her if she was satisfied with how it went. She replied, 'It was fine, but I couldn't find the knives' and 'I'm very satisfied. My husband will like this'.

After the observation, Jarod used the Motor and Process Skills Rating Form and rated Margaret's overall quality of performance and the quality of each observed motor and process skill using the detailed criteria provided by Fisher and Marterella (2019). When Jarod rated Margaret's overall quality of occupational performance, he used the criteria proposed by Fisher and Marterella (2019). Although

PERFORMANCE ANALYSIS FOR MARGARET—cont'd

she performed the task safely and independently, he had observed an overall minimal increase in physical effort and overall moderate to marked inefficiency.

Some of the performance skills Jarod considered when rating the quality of Margaret's performance included: bending and reaching for the bowl; grasping the bowl; lifting the bowl, transporting the bowl to the counter; searching for the different fruits in the refrigerator; gathering the fruits, cutting board and knife to the counter where the bowl was placed; initiating each step in the task without hesitation (e.g., peeling the fruit and cutting the fruit); terminating the chopping of the fruit; noticing and responding when the bowl was full but without fruit spilling out. Jarod was aware that rating the quality of each skill is what leads to a sensitive evaluation. Jarod's performance analysis ratings for Margaret when making a fruit salad are provided in Fig. 9.2.

Jarod knew that when conducting a performance analysis, he was to stay focused on the actions observed, not any of the situational elements that might influence occupational performance. For example, Jarod did not focus on the size or weight of the bowl Margaret was lifting or where the fruits were located when she gathered them. These elements likely influenced or shaped her occupational performance but they were not the proximal focus of a performance analysis. Jarod made sure that his performance analysis focused on the observable actions during the task performance. His intent was to remain occupation focused.

Jarod then compared his performance analysis with what Margaret had reported at the end of the task, to determine the extent of the discrepancy of the two perspectives. He had observed moderate to marked inefficiencies, but Margaret reported only that she had problems finding the knives. He rated the extent of discrepancy as being moderate.

Motor and Process Skill Ratings
Rating (based on level of observed problems): No = none, Mi = mild, Mo = moderate, or Ma = marked

Motor skills –within the context of performing a chosen and ecologically-relevant task, observable task actions related to effectively moving self and tangible task objects

	Rating				Observed performance/rationale
Walks	(No)	Mi	Mo	Ma	Walked easily around the kitchen
Reaches	No	(Mi)	Mo	Ma	Effort reaching for bowl

Process skills –within the context of performing a chosen and ecologically-relevant task, observable task actions related to effectively selecting, interacting with, and using tangible task objects; and carrying out individual actions and steps in a timely manner

Heeds	No	Mi	(Mo)	Ma	Fruit salad had extra ingredients, different than specified
Chooses	No	Mi	(Mo)	Ma	Choose extra fruit (grapes & blueberries)
Initiates	No	Mi	(Mo)	Ma	Hesitated before starting to peel or cut each fruit
Continues	No	Mi	(Mo)	Ma	Paused when peeling and cutting fruit
Searches/locates	No	Mi	Mo	(Ma)	Long delay to find bowl and knife
Notices/responds	No	Mi	Mo	(Ma)	Not noticing and responding to overflowing fruit bowl

Fig. 9.2 Selected performance skill ratings from Jarod's rating form for Margaret.

Finalize Evaluation

In the third ribbon under the evaluation and goal-setting phase in Fig. 9.1, the occupational therapist synthesizes information from the preceding steps and uses the findings to document the results of the initial evaluation. The occupational therapist considers the rating of the observed performances and identifies the actions that were strengths and those that were challenging during the observed occupational performances. The occupational therapist also considers the discrepancy between what the client reported and what was observed. The occupational therapist shares this information with the client and collaborates to finalize the client's goals that focus on occupation, supporting client-centred and occupation-focused reasoning.

SYNTHESIS OF MARGARET'S PERFORMANCE ANALYSIS

Jarod began his documentation with a global baseline statement, reflecting the overall quality of Margaret's performance when making the fruit salad. He had limited space for documentation, so he wrote only short phrases in Margaret's record:

- Fruit salad for two: Performed with moderate to marked inefficiency and minimally increased physical effort; safe and independent.

Jarod then considered the skills that supported Margaret's task performance and those skills that limited her task performance. Because he was aware that the health-care provider might not want to fund services if she was safe and independent, he wanted to be sure to stress her moderate to marked inefficiencies.

Jarod started by clustering the skills that best reflected Margaret's challenges with task performance:

- Inquires and searches/locates
- Chooses and heeds
- Initiates and continues
- Terminates and notices/responds
- Restores

Jarod wrote the following phrases to document the observed challenges in Margaret's task performance:

- Moderate to marked difficulty searching for and finding task objects (e.g., bowl, knife)

- Did not perform the task as she had said she would (e.g., added two fruits that were not preplanned)
- Frequently hesitated before starting and during task actions
- Prepared enough fruit salad for four to five people, filling bowl until fruit was spilling out of the bowl
- Did not tidy up workspace (i.e., she failed to replace items to their original locations, left utensils and fruit scraps on the counter)

Next, Jarod clustered the following skills to reflect Margaret's strengths in her task performance:

- Walks and transports
- Sequences and uses

Jarod put these skills together into two short phrases to describe Margaret's strengths in performance. Again, he used everyday language:

- Easily walked and carried task objects around her kitchen
- Performed task actions in a logical order, using appropriate tools

Jarod's documentation of Margaret's overall quality of performance and specific problems he observed used words to indicate the quality of her performance in an observable, measurable way (e.g., noting she had moderate to marked difficulty finding task objects, frequently hesitated during her task performance).

Next in the OTIPM process, the occupational therapist collaborates with the client to finalize the client's goals. Recall that the client initially indicated occupations that were challenging and prioritized these during the initial information gathering portion of the evaluation and goal-setting phase. At that point, the client also indicates their initial desired outcomes. The observations and performance analyses of the client's prioritized tasks provide specific indications of their challenges with occupational performance. These can be used to collaborate with the client to finalize their goals.

This collaboration can begin as the occupational therapist shares the results of the performance analyses with the client. If the occupational therapist gathered information about the client's perspective regarding the task performance, they can compare the occupational therapist's observed rating with what the client reported just after completing each task. When there is a shared perspective (i.e., there is no more than a minimal discrepancy), the client and occupational therapist are able to more easily identify goals based on what they agreed was challenging. But when the discrepancy is moderate

or larger, the occupational therapist may need to work with the client to try to minimise the discrepancy before proceeding. Otherwise, the risk is that the decision-making related to the client's goals becomes driven by the therapist.

Typically, the occupational therapist and the client collaboratively use the evaluation results to write the client's occupation-focused goals. More specifically, the client specifies what the client wants to achieve, and the occupational therapist formulates the client's goals in terms that are observable and measurable. Thus goals should include what the client will do and how well the client will perform the task.

Speculation of Reasons for Occupational Challenges

After the occupational therapist and the client have finalized the occupation-focused goals, the occupational therapist is ready to speculate about possible reasons for the client's challenges in occupational performance. The occupational therapist uses the Transactional Model of Occupation (Fisher & Marterella 2019) to consider how

COLLABORATIVE GOAL WRITING WITH MARGARET

Jarod returned to Margaret's home a few days later and shared his documentation with Margaret and her daughter. He reflected on what Margaret had reported regarding her perspective on the task performance just after completing each task to highlight areas of agreement on her difficulties and the aspects where they did not agree. Together, Jarod and Margaret identified goals. For example, Margaret had reported she had difficulty finding the knives; she did not mention her moderate to marked difficulty finding the bowl. Jarod had observed difficulty with both. Nevertheless, their shared perspective related to finding knives easily led to their collaboratively writing a goal related to more efficiently finding frequently needed tools. Because Jarod had included language that reflected measurable terms in his documentation, he suggested that these words could help them write specific goals. Jarod had reported that Margaret had 'moderate to marked difficulty searching for and finding task objects'. Jarod suggested that a realistic goal might be for Margaret to find needed tools in her kitchen without any difficulty.

After the task performance, Margaret had not mentioned that she had demonstrated a minimal increase in physical effort (e.g., clumsiness). This did not concern Jarod because the discrepancy was mild. More importantly, Margaret had not reported that she had added extra ingredients, that she cut too much fruit for the size of the bowl or tidied up her workspace. When Jarod explained what he had observed, Margaret denied they were problems and made a statement that more salad would give her husband and her something to eat later. Jarod realized that the goals needed to be Margaret's goals and not his, to maintain client-centred services, so he did not push to add a goal related to these observed problems.

In contrast, Margaret also had not reported that she frequently hesitated when making the fruit salad, something that Jarod had observed. When hearing what Jarod had observed, Margaret agreed that she did work slowly but had not thought of it as hesitations. Their now shared perspective led them to write a goal to address Margaret making a simple meal, such as a salad, with only occasional hesitations during the task performance. They also wrote goals related to vacuuming, the other task that Jarod had observed.

the situational and occupational elements might be mutually influencing one another and interacting with the client's occupational performance. After considering all of the elements in the Transaction Model of Occupation, the occupational therapist can determine if there is need to further evaluate any of the elements, situational or occupational, using other assessment tools. In true top-down reasoning, this is the time in the evaluation process to consider assessments specific to the environment, activity demands, and client elements such as motivation and body functions (e.g., memory, executive function, strength). Occupational therapists who maintain an occupation-centred perspective often find that further evaluation is not needed.

CONSIDER NEED FOR FURTHER EVALUATION

Jarod considered different situational and occupational elements that possibly interacted with Margaret's quality of occupational performance. Those elements that Jarod speculated as supportive of Margaret's performance included social environmental elements: she has a supportive husband at home, friends whom she sees regularly and who expressed caring about her, someone to help with weekly cleaning and a daughter who visits monthly. The geopolitical elements and sociocultural elements supported one another and, in turn, Margaret's overall situation: Margaret lives where services and supports are available and there are regulations and norms to obtain needed support. Jarod speculated that physical environmental elements might not be supporting Margaret's occupational performance, thinking specifically of the location of tools and materials. Jarod observed that Margaret had not tidied up and put the tools and materials away, and thus her occupational performance may be influencing the physical and social environments. Jarod made a mental note to talk to Margaret's husband – was her husband feeling a need to put things away and might he be putting them in locations different from ones she was familiar with? Perhaps all of these elements were interacting with Margaret's embodied habits and routines. Yet, Jarod had ensured that Margaret had placed all needed tools and materials where she wanted them before she made the fruit salad.

Jarod recognized that client elements related to a lack of routine and body functions, particularly memory, likely contributed to Margaret's diminished quality of task performance. Jarod reasoned that using the Transactional Model of Occupation to reflect on the transactional relationships among all of the occupational and situational elements and Margaret's occupational performance enabled him to consider the transactional whole as he speculated about Margaret's biggest challenges. Jarod determined that he did not need to evaluate any elements further; he was confident in his analysis of the transactional whole.

Intervention Phase

The next phase of the OTIPM, intervention, is represented by a single ribbon in Fig. 9.1 and indicates there are four models of intervention (Fisher & Marterella 2019). When using the compensatory model, the occupational therapist provides modifications to the way in which a client performs tasks or adapts aspects of the situational context to make task performances easier for the client (i.e., to compensate for diminished performance skills). An example might be to suggest a client use a rocker knife to cut food with less effort or obtain help from another to locate needed supplies. When using the acquisitional model, the occupational therapist engages the client in occupation to enable the client to acquire or reacquire the performance skills needed to perform desired tasks, for example, supporting a client to acquire manipulating or searching skills needed to more easily manipulate task objects or find needed tools and materials. When using the restorative model, the occupational therapist engages the client in occupation to enhance client factors, including body functions. When using any of the intervention models noted above, the intervention should be occupation-based—that is, the client should be engaged in occupation (Fisher & Marterella 2019).

The fourth model of intervention in the OTIPM is the education and teaching model. As Fisher and Marterella (2019) pointed out, occupational therapists educate clients when using each of the previously identified intervention models. Such education is not part of the education and teaching model. Rather, they explained that when using the education and teaching model, occupational therapists provide education, focused on occupation, to groups of people. This education is always provided in the form of in-service training, workshops or other more lecture-like formats, for example, an occupation-focused workshop given to a group of caregivers who support others to more easily engage in personal activities of daily living, or an occupation-focused in-service training to a group of teachers or teaching assistants who provide support to children with identified needs.

The occupational therapist and the client collaborate to choose one or more types of intervention. The occupational therapist uses evidence and professional reasoning while clients provide their personal perspectives on which interventions they want to try (Fisher & Marterella 2019). Professional reasoning includes considering everything that was summarized in the synthesis of the completed evaluation and goal-setting phase.

Fisher and Marterella (2019) clearly promoted the use of occupation-based intervention when using the first three intervention models, that is, interventions in which the client is engaged in a real occupation in a real situation. Compensatory and acquisitional interventions are also occupation focused. When providing intervention using the education and teaching model, the intervention is focused on occupation, but not occupation based. Furthermore, Fisher and Marterella boldly argued that preparatory and rote practice/exercise are not 'legitimate *occupational* therapy intervention types' (p.220). They supported their position based on the lack of evidence on the effectiveness of these intervention types to improve occupational performance, and because of the lack of alignment of these intervention types with 'authentic *occupational* therapy services' (p.220).

To support their perspective on legitimate intervention methods and to guide occupational therapists in self-critique of their occupational therapy services, Fisher and Marterella (2019) suggested four continua for occupational therapists to use when reflecting on their practice. These continua pertain to the degree to which the evaluation or intervention is client-centred, ecologically relevant, occupation-based and occupation-focused. More specifically, occupational therapists will consider (1) how collaboratively decisions are made between the client and occupational therapist, (2) the ecological relevance of the method used for intervention (i.e., contextualized vs. decontextualized situation), (3) the occupation-based nature of the intervention (i.e., whether or not the client is engaged in occupational performance), and (4) the focus of the intervention (e.g., proximal focus on occupation vs. proximal focus on contextual factors).

INTERVENTION PLAN

To plan intervention, Jarod reflected on Margaret's goals related to simple cooking tasks and vacuuming, the two tasks that she had identified as important during her initial conversation. Jarod also considered the results of the performance analyses of the two tasks he had observed: making a fruit salad and vacuuming. Jarod then used his professional reasoning, guided by the Transactional Model of Occupation and the OTIPM, and recalled his speculations of how the occupational and situational elements mutually influenced one another to determine what intervention model(s) to suggest. He speculated that primary reasons for Margaret's lack of routine for the two tasks she performed and declining memory were hindering her performance. Jarod did not believe the client elements related to routine or memory were going to be easily improved. This realization helped Jarod rule out using restorative occupation for intervention. Similarly, he did not think that Margaret would readily re-acquire skills, ruling out acquisition occupation for intervention. He thought that having

INTERVENTION PLAN—cont'd

specific drawers and cupboards for frequently needed tools and materials would support Margaret's occupational performance. He also wondered if labelling these would help Margaret find what she needed more easily and help Margaret and her husband put them away in the designated location to find them the next time she needed them. Margaret and her husband both thought labelled drawers would help them put needed tools in the same place so that she could find them the next time she needed them. Regarding the hesitations observed during task performance, Margaret said she often 'lost track of what she was doing'. Jarod suggested that a list of steps for frequently desired tasks might help her 'stay on track' when performing tasks. Jarod explained to Margaret's husband and daughter, Christine, that the intervention model he would use is compensatory. Christine said she wanted her mother to continue to do tasks she enjoyed and thought the strategies Jarod suggested would allow her to continue to do those tasks, as long as her dad agreed to support her mom. Jarod also suggested that Christine and her father attend an upcoming evening seminar that he and his colleagues were giving to provide general strategies to support people with memory challenges to avoid decreased occupational performance—as example of an intervention based on the education and teaching model.

Re-Evaluation Phase

In the last phase of the OTIPM, re-evaluation, shown as the final ribbon in Fig. 9.1, the occupational therapist determines if the client has reached the desired outcomes. More specifically, the occupational therapist and the client determine if there has been a change in the clients' observed quality of occupational performance, if there has been a change in the discrepancy between the perspective of the clients and the observed performance, if the clients' satisfaction with occupation has changed, and if their level of participation has changed. The occupational therapist also evaluates if the client's goals have been met. All of these are different ways to ascertain outcomes. Such determinants of change remain occupation-focused as well as client-centred.

Although re-evaluation and determining if a change has occurred are obviously important to clients, building professional evidence is critical to support occupational therapy practice. Nonstandardized assessment methods, such as the informal performance analyses guided by OTIPM

(Fisher & Griswold 2019, Fisher & Marterella 2019), allow occupational therapists to document change in a client's occupational performance. Accurately describing a client's performance of skills using observable terms (e.g., none, minimal, moderate, marked; rarely, occasionally, frequently, consistently) provide the opportunity to gather practice-based evidence (Fisher & Marterella 2019).

After the re-evaluation phase, the occupational therapist and the client collaboratively determine if occupational therapy services are to be discontinued or if the client has new goals and wishes to continue to receive occupational therapy services, if allowed by the healthcare provider. If services are to be continued, the occupational therapist and the client would re-enter the OTIPM process at any point in the cycle.

RE-EVALUATION AND OUTCOMES

Jarod re-evaluated Margaret near the end of the approved intervention time period. Recall that Margaret's goals had been to 'find needed tools in her kitchen without any difficulty' and 'make a simple meal with only occasional hesitations during the task performance'. Jarod again implemented performance analyses, observed Margaret doing meal preparation tasks that were relevant and important for her. He again evaluated her quality of occupational performance. He used these results, and compared them with her initial performance analyses and her goals, to determine if Margaret had made progress and, more importantly, to see if Margaret had met her goals. Margaret chose to make soup from a can for lunch and make a pot of tea. Her performance was now only minimally inefficient. She continued to demonstrate minimal increase in physical effort, but that had not been a target of the intervention. After each task, Margaret reported that she felt more confident in her ability to do these tasks. Her husband said he thought Margaret was 'doing a better job and without help'. These findings support that Margaret was satisfied with her occupational performance and participating in desired instrumental activities of daily living. Margaret said she was pleased with her progress. She commented that she would like Jarod's help in supporting her in her volunteer work. Jarod then re-entered the OTIPM cycle again, and for his last approved occupational therapy session he focused on tasks Margaret did at the food pantry.

Standardized Assessment for Re-Evaluation

Although using nonstandardized assessment can help determine progress, the occupational therapist cannot say with any certainty that change has been made. Using assessments that are standardized, with strong reliability and validity, are essential to support evidence-based occupational therapy practice. As Fisher and Marterella (2019) pointed out, assessment tools like the Canadian Occupational Performance Measure that provide a numeric score may in fact merely represent descriptive data, not true quantitative data in the form of linearized measures with standard errors needed to determine if a statistically significant change has occurred, to provide evidence of a change over time or between groups of people. Had Jarod used a standardized assessment of occupational performance such as the AMPS (Fisher & Jones 2012, 2014), he would have been able to determine if Margaret had experienced a significant change in her Instrumental activities of daily living performance. The standardized measures from the AMPS would have also supported his decision about Margaret's ability and her need for assistance from others and to determine the most appropriate intervention model to select.

CONCLUSION

The OTIPM, first described by Fisher in 1998 and revised over time, most recently in 2019 by Fisher and Marterella, offers a clear process model for evaluation and intervention. The process represents true top-down reasoning, and thereby differs from other process models by including performance analyses—occupation-based and occupation-focused evaluations of quality of occupational performance. The OTIPM has the added advantage of being intimately linked to detailed occupation-based and occupation-focused intervention models and the Transactional Model of Occupation. The OTIPM promotes the value of occupational therapy and helps us realize our unique contribution to the professional team—occupation.

✳ REFLECTIVE LEARNING

- How would Margaret's goals and intervention plan been different if Jarod had not included a performance analysis?
- How does the Transactional Model of Occupation influence the approach chosen for intervention?
- How does the true top-down approach of the OTIPM differ from what you have seen in occupational therapy practice? What changes could be implemented to facilitate occupational therapy practice?

REFERENCES

Aldrich, R. M. (2008). From complexity theory to transactionalism: Moving occupational science forward in theorizing the complexities of behavior. *Journal of Occupational Science, 15,* 147–156.

Dickie, V., Cutchin, M. P., & Humphrey, R. (2006). Occupation as transactional experience: A critique of individualism in occupational science. *Journal of Occupational Science, 13,* 83–93.

Fisher, A. G. (1998). Uniting practice and theory in an occupational framework – 1998 Eleanor Clarke Slagle Lecture. *American Journal of Occupational Therapy, 52,* 509–521.

Fisher, A. G. (2009). *Occupational Therapy Intervention Process Model: A model for planning and implementing top-down, client-centered, and occupation-based interventions.* Ft. Collins, CO: Three Star Press.

Fisher, A. G. (2013). Occupation-centred, occupation-based, occupation-focused: Same, same or different? *Scandinavian Journal of Occupational Therapy, 20,* 1620173.

Fisher, A. G., & Jones, K. B. (2017). Occupational therapy intervention process model. In J. Hinojosa, P. Kramer, & C. B. Royeen (Eds.), *Perspectives on human occupation: Theories underlying practice* (2nd ed.) (pp. 237–286). Philadelphia: Wolters Kluwer|Lippincott Williams & Wilkins.

Fisher, A. G., & Marterella, A. (2019). *Powerful practice: A model for authentic occupational therapy.* Ft. Collins, CO: center for innovative OT solutions.

Fisher, A. G., Bryze, K., Hume, V., & Griswold, L. A. (2007). *School AMPS: School version of the assessment of motor and process skills* (2nd ed.). Ft. Collins, CO: Three Star Press.

Fisher, A. G., & Griswold, L. A. (2018). *Evaluation of social interaction* (4th ed.). Fort Collins, CO: Three Star Press.

Fisher, A. G., Griswold, L. A., & Kottorp, A. (2017). *Assessment of compared qualities – occupational performance* (3rd ed.). Fort Collins, CO: Three Star Press. Retrieved August 28, 2018 from https://www. innovativeotsolutions.com/acq-manual.

Fisher, A. G., Griswold, L. A., & Kottorp, A. (2017). *Assessment of compared qualities – social interaction* (3rd ed.). Fort Collins, CO: Three Star Press. Retrieved August 28, 2018 from https://www. innovativeotsolutions.com/acq-manual.

Fisher, A. G., & Jones, K. B. (2012). Development, standardization, and administration manual, revised (7th ed.). *Assessment of motor and process skills* (vol. 1). Fort Collins, CO: Three Star Press.

Fisher, A. G., & Jones, K. B. (2014). User manual (8th ed.). *Assessment of motor and process skills* (vol. 2). Fort Collins, CO: Three Star Press.

Fisher, A. G., & Griswold, L. A. (2019). Performance skills: Implementing performance analyses to evaluate quality of occupational performance. In B. A. B. Schell, & G. Gillen (Eds.), *Willard and Spackman's occupational therapy* (13th ed.) (pp. 335–350). Philadelphia, PA: Wolters Kluwer.

10

The *Kawa* (River) Model

Kee Hean Lim, Michael Iwama

OVERVIEW

Occupational therapists are employed within increasingly diverse and complex local and global spheres of practice. Client-centred and culturally safe practice is a key priority in providing meaningful, valued and appropriate occupational therapy (Lim & Iwama 2011). The intricate lived experiences and challenges faced by service users/clients require occupational therapists to focus beyond cost efficiency towards providing culturally relevant and effective healthcare. The Kawa

(River) Model provides a framework within which service users/clients and occupational therapists alike can engage in examining the self and appreciate how participation in meaningful occupation enhances health and well-being. The Kawa Model focuses on the distinctive and diverse nature of each person's occupational narrative and provides a structure within which the occupational therapists can develop insight and understanding of each person's unique lived experience and occupational world within their wider context.

HIGHLIGHTS

- Each person's experience of and the meanings they attach to daily life are unique.
- Service users/clients and occupational therapists alike carry diverse interpretations of occupation and of occupational therapy.
- Context and personal experience are important and central to understanding and shaping one's occupational world and daily life narratives.
- Professional culture, standard practice frameworks and prescriptive assessments based on universal criteria can exclude as well as reinforce power differentials between client and professional.
- In the current climate of evidence-based practice there can be an overemphasis on standardized clinical assessment

and measurement, at the expense of appreciating clients' lived experiences and wellness narratives.
- Person-centred occupational therapy begins, is based on, and ends with the client's narrative of daily life experience.
- To be meaningful and relevant, occupational therapy must be both person and context-focused, inclusive, enabling and culturally safe.
- The Kawa Model has the potential beyond clinician application to be used as a research tool in eliciting both personal narratives and lived experience, and as a reflective tool for the researcher.
- The Kawa Model has the potential to be used in the education of students for their personal development, and in developing their reflective skills and knowledge.

INTRODUCTION

Occupational therapy endeavours to enable people from all walks of life to engage and participate in occupations and activities that enhance their health and well-being. However, to discover and appreciate what individuals' and communities consider meaningful, valued and purposeful is a far more complex undertaking (Iwama 2007). Indeed occupational therapists have

been challenged to provide occupational therapy that is relevant and responsive to the day-to-day realities of their diverse clientele. An examination of current occupational therapy models reveals that the meanings and interpretations attached to such concepts as occupation, autonomy and independence, like other socially situated constructs, have been prescribed mainly by people situated in the English-speaking Western world, distinct from the experiences of those who inhabit a different socio-cultural context (Iwama 2006, Lim 2008a, Whalley Hammell 2018).

The meanings of human occupations are uniquely tied to socio-cultural contexts, varying from group to group, from person to person and from situation to situation. Given this degree of diversity and cultural relativity in occupation's fundamental meaning, a single or universal interpretation of this core construct of occupational therapy is virtually impossible to maintain. How then, will specific conceptual models in occupational therapy, largely constructed on such universal premises, explain, describe and guide occupational therapy approaches and processes for diverse clientele in varied contexts? How well do the tacitly held ideals that essentially reflect middle-class, North American and Western European ideals of self-determinism, competence and individual agency explain the day-to-day realities and meanings of occupation for clients that do not fit these socio-cultural ideals (Iwama 2006, Whalley Hammell 2018).

Although many aspects of contemporary occupational therapy and its locations of practice have been aligned with biomedicine, numerous occupational therapists have been resolute in ensuring that occupational therapy practice is closely aligned with their clients' daily realities and experiences (Iwama 2005a), with a focus beyond pathology, symptoms and functional limitations and towards addressing personal goals, challenges, creating opportunities and meeting the needs of a diverse clientele. This is where the power of occupational therapy lies: to enable people from all walks of life to engage and participate in activities and processes that have personal meaning, value and relevance (Lim & Iwama 2006, 2011).

Occupation-based occupational therapy is challenging to deliver, especially when diversity and cultural relativity are brought into the equation. Cultural variation and the challenges of diversity negate the applicability of a one-size-fits-all worldview or single framework in explaining personal phenomena and human experience (Iwama 2005a, Lim 2008b). What may be appropriate for clients whose experiences fall within minor deviations from the norm may possess limitations for 'other' clients outside of the demographic mean curve, who may be effectively excluded or disadvantaged by the same standard. What happens when norms and imperatives of autonomy, personal causation and self-determinism are also imposed on to 'other' clients who come from a sphere of shared learning and experience that idealizes dependency, group harmony and collective determinism? How does the single parent with four young children, a refugee who lives in a hostel, a young man with mental illness and others who have survived circumstances of abject poverty and social marginalization relate to occupational therapy's middle-class, Western principles and

ideals of competence, self-agency and self-reliance (Whalley Hammell & Carpenter 2004, Iwama 2006)?

Delivering an occupation-based service for a diverse client population that makes sense of the value of activities and processes of daily life (occupation) in unique and diverse ways remains a daunting task for occupational therapists. Catering to the uniqueness of each client's day-to-day occupational issues is difficult to enact when conventional theory and the approaches that these theories guide and explain are based on questionable premises of homogeneity of clientele, their needs and universality of a given occupational therapy model. An appreciation of the personal impact of disability, impairment and exclusion is a central to understanding how those that are restricted by their health condition or marginalized by society can be assisted through providing relevant, comprehensive and quality care.

Issues of Culture and Cultural Safety in Occupational Therapy Theory and Practice

Culture is more than individual-embodied features of ethnicity and race. It is broadly defined here as spheres of shared experience and the ascription of meaning to phenomena and objects in the world (Iwama 2007, Lim, 2008a). Indeed the occupational therapy profession itself could be regarded as a cultural group or entity, with its own unique sphere of shared experiences, specialized language, tacit rules of professional conduct and acceptable rules for knowledge production and theory development. For many occupational therapists, the cultural features and imperatives concealed within conventional occupational therapy theory may go problematically unnoticed (Iwama 2005a). The preference for individual centric views of daily life occupations, the imperatives of autonomy and independence in daily living skills and de-emphasis on contexts that shape occupational meanings are often taken for granted and accepted as 'normal'—especially by those who have shared experiences in Western contexts of daily living (Lim 2008b). Unwittingly, this can lead to occupational therapists enquiring and filtering each client's unique lived experience and personal narratives through predetermined concepts and principles belonging to someone else's (unfamiliar) worldview and interpretation of human occupation and experience (Lim & Iwama 2011). Problems are identified and plans for intervention are then determined that can potentially stray or diverge from what the client actually regards to be meaningful, valued, worth knowing and worth doing. Often, the ideals of client-centred occupational therapy fail to extend far enough into the rich, contextual cultural world of the client (Iwama 2005b, Lim 2006).

For many occupational therapists and their clients who fall outside of such mainstream cultural norms, universal models that have risen out of a dominant mainstream culture, infused with its own tacit standards and ideals of what is considered 'normal', 'acceptable' and 'good', can be regarded in some instances as being culturally unsafe (Lim & Iwama 2006). Ramsden (1990) highlights the importance and principles of cultural safety: a framework by which power relationships between health professionals and the peoples they serve are critically considered. The impact of historical, social and political processes on minority health groups holds important implications for equity wherever health issues of a particular group are being described, explained, mediated and evaluated by other people within their own standards (Jungerson 1992). This idea of cultural safety is especially pertinent to occupational therapists when taking their ideas and processes into new cultural domains, including into the lives of their diverse clients and contexts (Gray & McPherson 2005, Iwama 2006). Often the recipients may be in weaker, disadvantaged positions and are discriminated against further by being compared and evaluated against standards and norms belonging to a different cultural context. Further, they may also lack the experience, knowledge and means to examine critically the veracity, utility and cultural safety of the procedures and materials imposed upon them (Lim 2008a).

There are also relevant issues of cultural safety in the interface between theory construction and theory application. When critical questions are asked about where the ideas have come from, on what realities these materials and ideas have been based, and about who has participated in the production of such knowledge, valuable insight is gained into the cultural features of the epistemology and theory of a profession. Theories and models, often developed in academic settings, can be far removed from the very people, situated in diverse, dynamic and changing practice contexts, for whom these theoretical materials and models are universally intended and considered appropriate (Lim & Iwama 2006).

Empowering Occupational Therapy Clients—The Way Forward

Reconfiguring client-centred practice may be difficult for both the seasoned therapist and conditioned client to come to terms with, as the current way of top-down delivery of occupational therapy often privileges the professional as 'knowing best' and the client submitting to the role of 'patient' (Lim & Iwama 2011). The reliance on certain (universal) frameworks and the standardized tests that reify and accompany them can take some of the guesswork out of professional decision-making and enhance the efficiency of occupational therapy processes, but the occupational therapist must ultimately understand whether the client and their 'story' of day-to-day living and circumstances are being comprehended and that the ensuing occupational therapy is truly client-centred and based on factors that are meaningful to the client.

Occupational therapists stand to benefit from theory, instruments, methods and approaches that enable clients to translate their real experiences of daily living into the therapeutic process, to form the basis on which occupational therapy is fashioned. Ideally, the client's 'story' of their day-to-day occupational issues, constructed and told by the client, in their own words, ought to be enabled and centralized to form the basis to the occupational therapy process (Iwama 2006, Lim 2006). Achieving this to any degree is not an easy or a simple undertaking, for it involves a series of difficult transitions for the professional therapist. A change in power relation between the therapist and client is required. The familiar hierarchical power structure of professional and client is upended, and the heterogeneity and diversity of clients and their 'stories' become normal. The skills necessary for those engaged in occupational therapy will change from being technical experts capable of delivering standard procedures of assessments and interventions, to health professionals who are able to apply their knowledge and skills effectively according to the unique and diverse clients and their contexts that emerge in each complex therapeutic instance (Lim & Iwama 2011).

Achieving this will move occupational therapy further towards becoming client-centred and more equitable with regard to the power differential that commonly exists in therapeutic relationships, where the occupational therapist is situated as expert and the service user/client is regarded as 'patient' (Ramsden 1990). Rather than forcing the individual to adapt to some standard requirements of occupational therapy, such an approach requires occupational therapy and occupational therapists to adapt and fashion their occupational therapy to the unique needs and specific requirements of the client. Imagine a process whereby the service user/client 'names' the concepts of their occupational therapy model and explains the principles that tie these highly personal concepts together, in which the occupational therapy process is transformed into a collaborative one in which it is bound by the individual's occupational narrative (Lim & Iwama 2011). The service user/client is now (acknowledged and respected as) the 'expert' of their own occupational narrative and the therapist becomes a partner or facilitator to enable better life flow.

THE KAWA (RIVER) MODEL

The Kawa Model represents a significant departure from the tacit ways in which theory is normally structured and translated into occupational therapy practice. The empowering of service users/clients and attention to their occupational narratives forms the basis of the occupational therapy processes and interventions to follow and represents a radical breakthrough from conventional occupational therapy practice (Lim & Iwama 2011). The Kawa Model adopts an approach more in line with the client's day-to-day realities and experiences of disablement rather than set predetermined concepts, principles and prescribed narrative (Iwama 2006, Lim & Iwama 2011).

Philosophical Underpinnings: A Social Constructionist Perspective

The primary philosophical orientation underlying the Kawa Model is one of social constructionism. Burr (1995) highlights that from a social constructionist perspective, knowledge and the meanings of phenomena and their explanations (theory) are understood to be created between people who share common experiences and agree on interpretations of those phenomena. This is in opposition to the dominant view in the scientific and empirical traditions that truth and reality are singular (universal) and lie external to (or outside of) the self and are knowable through rational enquiry (Gergen 1999). Burr (1995) argues that our current accepted ways of understanding the world are a product not of objective observation of the world, but of the social processes and interactions in which people are constantly engaged with each other. The implication of this alternative way of conceptualizing phenomena is that people's understandings of issues, such as occupation and occupational performance, are said to be historically and culturally situated (Ramugondo 2018). Occupation and its enactment will therefore mean different things to different people situated in differing spheres of experience and circumstances (Iwama 2006, Lim 2008a).

Ontological Views: Self in Relation to Context, Environment and Time

Culture can be identified at the core of most contemporary conceptual models of rehabilitation, and is particularly observable in how the 'self' is socially constructed and situated in relation to the surrounding environment or context. The interpretations and meanings we derive through what we do in the world may vary according to how this dualism of self vis-a-vis the environment is regarded and understood. Conventional occupational therapy models construe the self as being not only focally situated in the centre of all concerns, but also understood to be rationally separate and superior in power and status to the environment and nature (Iwama 2006). Well-being is constructed to be contingent on the extent to which the self can act on and demonstrate its ability to control one's perceived circumstances located in the environment. Failure or compromise in controlling the environment is construed with such terms as *dysfunction* and *disability*. These terms are often pejorative in a socio-cultural context in which the self is required to be competent,

able and in control (of one's environment and circumstances). In these worldviews, dependency can often represent an undesirable state of disability (Lim & Iwama 2011).

An independent self, centrally situated and agent upon a separate and subordinated environment, also appears to coincide with a particular sensation of time. When the self is centrally located in relation to the environment at large, one's sense of entitlement to doing in the present (here and now) can also extend temporally into one's future. The relation between intention, one's immediate action on the environment, and some specific (future) objective is often rationally connected. It is not uncommon for people situated in the Western world to believe that they carry primary responsibility for their own destinies. 'You make your bed and lie in it' and 'you get what you pay for' are familiar adages, particularly in Western social contexts. It should come as little surprise, then, to see that independence, autonomy, equality and self-determinism are celebrated ideals that point to a common worldview and value pattern shared between mainstream rehabilitation ideology and the broader Western social contexts from which they emerged (Iwama 2006). In contrast to this worldview is the East Asian and Aboriginal one. In the primitive cosmological myth (Bellah 1991), the 'self' is not central nor unilaterally empowered but rather construed to be just one of many parts of an inseparable whole (Bellah 1991, Gustafson 1993). In this view of reality, one does not need to occupy or wrest control of anything because in an integrated view of self and nature, one is already there amongst others. In this view of reality, health and disability states are also not imagined nor believed to be an individual-centred matter.

Life circumstances are dependent on a broader whole, determined by a constellation of factors and elements located both within and outside of the physically defined body (Shakespeare 1994). The self is decentralized and not accorded an exclusive privilege to exercise stewardship, nor unilateral control, over one's environment or circumstances. Hence, conceptual models in occupational therapy that are based on a tacit understanding of a central individual separate from a discrete environment are often incongruent with experiences of disability and well-being for many who are situated outside of mainstream Western social norms (Iwama 2006, Ramugondo 2018). The Kawa Model follows the more 'primitive' ontological view of people and nature, drawing no clear distinctions or separations between selves and their contexts of reality. This is a dynamic view of human experience and meanings. The self and surrounding context share an inseparable co-existence in which changes to any one aspect of the self-context complex will affect the entire frame. *Kawa* is the Japanese term for 'river', and is employed as a metaphor for 'life flow'. The river's rocks, configuration of the river banks and driftwood in the Kawa Model combine uniquely, from instance to instance, to shape and determine the quality of the ensuing river flow. Such is the flow of life, as self and context fluidly change from instance to instance. Problems, the social and physical environments and one's own personal attributes, strengths and limitations all combine to render a particular quality of one's life flow. This is the Kawa Model, and occupational therapy's subsequent mandate is to help the client enhance and balance the flow within their lives (Iwama 2006, Lim 2018).

The Power of Metaphor

The power of metaphor can be understood to be a figure of speech in which an expression or symbolic image is used to refer to something that it does not literally denote, to suggest a similarity. 'Life is a river' or 'people are complex machines' are just two common examples of metaphors. Models can also be seen as metaphors, whether they be of 'systems' like machines, or 'rivers' of nature. Lakoff and Johnson's (1980) seminal work in *Metaphors We Live By*, illuminates the degree to which metaphor plays a fundamental role in matters of self-identity and one's relation to the world. We not only communicate through metaphors, but we also think through them. The occupational therapeutic relationship is structured and mediated through metaphor (Iwama 2006), and the Kawa Model serves as one particular metaphor through which the powerful processes of occupational therapy can be enacted.

When the Kawa Model was first developed, there was a tendency to situate the model in Japanese culture, and therefore it was assumed to be applicable to 'Eastern' clients and others located in East Asian contexts. Since its development, the metaphor of the river, used to depict life flow or the life journey, has been found to resonate with people beyond Asian societies (Iwama 2006). When the 'kawa' metaphor is found to be a common link spanning the therapist's and client's spheres of shared experience, it can be exploited as an effective medium through which the process of occupational therapy can flow (Lim & Iwama 2011). The authors speculate that the explanatory power of conceptual models in occupational therapy has much to do with the power and resonance of the metaphor that underpins the model, in relation to the spheres of shared experience (culture) of the client and occupational therapist. The resonance of the river metaphor to diverse occupational therapy practice contexts, in a relatively short period of time

since its publication, has been remarkable. The Kawa Model has been translated into several languages and utilized by occupational therapists located across six continents.

The occupational therapeutic relationship is structured and mediated through metaphor (Iwama 2006), and the Kawa Model serves as one particular metaphor through which the powerful processes of occupational therapy can be enacted. The use of the 'river' metaphor within the Kawa Model illustrates a dynamic, fluid and more integrative image which represents the complexity and harmony of the client's occupational life flow. Each individual is perceived to have their own unique 'personal river' that symbolizes their life journey, flowing through time and space as observed in Figure 10.1, with a beginning and an eventual end. The upstream of one's river represents the past, the lower stream represents the future, and personal health and well-being are expressed by the free and unrestricted flow of one's river. During different points in time, potential barriers and enablers that influence the flow with an individual's river journey can be ascertained. An optimal state of well-being in one's life or river can therefore be metaphorically portrayed by an image of strong, deep, unimpeded flow.

Aspects of the environment and phenomenal circumstances, like certain structures found in a river, can influence and affect that flow. Rocks (life circumstances), walls and bottom (environment), and driftwood (assets and liabilities) are all inseparable parts of a river that determine its boundaries, shape and flow (Fig. 10.2). Occupational therapy's purpose in this metaphorical representation of human being, then, is to enable and enhance life flow.

COMPONENTS OF THE KAWA MODEL

A fuller description of the Kawa Model can be studied in main text *The Kawa Model: Culturally Relevant Occupational Therapy* (Iwama 2006). However, highlighted here are the four basic (categories) concepts outlined within the Kawa Model and their metaphorical counterparts, listed in both the original Japanese and their English equivalents.

Mizu (Water)

Mizu, Japanese for 'water', metaphorically represents the individual's life energy or life flow. Fluid, pure, spirit, filling, cleansing and renewing are only some of the meanings and functions commonly associated with this natural element. Just as people's lives are bounded and shaped by their surroundings, people, experience

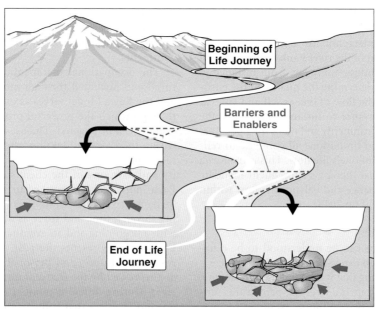

Fig. 10.1 Personal rivers and life journey. Each individual has their own life journey 'river' which has a beginning and end. At any point in time it is possible to examine the barriers and enablers that influence one's life flow.

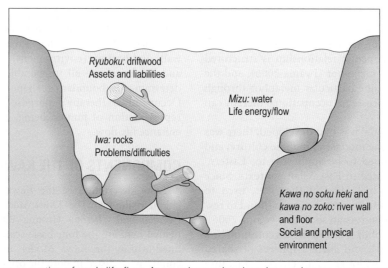

Fig. 10.2 A cross-section of one's life flow. At any given point along its continuum, a cross-section view of the river can be considered as understanding life's condition from the client's vantage point. The quality of water flow is affected by the river walls and bottom, and by rocks and driftwood. Wherever there is a need to enhance life flow, there is a need for occupational therapy.

and circumstances, the water flowing as a river touches the rocks, sides and banks and all other elements that form its context. The volume, direction and rate of flow can reflect the state of one's health; that is, when life energy or flow weakens, the individual may be said to experience a state of ill health or disharmony. Just as water is fluid and adopts its form from its container, people in many collective-oriented societies often interpret the social as a shaper of individual self. There is greater value in 'belonging' and 'inter-dependence' than in unilateral agency and individual determinism (Doi 1973, Lebra 1976). In such experience, the inter-dependent self is deeply influenced and even determined by the surrounding social context, at a given time and place (Iwama 2006).

Kawa No Soku-Heki (River Sidewall) and *Kawa No Zoko* (River Bottom)

The river's sides and bottom, referred to in the Japanese lexicon respectively as *kawa no soku-heki* and *kawa no zoko*, are the structures/concepts from the river metaphor that stand for the client's environment. These are perhaps the most important determinants of a person's life flow in a collectivist social context because of the primacy afforded to the environmental context in determining the construction of self, experience of being and subsequent meanings of personal action. In the Kawa Model, the river walls and sides represent the subject's social context/frame or *ba* (Nakane 1970). This comprises mainly the 'others' who share a direct relationship with the subject. Depending upon which social frame is perceived as being most important in a given instance and place, the river sides and bottom can represent family members, workmates, friends in a recreational club or classmates.

The shape and status of water, or life flow, are determined by the compounding interplay of rocks (problems), driftwood (assets/liabilities) and the river walls and floor (environment). Rocks increase in size, shape and number, and exist in a dynamic, enclosing environment, trapping driftwood (Fig. 10.3). Life flow is compromised, indicating a need for occupational therapy. In societies like those of Japan, social relationships are regarded to be the central (Nakane 1970) determinant of individual and collective life flow. Aspects of the surrounding social frame on the subject can affect the overall flow (volume and rate) of the *kawa*. Harmonious relationships can enable and complement life flow. Increased flow can have an agent effect upon difficult circumstances and problems, as the force of water displaces rocks in the channel and even creates new courses through which to flow. Conversely, a decrease in flow volume can exert a compounding, negative effect on the other elements that take up space in the channel. If there are obstructions (rocks and driftwood) in the watercourse when river walls and bottom are constricting, the flow of the river is especially compromised (Fig. 10.3). The rocks in this river can directly butt up against the river walls and bottom, compounding and creating larger impediments to the river's usual flow. When applying the Kawa Model in collectivist-oriented populations, these components and the perceptions of their importance are paramount.

Iwa (Rocks)

Iwa (Japanese for 'large rocks') represent discrete circumstances that are considered to be impediments to one's life flow. They are life circumstances perceived by the client to be problematic and difficult to remove. Most rivers, like people's lives, have such rocks or impediments, of varying size, shape and number. The impeding effect of rocks by themselves or in combination with other rocks, jammed against the river walls and sides (environment), can profoundly impede and obstruct flow. The client's rocks may have been there since the beginning, such as with congenital conditions. They may appear instantaneously, as in sudden illness or injury, and even be transient (Lim & Iwama 2006).

A person's bodily impairment becomes disabling when interfaced with the environment. For example, the functional difficulties associated with a neurological condition can change according to the environmental context. A (physically) barrier-free environment can decrease one's disability, as can social and/or political/organizational environments that are accepting of people with disabling conditions. Once the client's perceived rocks are known (including their relative size and situation), the therapist can help to identify potential disabling circumstances and areas of intervention and strategies to enable better life flow. Occupational therapy intervention can therefore include treatment strategies that expand beyond the traditional patient, to their social network and even to policies and social structures that ultimately play a part in setting the disabling context (Lim & Iwama 2011). The subject, be it an individual or a collective, ideally determines specific rocks and their number, magnitude, form and situation in the river. As with all other elements of the model, if the client is unable to express their own river, family members or a community of people connected with the issue at hand may lend assistance.

Ryuboku (Driftwood)

Ryuboku is Japanese for 'driftwood', and represents the subject's personal attributes and resources, such as values (e.g., honesty, respects), character (e.g., optimism, stubbornness), personality (e.g., reserved, outgoing), special skill (e.g., carpentry, public speaking), and immaterial (e.g., friends, siblings) and material assets (e.g., wealth, special equipment) that can positively or negatively affect the subject's circumstance and life flow. Like driftwood, they are transient in nature and carry a certain quality of fate or serendipity. They can appear to be inconsequential in some instances and significantly obstructive in others, particularly when they settle

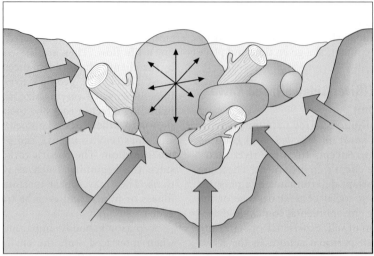

Fig. 10.3 Restrictions within the life flow. The shape and status of water, or life flow, are determined by the compounding interplay of rocks (problems), driftwood (assets/liabilities) and the river walls and floor (environment). Rocks increase in size, shape and number, and exist in a dynamic, enclosing environment, trapping driftwood. Life flow is compromised, indicating a need for occupational therapy.

in amongst rocks and the river sides and walls. On the other hand, they can collide with the same structures to nudge obstructions out of the way. A client's religious faith and sense of determination can be positive factors in persevering to erode or move rocks out of the way. Receiving a grant to acquire specialized assistive equipment can be the piece of driftwood that collides against existing flow impediments and opens a greater channel for one's life to flow more strongly. Driftwood is a part of everyone's river and often resembles intangible components possessed by each unique client of occupational therapy. Effective therapists pay particular attention to these components of a clients' or community's assets and circumstances, and consider their real or potential effect on the client's situation.

Sukima (Space Between Obstructions): The Promise of Occupational Therapy

In the Kawa Model, spaces are the points through which the client's life energy (water) evidently flows, and these spaces represent 'occupation'. When the metaphor of a river depicting the client's life flow becomes clearer, attention turns to the *sukima* (spaces between the rocks, driftwood, and river walls and bottom). These spaces are as important to comprehend in the client as are the other elements of the river when determining how to apply and direct occupational therapy. For example, a space between a functional impairment such as arthritis (an *iwa*/rock) and a social group or

person (in the river sides and walls) may represent a certain social role, such as parent, company worker, neighbour and friend.

Water coursing naturally through these spaces can work to erode the rocks and river walls and bottom, and over time can transform them into larger conduits for life flow. This effect reflects the latent healing potential that each subject naturally holds within themselves and in the inseparable context. Thus occupational therapy in this perspective retains its hallmark of working with the client's abilities and assets, and seizing upon opportunities to bring about change and promoting health. It also directs occupational therapy intervention towards all elements (in this case, a medically defined problem, various aspects and levels of environment) in the context (see inner image, Fig. 10.4).

Spaces, then, represent important foci for occupational therapy. They occur throughout the context of the self and environs, between the rocks, walls and bottom, and driftwood. Spaces are potential channels for the client's flow, allowing client and therapist to determine multiple points and levels of intervention (Fig. 10.4). In this way, each problem or enabling opportunity is bounded by and appreciated in a broader context. Rather than attempting to reduce a person's problems (i.e., focusing only on rocks) to discrete issues, isolated from their particular contexts, similar to the way in which rational processes in which client problems are identified and discretely named/diagnosed in conventional Western health practice, the Kawa Model framework compels the

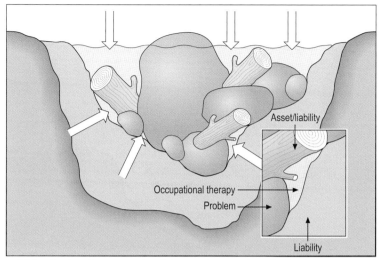

Fig. 10.4 Potential focal points for occupational therapy intervention. *Sukima*/spaces: potential focal points for occupational therapy. Intervention can be multi-faceted and include breaking or eroding away the (medical) problem, limiting personal liabilities and/or maximizing personal assets, as well as intervening on elements of the greater environment (including the social and physical). Focusing water on these objects to erode or move them is metaphorical of the client using their own abilities or 'life force'.

occupational therapist to view and treat issues within a holistic framework, seeking to appreciate the clients' identified issues within their integrated, inseparable contexts. Occupation is therefore regarded in wholes, to include the meaning of the activity to self and to the community to which the individual inseparably belongs, and not just in terms of biomechanical components or individual pathology and function. Indeed, phenomena and life circumstances rarely occur in isolation. By changing one aspect of the client's world, all other aspects of their river change. The river's spaces represent opportunities to problem-solve and to focus intervention on positive opportunities, which may have little direct relation to the person's medically defined condition.

By using the Kawa Model, occupational therapists, in partnership with their clients, are directed to stem further obstruction of life energy/flow and look for every opportunity in the broader context, to enhance it (Fig. 10.5). Through the vantage point of the Kawa Model, a subject's state of well-being coincides with life flow. Occupational therapy's overall purpose in this context is to enhance life flow, regardless of whether it is interpreted at the level of the individual, institution, organization, community or society. Just as there are constellations of inter-related factors/structures in a river that affect its flow, a rich combination of internal and external circumstances and structures in a client's life context inextricably determine their life flow.

RESEARCH, DEVELOPMENT AND APPLICATIONS OF THE KAWA MODEL

Since the publication of *The Kawa Model: Culturally Relevant Occupational Therapy* in 2006, the Kawa Model book has been translated into several languages. The Kawa Model has also been published in peer-reviewed journal articles in several languages, including German, French, Arabic and Spanish, in addition to English and Japanese. The Kawa Model's presence across electronic resources has also increased over the last few years, with a Facebook page https://www.facebook.com/KawaModel/ and a website (http://www.kawamodel.com/v1/), where a healthy and lively discussion forum attracts worldwide dialogue, discussion and critique around the utility, limitations and innovative use of the Kawa Model within research, clinical practice and education.

Many clinicians have incorporated the use of the Kawa Model within various aspects of their practice, whether as a framework to guide their interactions and discussions, to inform their goal setting and planning of interventions. This has included the use of the Kawa Model within paediatrics and school context, to physical health, mental health and nontraditional practice context such as with refugees and in forensic practice. The Kawa Model has also been implemented within several research studies from master level dissertations to doctorate theses to further examine the scope, utility and value of the Kawa

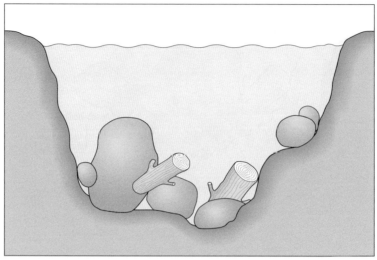

Fig. 10.5 Promoting life flow through minimizing obstructions and restrictions. The power of occupational therapy: increased life flow. All obstacles may not have been completely eliminated; some may have even remained unchanged. However, life flows more strongly, despite obstacles and challenges.

Model. Research has included the use of the Kawa Model to explore the perspectives of women who have overcome intimate partner violence (Humbert et al 2013); the experiences and perspectives of military personnel who have experienced posttraumatic stress disorder as a consequence of combat stress (Gregg et al 2015); and the contribution and the value of the Kawa Model in exploring mental health recovery (Lim 2018).

To promote the use of the Kawa Model, several academics and clinicians have developed applications and online materials to support its use. One example is this link (developed by Helen Mason, Animations Therapy Ltd.) introducing the key concepts and demonstrating the application of the Kawa Model: https://www.youtube.com/watch?v=ZxT-VH049MNU. Another is the Kawa Model application, available from appstore.com. The app enables an individual to engage in creating their own river map, depicting what their lived experience is like and what they might be able to do to challenge the difficulties they might face.

Client Feedback on the Kawa Model

Joan mentioned that she liked the simplicity of the Kawa Model and could relate to its naturalistic qualities, having lived near a river for many years. She found the concepts easy to grasp and was able to sketch her recent journey to the point she was admitted to hospital. She mentioned that by looking at the wider context as highlighted within the Kawa Model, she could see how the various individuals and groups around her, that is, family, friends and health professionals, could support her rehabilitation and return home.

> **CASE STUDY JOAN**
>
> This case vignette and the following one illustrate the use of the Kawa Model in practice.
>
> Joan is a 78-year-old female who has had a recent stroke. She is optimistic and has led an active life.
>
> She can walk slowly using a cane but needs to use a wheelchair for longer distances. She has some difficulties with her personal activities of daily living (ADLs) and her mobility. She enjoys socializing, gardening and swimming.
>
> Joan currently lives in her own ground floor flat, which would need adapting. She has a good network of friends and family. She is currently attending the in-patient rehabilitation unit and is due for discharge in 2 weeks.
>
> The focus of Joan's occupational therapy intervention is shown in Figure 10.6 and Table 10.1.

Stewart mentioned that he found the Kawa Model really helpful as a framework in assisting him to visualize and understand his recovery journey. He was able to identify with and relate to the metaphor of his life's journey, represented as a river. Stewart felt that the depictions within his own river indicated that, despite his health condition, he did lead an active life, meeting up with friends, attending football games and community art classes, visiting his brother and helping as a volunteer, and that all these occupations of meaning contributed to and supported his personal journey of recovery through mental health.

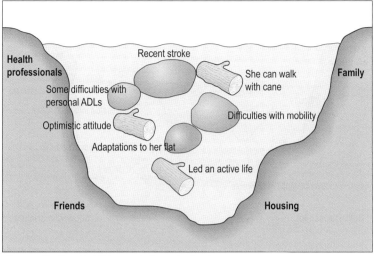

Spaces: She likes Socializing, gardening and swimming

Fig. 10.6 Cross-section of Joan's river before therapy.

TABLE 10.1	Joan's Occupational Therapy Intervention
Break the rocks	Remove the obstacles by providing activities of daily living skills, working on gait and balance. Tackling housing adaptation.
Maximize the spaces	Promote the inner strength, interest and skills that Joan possesses (gardening, swimming and socializing, active lifestyle, etc.).
Utilize the driftwood	Enhance the positive aspects of her character and attributes (optimism, desire for independent living, ability to walk with cane, etc.).
Widen the river walls and bed	Assisting with housing through home adaptation or looking at alternative housing. Provide wheelchair to promote independence. Engage with her friends and family to help in her recovery and in achieving her goals. Involve the multi-disciplinary team in her discharge planning and return home.

STEWART

Stewart is a 32-year-old white male. He lives on his own, in a rented flat in a suburb of London. He has a long-term mental health condition and is preoccupied with his benefits situation. He does not cope well with change and was bullied at school. His strengths are as follows: he is friendly and sociable, has supportive friends and brother, has an interest in football, is involved in art classes and is a local volunteer. His difficulties are poor concentration affecting his reading ability and low self-esteem. He has some interest in seeking work but is concerned about whether he would manage.

The focus of Stewart's occupational therapy intervention is shown in Figure 10.7 and Table 10.2.

QUALITIES OF THE KAWA MODEL

The Kawa Model represents a vital addition to conventional occupational therapy conceptual model development. The Kawa Model was developed by occupational therapy practitioners within clinical practice who desired a guiding framework that could be easily understood by both service users/client and therapist (Lim & Iwama 2011). The use of a simple and common 'river' metaphor means the Kawa Model can easily be understood while providing a radically different perspective on how occupation and the self is conceptualized. The Kawa Model emphasizes the importance and centrality of context to an occupation-based occupational therapy, ascribing an ontological basis of viewing the 'self' as inextricably imbedded in the environment rather than as a discrete, centrally situated

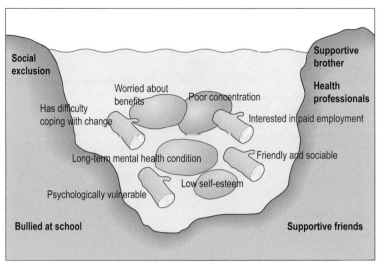

Spaces: He enjoys football, art, volunteer work and reading

Fig. 10.7 Cross-section of Stewart's river before occupational therapy. Potential focal points for occupational therapy intervention. *Sukima*/spaces: potential focal points for occupational therapy. Intervention can be multi-faceted and include breaking or eroding away the (medical) problem, limiting personal liabilities and/or maximizing personal assets, as well as intervening on elements of the greater environment (including the social and physical). Focusing water on these objects to erode or move them is metaphorical of the client using their own abilities or 'life force'.

concern. Users of this Kawa Model are enabled to appreciate better the complexities and transactional qualities of the client within their occupational context. Harmony and balance in this fluid, comprehensive integration of person(s) in context are not based on individual determinism or causation but on all elements that share the complex. The individual within the framework of the Kawa Model is visualized within a wider context, inclusive of their family, community and socio-cultural context.

The Kawa Model can potentially assist the clinician and client to focus on the holistic interplay of strengths, difficulties, assets, circumstances, pressures and so on that may have an impact on the individual (Lim 2006). Such a framework, which harmonizes the status of self vis-a-vis context, is also mirrored in the Kawa Model's view of client-centred occupational therapy. The conventional top-down, hierarchical pattern to therapeutic interactions is upended to enable the client to be the 'expert' in their own occupational narrative (Lim 2018). Although certain categories of concern (life flow, environment, assets and liabilities, difficulties and circumstances) are suggested, ultimately the client names (in their own words) the concepts of the model and explains the principles that relate these concepts. The occupational therapist therefore acts as a facilitator and looks for ways in which their skills and knowledge can contribute towards enabling the client's life

to flow better. The quality of this framework and its philosophical leanings encourages the occupational therapist to 'come alongside the client' and to regard the individual client as the expert in their own lives (Lim 2008, 2018).

This represents a stark difference from the usual practice of 'expert professional knows best' and forcing clients' occupational narratives through (universal) frameworks/instruments containing predetermined sophisticated concepts and principles that are likely to have originated in a different sphere of experiences or culture. How many clients of occupational therapy can readily understand the concepts of occupational therapy models? The Kawa Model challenges the existing hidden power relations embedded in occupational therapy model structures and applications (Lim & Iwama 2011). The representation of a pictorial image that includes the client not only as a stand-alone individual who has difficulties or needs to be addressed, but also as one who possesses strengths, assets and the innate potential to recover. It also helps in focusing attention beyond the individual to include the collective strengths of the individual within their wider context. The visual qualities of the Kawa Model are another asset. They promote greater understanding of the model for those who might otherwise be unable to understand the concepts of existing occupational therapy models that require the mastery of

TABLE 10.2	Stewart's Occupational Therapy and Recovery Process
Water	The aim of occupational therapy is to maximize Stewart's life flow and thereby support his personal recovery.
	This involves reducing and removing elements that impede his river flow and maximizing existing channels where his water currently flows thereby promoting his health and well-being.
Rocks	Identify the difficulties (rocks) and work towards reducing these obstacles. This involves enhancing Stewart's concentration through him engaging in regular focused adult education art and pottery sessions, which also promotes his self-esteem whilst supporting his health and recovery.
	Working with his anxiety positively through exploring his concerns and arranging for him to see a benefits adviser who can answer his questions, whilst teaching him techniques for coping with stress and anxiety.
	Providing psycho-education sessions so that Stewart understands his condition better, how the medication and other therapies can help and also how his existing lifestyle and occupations may support his recovery.
River bed and sides	Widen the river's walls and deepen the river bed, through supporting Stewart in his relationships with his brother and friends and involving them more in supporting his goals, interests and recovery.
	Ensure that the health professionals involved with Stewart are aware and supportive of his goal of engaging in adult education classes, football sessions and exploring the opportunities for paid employment.
	Work with the adult education institutions and course leaders to ensure support and inclusion for Stewart in the art, pottery and voluntary work sessions.
	Offer Stewart the opportunity to be referred for psychological help to explore his experience of being bullied at school.
	Examine his socio-cultural context to understand such factors as his educational experience, personal beliefs and values, family relationships, and cultural perspectives that may influence his health, recovery and well-being.
Driftwood	Identify positive aspects of Stewart's character and attributes that may enhance his life flow and recovery, like his friendliness, sociability and potential interest in paid employment.
	Work on areas like his psychological vulnerability and difficulties with change to equip him with more confidence, skills, knowledge and coping strategies to manage with his anxiety and negative ideas.
Spaces/channels	Identify potential spaces and the context of Stewart's river, whilst determining the areas most important to him.
	Maximize spaces through supporting his engagement in art and pottery classes and exploring opportunities for him to join a book club.
	Maximize the support of his friends in helping him to continue with voluntary work in his local charity shop and to engage in fortnightly five-a-side football to enhance his physical health.

a series of technical terms and professional jargon and terminology understood by few clients or carers that we encounter (Iwama 2006, Lim 2018).

All universal assumptions and proprietary interpretations of the model and its applicability are discouraged, permitting and encouraging occupational therapists to alter and adapt the model in conceptual and structural ways to match the specific social and cultural contexts of their diverse clients. Although the Kawa Model may appear to favour Japanese cultural contexts, it should not be viewed as culturally exclusive. The utility and safety of this model for varying populations depend on the river metaphor's familiarity and relevance to its users. The Kawa Model has been introduced to groups of practitioners in

a variety of cultural settings spanning six continents, with encouraging results (Okuda et al 2000, Hibino et al 2002, Fujimoto et al 2003, Iwama et al 2003, Iwama 2006, Lim 2008).

Occupational therapists should view the Kawa Model as a tool for better understanding and appreciation of their clients' complex occupational worlds. This model is only as powerful as the metaphor that represents it in the client's own cultural context of meanings. Therapists applying the Kawa Model in new or unfamiliar settings or with diverse individuals are advised to refrain from transferring their own views of the metaphor onto the client. Instead the Kawa Model welcomes the search for and use of metaphors that have meaning and relevance for the individual service user/client and discovering metaphors that have meaning and relevance are key to successfully applying the Kawa Model.

DISCUSSION

The Kawa Model was introduced to provide occupational therapists with an alternative perspective aimed at understanding the experiences of their patients and clients. It recognizes the uniqueness, dynamic nature and diversity of each client's occupational narrative and provides a framework within which occupational therapists can appreciate each client in the unique context of their day-to-day realities and circumstances (Lim & Iwama 2011). Hagedorn (2001) highlighted how important it is for occupational therapists to be educated in learning how to think, as opposed to being told what to think or what to do. The Kawa Model fulfils this objective, as it encourages exploration, debate and discussion, and does not prescribe a fixed and predominant view or way of understanding the situation in hand. Ultimately, the model seeks to empower the client by giving credence to their occupational life and issues in the context of the client's perspective of reality rather than imposing a prescribed framework of concepts and principles raised out of another experiential context (Iwama 2006).

The Kawa Model is based on a fluid construction of lived experience with the individual participant provided with the tools to engage in a process of representing his/ her own lived experiences and life world within the visual creation of their Kawa maps. These pictorial and symbolic representations enabled the individual to visually examine and verbally discuss how the different component within their Kawa maps influenced and contributed to their lived experiences. Participants are also encouraged through the use of the Kawa Model to look beyond their presenting challenges and difficulties (rocks) and to consider the different personal assets within their lives which they were drawing upon to positively and proactively enhance their lived experiences and recovery. The Kawa Model also considers the wider range of contextual and environmental influences like family, social support, the physical environment and the cultural norms that may influence both individuals and communities in an increasing diverse and culturally dynamic and vibrant world.

As occupational therapy continues its foray into new cultural frontiers, the diversity of contexts in which people define what is important and of value in daily life in relation to their states of well-being will continue to broaden. Beyond race and ethnicity, conditions of poverty, limited access to technology, a global economy, diversity in health policy, continuation of population migration and deprivation of meaningful participation in society, to name but a few, represent some real-world contexts for the lives of millions of people. These increasingly familiar contexts will challenge the meaning and efficacy of occupational therapy in this era. Occupational therapy proceeds when the client privileges the occupational therapist to develop an interest in their day-to-day circumstances and world of meaning (Iwama 2006). To appreciate the complex dynamic of people's lives and to deliver meaningful interventions that support a better state of harmony, occupational therapists require approaches that are guided and informed by theories and conceptual models that are culturally responsive and safe for their clients. Existing occupational therapy theories and methods of application must be adequate to meet these diverse societal conditions, and blindly applying social-theoretical precepts with universal intent may result in compromising the client's capacity to participate fully in their unique social context and requirements of everyday life (Lim & Iwama 2011).

The Kawa Model challenges the therapist to recognize and respond to the uniqueness of each subject's situation/ context. The structure and meanings of the river metaphor take shape according to the subject's views of their circumstances, in an appropriate cultural context (Lim & Iwama 2006, 2011). The Kawa Model facilitates an examination and understanding of the complex dynamic between people's day-to-day realities and their contexts, and the need to deliver meaningful interventions that support a better state of harmony in people's lives. Occupational therapists require approaches that are guided and informed by theory that is culturally relevant and safe for their clients.

The Kawa Model represents one example of the kind of theoretical material that occupational therapy may need to develop if it is to retain its relevance and effectiveness as it transcends cultural borders (Iwama 2003). Along with the acknowledgement of the primacy of nature in human experience, the Kawa Model also serves as a prototype for a new way of regarding and employing theoretical material in our profession. In this postmodern era of recognizing cultural relativity and variation in worldviews and interpretations of life, the notion of one rigid explanation of occupation and well-being will be increasingly difficult to maintain. That notion would limit occupational therapy's cultural relevance and meaning to a narrower exclusive scope of practice. In many cases, occupational therapists have grown accustomed to wielding their professional license to enforce clients to abide by their own culturally bound assumptions for normal occupational performance.

Occupational therapy, in an ideal sense, should be as unique as its clients—changing its form and approach according to the clients' diverse circumstances and meanings of well-being. To move closer to that ideal, conceptual

---

⁂ **REFLECTIVE LEARNING**

- What socio-cultural norms are embedded in occupational therapy models and frameworks? Do these theoretical materials privilege one cultural group or individual profile over another?
- To what extent are current occupational therapy models and practice frameworks sensitive and relative to the actual, unique, day-to-day contexts and lived realities of your clients?
- Can occupational therapy models, practice frameworks and professional culture end up excluding certain client groups?
- How can we make use of metaphor to better appreciate and understand the service users/clients' life world?
- How do we address issues of diversity, cultural safety and power differentials between professionals and their clients when examining issues of the socio-cultural context, interpretations of occupation, assessments and interventions?
- How do the power relations and dynamics between client and therapist as depicted in the Kawa Model differ from other contemporary models?
- How might implementing the Kawa Model into my practice affect my understanding of my client's occupational world, narrative and lived experience?

---

models and theory should be better informed and drawn, at least in part, from diverse social landscapes and profound contents of the occupational therapist–client practice context. Unless occupational therapists themselves acknowledge and understand the cultural boundaries of their occupational therapy, they may never fulfill occupational therapy's magnificent promise: to enable people from all streams to life to engage and participate in activities and processes that have meaning, value and relevance to their daily lives.

ACKNOWLEDGEMENTS

We would like to acknowledge several individuals who have contributed to this chapter. They are Beki Dellow, May Lim Sok Mui, Helen Mason, Linda Renton, Jouyin Teoh and Natalia Rivas Quarneti.

REFERENCES

Bellah, R. N. (1991). *Beyond belief: Essays in a post-traditionalist world*. Berkeley: University of California Press.
Burr, V. (1995). *An introduction to social constructionism*. London: Routledge.
Doi, T. (1973). *The anatomy of dependence*. Tokyo: Kodansha International.
Fujimoto, H., Yoshimura, N., & Iwama, M. (2003). *The Kawa (River) Model Workshop addressing diversity of culture in occupational therapy*. Singapore: 3rd Asia Pacific Occupational Therapy Congress.
Gergen, K. J. (1999). *An invitation to social construction*. Thousand Oaks: Sage.
Gray, M., & McPherson, K. (2005). Cultural safety and professional practice in occupational therapy: A New Zealand perspective. *Australian Occupational Therapy Journal*, 52(1), 34–42.
Gregg, B. T., Howell, D. M., Quick, C. D., & Iwama, M. K. (2015). The Kawa river model: applying theory to develop interventions for combat and operational stress control. *Occupational Therapy in Mental Health*, 31(4), 366–384.
Gustafson, J. M. (1993). *Man and nature: A cross-cultural perspective*. Bangkok: Chulalongkorn University Press.
Hagedorn, R. (2001). *Foundations for practice in occupational therapy*. Edinburgh: Churchill Livingstone.
Hibino, K., Tanaka, M., & Iwama, M. (2002). *Applying a new model of Japanese occupational therapy to a client case of depression*. Stockholm: 13th International Congress of the World Federation of Occupational Therapists.
Humbert, T. K., Bess, J. L., & Mowery, A. M. (2013). Exploring women's perspectives of overcoming intimate partner violence: A phenomenological study. *Occupational Therapy in Mental Health*, 29(3), 246–265.
Iwama, M. (2003). The issue is...toward culturally relevant epistemologies in occupational therapy. *American Journal of Occupational Therapy*, 57(5), 582–588.
Iwama, M. (2005a). Situated meanings: An issue of culture, inclusion and occupational therapy. In F. Kronenberg, S. A. Algado, & N. Pollard (Eds.), *Occupational therapy without borders – Learning from the spirit of survivors*. Edinburgh: Churchill Livingstone.
Iwama, M. (2005b). Meaning and inclusion: Revisiting culture in occupational therapy. *Australian Occupational Therapy Journal*, 51, 1–2.
Iwama, M. (2006). *The Kawa Model: Culturally relevant occupational therapy*. Edinburgh: Churchill Livingstone.
Iwama, M. (2007). Culture and occupational therapy: Meeting the challenge of relevance in a global world. *Occupational Therapy International*, 14(4), 183–187.
Jungerson, K. (1992). Culture, theory and the practice of occupational therapy in New Zealand/Aotearoa. *American Journal of Occupational Therapy*, 46, 745–750.
Lakoff, G., & Johnson, M. (1980). *Metaphors we live by*. Chicago: University of Chicago Press.
Lebra, S. (1976). *Japanese patterns of behavior*. Honolulu: University of Hawaii Press.
Lim, K. H. (2006). Case studies in the application of the Kawa Model. In M. K. Iwama (Ed.), *The Kawa Model: Culturally relevant occupational therapy*. Edinburgh: Elsevier.
Lim, K. H. (2008a). Cultural sensitivity in context. In E. A. McKay, C. Craik, K. H. Lim, et al. (Eds.), *Advancing occupational therapy in mental health Practice* (pp. 30–47). Blackwell.

Lim, K. H. (2008b). Working in a transcultural context. In J. Creek, & L. Lougher (Eds.), *Occupational therapy and mental health* (4th ed.) (pp. 251–274). Edinburgh: Churchill Livingstone.

Lim, K. H., & Iwama, M. (2006). Emerging models – an Asian perspective: The Kawa (River) Model. In E. Duncan (Ed.), *Foundations for practice* (4th ed.). Edinburgh: Elsevier.

Lim, K. H., & Iwama, M. (2011). The Kawa (River) Model. In E. Duncan (Ed.), *Foundations for practice* (5th ed.). Edinburgh: Elsevier.

Lim, K. H. (2018). *Personal journeys of recovery: Exploring the experiences of mental health service users engaging with the Kawa 'River' model. Doctoral dissertation.* London: Brunel University.

McKay, Craik, C., Lim, K. H., & Richards, G. (2008). *Advancing occupational therapy in mental health practice.* Oxford, UK: Blackwell Publishing.

Nakane, C. (1970). *Tate shakai no ningen kankei [Human Relations in a Vertical Society].* Tokyo: Kodansha.

Okuda, M., Iwama, M., Hatsutori, T., et al. (2000). A Japanese model of occupational therapy. One: the 'river model' raised from the clinical setting. *Journal of the Japanese Association of Occupational Therapists, 19*(Suppl), 512.

Ramsden, I. (1990). *Kawa Whakaruruhau—Cultural safety in nursing education in Aotearoa: Report to the Ministry of Education.* Wellington: Ministry of Education.

Ramugondo, E. (2018). Healing work: Intersections for decoloniality. *World Federation of Occupational Therapists Opening Keynote Address* https://www.youtube.com/watch?v=S96IIytPG9I.

Shakespeare, T. (1994). Cultural representation of disabled people: dustbins for disavowal? *Disability and Society, 9*, 283–299.

Whalley Hammell, K., & Carpenter, C. (2004). *Qualitative research in evidence-based rehabilitation.* Edinburgh: Churchill Livingstone.

Whalley Hammell, K. (2018). *World Federation of Occupational Therapists Final Day Plenary.* https://www.youtube.com/watch?v=9WipUPXx_Kk.

Frames of Reference

11

The Person-Centred Frame of Reference

Davina M. Parker, Catherine Sutherland

OVERVIEW

The core principle of practice in occupational therapy across many countries worldwide places the person at the centre of all intervention. This approach has been articulated variably as client-centred practice (Sumsion & Law 2006) or person-centred occupational practice (Brown 2013). Professional bodies have affirmed this approach by incorporating it into codes of conduct and standards of practice, as in the United Kingdom, for example, where the Royal College of Occupational Therapists (RCOT) sets the benchmark for practice by stating that 'the College is committed to person-centred practice and the involvement of the service user as a partner in all stages of the therapeutic process, (College of Occupational Therapists 2015).

Theory-based models have done much to provide occupational therapists with a rationale for their thinking, but little has been done to explore the application of a person-centred approach as a frame of reference with which to mould and shape practice. This chapter guides the therapist and aspiring practitioner through the occupational therapy process to connect the theory of person-centred practice with the reality of everyday service delivery, using an individual case to illustrate converting theory into practice.

For the purpose of this chapter and to provide the reader with consistency, those engaging in occupational therapy will be referred to as 'the person' or 'the individual'. However, in terms of the language used and the range of organizations where occupational therapy is delivered, other terms may be in use: *client, service user* or *patient*.

INTRODUCTION

Person-centred care is considered the optimum way of delivering healthcare, as the individuals' perspectives are regarded as important indicators of quality in healthcare (Gan et al 2008). It is defined as care provision that is consistent with the values, needs and desires of patients, and is achieved when clinicians involve patients in healthcare discussions and decisions (Mead & Bower 2000). Person- or client-centred practice is advocated as the way ahead for occupational therapy internationally (Falardeau & Durand 2002, Palmadottir 2003, Conneeley 2004). The reality of being a person-centred therapist can, however, be demanding and sometimes bewildering, but also a rewarding way to practice. It requires a true understanding of how to deliver person-centred practice and a recognition that it permeates all aspects of interactions with people.

So, what is person-centred practice all about? Put simply, person-centred practice is a process in which occupational therapy revolves around the individual as the focal point of intervention (Maitra & Erway 2006); therapy is tailored to individual needs. This chapter will help you to understand and use a person-centred frame of reference in your practice. The chapter aims to

- define the person-centred frame of reference
- describe the context of person-centred practice
- explore the principles of a person-centred frame of reference
- provide examples of the application of the person-centred frame of reference in practice.

Using a vignette to illustrate ways in which person-centred practice can be achieved will help to link the theory of this frame of reference into practice. Throughout this chapter, the task for you, the reader, is to examine your own working style for evidence of the person-centred approach. Reflective questions at the end of the chapter will help you achieve this.

> ◎ **HIGHLIGHTS**
>
> This chapter
> - explores what being person-centred means in practice
> - describes the key elements of a person-centred frame of reference
> - applies the person-centred frame of reference throughout the occupational therapy process
> - emphasizes respect, partnership and communication
> - encourages self-reflection on practice.

Historical Roots of Person-Centred Practice

The person-centred approach is firmly rooted in the work of Carl Rogers, who used the term *client-centred practice* in his book, *The Clinical Treatment of the Problem Child* (Rogers 1939, 1951, Law et al 1995, Corring & Cook 1999). In this text he described a practice that was nondirective and focused on concerns expressed by the individual. He believed that people receiving services were capable of playing an active role in defining and solving problems, with the therapist as a facilitator to help solve their problems, enabling understanding and proposing solutions. Two of the most important points he made in the articulation of person-centred therapy were the skill of listening and the exploration of the quality of the therapist–individual interaction (Law et al 1995). Rogers, along with other theorists such as Abraham Maslow, tried to separate the humanistic approaches of human interaction from the more mechanistic and biological approaches favoured by the likes of Freud and Skinner (Simon & Daub 1993). His approach stressed the importance of some key elements: empathy, respect, active listening and an understanding of the person's self-actualization. These themes echo the structures underpinning a person-centred frame of reference in occupational therapy.

Background to Person-Centred Practice in Occupational Therapy

The person-centred approach is not a uni-professional domain, however; its development in occupational therapy took place in Canada and emerged as 'client centred practice'. During the 1980s Canadian occupational therapists explored and described the links between the theoretical framework of occupational performance and the core values of person-centredness. In the *Guidelines for the Client-centred Practice of Occupational Therapy*, which are still relevant (Canadian Association of Occupational Therapists & Department of National Health and Welfare 1983, 1991), the acknowledgement of the worth of, and the holistic approach to, the individual was explicit. The core elements of this person-centred approach, identified by Law (1998), were

- respect
- personal responsibility for decision making
- provision of information and communication
- participation in individualized service delivery
- personal enablement
- the person–environment–occupation relationship

Respect

Respect for the individual means consideration of their opinions, choices and values as well as their limitations and capabilities. In the therapist–individual relationship, negotiation is recommended as offering greater scope for achieving a balanced approach in person-centred care (Falardeau & Durand 2002). Listening and demonstrating empathy can provide the basis for a trusting relationship with the individual, as well as recognizing the strengths and resources that each person brings to the therapeutic encounter (Law et al 2001).

Personal Responsibility for Decision Making

Individual experiences and self-knowledge about one's own needs should be valued and used to enable the individual to make choices about which issues they need help with. People may be exposed to risks to their individual safety when defining their problems and seeking solutions. Risks and failure can be a valuable learning experience; however, this needs to be balanced within a safe environment (Moats 2007). The therapist should not support actions that are unethical, could lead to harm or be deemed as malpractice, as there is a professional responsibility to ensure that people are informed about risks and to advise them on techniques and activities that may support risk avoidance (Moats & Doble 2006).

Information and Communication

Providing choice means that person-centred care should address individual needs and values (Rebeiro 2000a); however, enabling people to make informed choices and set achievable goals means that individuals have the right to be given information in a manner they understand. Sharing information in a common language understandable by therapist and individual is both respectful and affirming of the therapeutic relationship (Lum et al 2004).

Individualized Service Delivery

Appreciating people as individuals means planning treatments and services which meet their needs rather than expecting them to slot into a set intervention programme. Using a person-centred frame of reference, jointly agreed goal-setting and individualized outcome measures to evaluate practice will ensure individualized service delivery is achieved.

Personal Enablement

Person-centred care means intervention is structured by the goals and expected outcomes agreed between the individual and the therapist. Achievement of these goals may come about as a result of changing roles or environment, skills or occupations rather than pure remediation. The emphasis throughout is on listening to the person and enabling them to explore, achieve and maintain their goals (Creek 2003).

Person–Environment–Occupation

The context of a person's life has been described as contextual congruence; in other words, it is the situation in which a person lives, their roles, expectations, interests and environments. It is about appreciating people as individuals rather than as a medical diagnosis or label. Part of the unique concept of the person-centred approach is the acknowledgement that people are not separate from their environments, which can present both challenges and potential solutions to problems in daily living (Sumsion 2006).

A DEFINITION OF PERSON-CENTRED PRACTICE

In the wider context of health and social care, person-centred care is about health and social care professionals working collaboratively with people who use services, both individuals and their carers (Morgan & Yoder 2012). This approach supports people to develop the knowledge, skills and confidence they need to more effectively manage and make informed decisions about their own health and healthcare (Fig. 11.1). It is co-ordinated and tailored to the needs of the individual, and, crucially, it ensures that people are always treated with dignity, compassion and respect (The Health Foundation 2016):

1. Affording people dignity, compassion and respect.
2. Offering co-ordinated care, support or treatment.
3. Offering personalized care, support or treatment.
4. Supporting people to recognize and develop their own strengths and abilities to enable them to live an independent and fulfilling life.

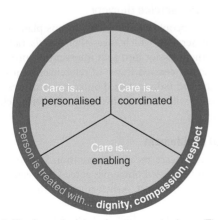

Fig. 11.1 The four principles of person-centred care (The Health Foundation October 2016. Person-centred Care Made Simple. The Health Foundation, 90 Long Acre, London WC2E 9RA. Reproduced by kind permission of The Health Foundation.)

In occupational therapy, person-centred practice is embedded in the Code of Ethics and Professional Conduct for Therapists (COT 2015) and in professional standards (COT 2017) where we are reminded that services should be person-centred and needs-led. These documents reinforce that therapists should demonstrate a commitment to person-centred practice involving the service user as a partner in all stages of the therapeutic process (COT 2017). Sumsion (2000) redefined 'client-centred practice' by recognizing the need to relate this approach to the realities of clinical practice. This definition clearly shaped person-centred practice within the context of resource-limited health services but reinforced a working respect for and real partnership with people, whilst recognizing that many factors influenced the successful implementation of client-centred practice.

To be comfortable using a person-centred frame of reference, the therapist should identify their own values and assumptions (Rebeiro 2000a) and check that they match the core values of person-centred practice: namely, respect, partnership and the ability to listen to the individual. Essentially, the foundation of person-centred practice is the capacity of the therapist to view the world through the individual's eyes (Jamieson et al 2006). To achieve this, it is vital that therapists understand the key elements of this frame of reference.

KEY ELEMENTS OF A PERSON-CENTRED FRAME OF REFERENCE

The Individual

The person-centred nature of occupational therapy acknowledges the individual as the central element in intervention (Donnelly & Carswell 2002). However, the therapist should be clear about who the person/client/patient/service user is and base planned intervention on their needs and with their full knowledge and co-operation. This is usually the individual who is referred to the service, but they may also be carers, family, support groups or others (Sumsion 1997).

Partnership

The importance of engaging in an effective partnership with an individual is vital. Understanding the meaning of partnership requires the therapist to recognize that achieving the end goal requires working together. Several studies have noted the dissonance that occurs when the therapist's and individual's expectations of the results of therapy are at odds (Law et al 1995, Banks et al 1997, Blank 2004, Sumsion & Smyth 2000). These studies found that the individual's perception of the problem was usually much more relevant than that of the therapist. Partnership is about working together to achieve goals—goals that are focused on individual issues and what the person wants to achieve. Those that are important to them and are framed within an agreed clear intervention plan are more likely to succeed. A practical way of achieving this is for the individual to have a copy of their goals and intervention plan. Another is to use an individualized outcome measure, for example, the Canadian Occupational Performance Measure (COPM) (Law et al 1990) (see Chapter 7). People whose views on intervention and service issues are sought are likely to experience increased confidence about engaging in a working partnership with therapists (Parker 2013).

Respect and Listening

Listening is vital to understand truly what is and what is not said (Whalley Hammell 2002). Bibyk et al (1999) suggest that a person-centred therapist is welcoming, that they are nonthreatening and nonauthoritarian. By being non-judgemental, they are in a better position to listen to the individual and engage in conversation. Respect is about demonstrating value for a person's views and opinions, not imposing your views on others. A person-centred therapist accepts a person for who and what they are and where they are at (Bibyk et al 1999). Falardeau and Durand (2002) suggest that respect of the individual goes beyond their opinions, choices and values; it includes their limitations and capabilities. Individual abilities and understanding may set limits on interaction, and in some circumstances it may be helpful to intervene against a person's will, especially when issues of risk and safety have been identified. Being able to show respect for an individual, to listen and to demonstrate empathy provide the basis for a trusting relationship with people. Such respect makes sense of this suggested definition, 'client-centred care means I am a valued human being' (Corring & Cook 1999). Brown (2013), however, suggests that a small change in professional terminology from client to person may seem trivial but is reflective of a more co-operative partnership with those to whom we provide occupation-focused services.

Empowerment

Bibyk et al (1999) suggest that the absence of a struggle for power and control is one of the most tangible indicators of how it feels to be with a person-centred therapist. Person-centred practice shifts power in the therapeutic relationship from the therapist as the expert, to the individual as a partner (Canadian Association of Occupational Therapists 2002). People are experts in their own condition and hold a wealth of knowledge about their own unique circumstances. Enabling the individual to recognize this knowledge base and use it to aid recovery is what makes the person-centred approach so unique (Lane 2000).

Goal Negotiation

One of the challenges of applying a person-centred frame of reference to practice is recognizing the shift from therapist-created goals to person-led ones. Many studies re-inforce the need for service users and therapists to work together at defining, clarifying and achieving goals (Peloquin 1997, Rebeiro 2000a). Negotiation can only start once a relationship has been forged and when listening to and communicating with each other are comfortable. Active engagement in problem identification and planning is a fundamental part of working in a person-centred way (Law et al 1997). The therapist should use clinical reasoning skills to evaluate performance and match individual skills with potential to achieve goals (Mew & Fossey 1996). Negotiation about how to achieve established goals, the risks involved and an agreed time frame demands constant attention and much sharing of information between therapist and client. The biggest barrier that prevents person-centred practice taking place occurs as a result of a therapist and individual having different goals (Sumsion & Smyth 2000). This barrier can often be resolved through effective communication.

Language

The use of language in communication is vital but do we speak the same language? In modern healthcare our service user population is diverse and varied, and comes from many ethnic backgrounds. It is inevitable that a therapist may not share the mother tongue of the people with whom they work. Therapists may need to access interpreters to assist, but that in itself may create a barrier to true person-centred working. The use of language is equally important: in other words, what and how things are said. Too often we as therapists hide behind our 'professional' language both to protect and to preserve a sense of our authority and knowledge. If we are really to apply a person-centred frame of reference to our practice, then we must consider the language we use when working with each individual. Clear information and simple explanations can go a long way to ensuring equality in the way we communicate. The way that language is used is also important. Check out this example:

- 'You must use your delta walker in the house or else you will fall and end up in hospital'—a non-person-centred approach
- 'You have told me you do not want to use your walking aid at home, and I understand why, but I have concerns about your risk of falling. Have you thought about that?'—a person-centred version

Informed Decision Making

It is unrealistic to expect anyone to make decisions about their lives if they do not have relevant information or do not understand how to interpret that information to inform their decision making. As people acquire more knowledge of their condition, this promotes self-esteem (Christiansen 1991); however, this may challenge therapists if they fail to understand about partnership in person-centred working (Parker 2013). Honest and factual explanations about risk and safety are another way of informing individuals and helping them to make safe and appropriate decisions about their care. The way we communicate is also important, backing up verbal explanations with clear and easily understandable written information, or clearly signposting them to other sources of information, for example, the World Wide Web.

DEFINITION OF A PERSON-CENTRED FRAME OF REFERENCE

A person-centred frame of reference is a framework that *guides* practice where the individual is the *focus* of *needs*-led occupational therapy, delivered with *respect* and in *partnership*. In short: *think person, plan practice*. Core beliefs of this frame of reference are
- assumed values of respect, partnership and enablement
- a shared belief that the person is the centre of all therapeutic activity
- the person's needs and goals directing how the occupational therapy process is delivered
- clinical reasoning and practice delivery structured to reflect those needs.

APPLYING THE PERSON-CENTRED FRAME OF REFERENCE IN PRACTICE

To understand how to apply a person-centred frame of reference in practice, it is necessary to appreciate the complexity and challenges of such practice and demonstrate this with confidence (Rebeiro 2000b, Chen et al 2002). Given that a frame of reference is there to provide structure to practice, it makes sense to consider how a person-centred approach can be applied throughout the occupational therapy process. Following the vignette, each stage includes questions to assist in the development of reasoning in the application of this frame of reference. Furthermore, support, training and the opportunity for reflection are crucial for therapists to undertake person-centred practice and to develop confidence and competence in it (Parker 2013, Lewin et al 2008).

The Occupational Therapy Process

Foster's (2002) occupational therapy process (i.e., gathering and analyzing data, planning and preparing for intervention, implementing intervention and evaluating outcomes) is a logical sequence. A variation of this process is followed by occupational therapists in most areas of practice. Its success is dependent on the rigour of data collection and its analysis at each stage. Frequently, the occupational therapy process is not a linear event but a cyclical one, which should be sensitive to the changing health and environmental needs of the individual. They should be engaged at all times throughout the process and should be guided by their occupational therapist's clinical reasoning ability and expert knowledge of the condition (Hong et al 2000). The occupational therapist's judgement and reasoning will, however, depend on experience, clinical expertise, data analysis and a true understanding and connection with the individual (Carpenter et al 2001, Turner 2002; see also Chapter 15).

The past decade has seen a change in how services are delivered to an individual. As an occupational therapist, it is rare to work in isolation from other health and social care professionals. Services tend to be multi-disciplinary or inter-disciplinary, with a focus on individual needs within a service specification outlined by the funding authority, which are modelled around the need to be person-centred for the individual to manage their condition. Experienced occupational therapists are well placed to lead on these services and demonstrate a true person-centred approach to intervention.

Referral, Data-Gathering and Analysis
Aim.
- To provide baseline information for assessment and intervention.

Data-gathering is continuous throughout the occupational therapy process and information is gained by assessment, observation, listening and analysis, all of which contribute towards the evaluation of progress and attainment of goals.
Process.
- Receiving a referral is the first information that the therapist has about the individual.
- The referral itself may provide little information about the person and should act as a reason for contact rather than directing what must take place.
- Gathering of data may be indirect, noting information from the medical records, or direct, when first contact is made with the individual.
- All information gathered should be accurate and reliable, and must meet professional requirements by being documented in the records to provide an honest, contemporaneous record of the history of the encounter.
Considerations.
How are referrals received?
- Is the occupational therapy provision part of a wider multi-disciplinary or inter-disciplinary team?
- Does the occupational therapist, team or service specification dictate who, when and how people are seen for occupational therapy or are users involved in that process?
- Can individuals self-refer? Do they have a choice?

Action:
- Review whether your service is clear about how people can access it.
- Change the process of referral, away from the traditional method of 'medical referral' by doctors, to a system based on personal need or self-referral.
- Consult with and involve user representatives, to ensure their opinion influences how occupational therapy is delivered.
- Publicize how people can access occupational therapy by means of information leaflets, posters, website, apps and audio-visual material.

When the referral is received, how do you name that person? Action:
- Always ask the individual how they wish to be addressed and then note that in their records. This reflects respect for, and recognition of, the individual as a person in their own right and prevents the likelihood of assumed superiority by the therapist.

Does the person understand the reason for the referral? Action:
- Ask the person referred whether they know and understand the reason for a referral to the service you are representing. Ensure you feel comfortable in representing your team of professionals as well as in your own role in the team as an occupational therapist.
- Check that they are comfortable with this and are happy to proceed.
- Check that you have told them how occupational therapy will be delivered.

Does the individual know why an occupational therapist needs to ask certain questions about their personal circumstances? Action:
- Data-gathering needs to be accurate and the source of that information noted.
- Be mindful that information taken from a third party may not truly reflect accuracy, or may be out of date or biased by individual views.
- Place the person at ease in what may be a stressful and bewildering situation by explaining each step clearly.
- Observation of how the individual responds to the therapist and the therapeutic environment is vital, as this will form part of the data-gathering for useful background information in planning intervention.
- Always start an initial assessment with an introduction and explanation about occupational therapy and the wider team involved.
- Giving information, both verbal and written, is part of achieving the person–professional balance and will empower the individual with knowledge.
- People may need time to reflect on the role that an occupational therapist plays in their care and so may have additional questions/issues to explore at future meetings.

Is the person able to give informed consent for occupational therapy? Action:
- Unless the individual has the information about what occupational therapy does and what support it can give them, they will not be able to give informed consent actively to participate in a course of therapy.

Do they have capacity or is this impaired? Can they make decisions for themselves (Department for Constitutional Affairs 2007)? Action:
- Provide accurate information about your service, for example, information leaflets.
- Consult with users of your service and invite feedback when developing service information, by establishing user focus groups.
- Take care with language, making sure the tone is 'right' without seeming patronizing and that the message is clear and accurate.
- For paediatric and learning difficulty services, a person-friendly information leaflet can be designed using characters or cartoons. Ask your speech and language colleagues for assistance in its design.
- Identify the most appropriate method to provide information for those with a visual impairment.
- Visual message boards can be used for the hearing-impaired.
- Check that mental capacity has been assessed if problems occur, but still include the client in all aspects of intervention even if capacity is impaired.

Case Study: Part 1. Charles is 45 and lives with his wife and 75-year-old mother, who has dementia, in an owner-occupied house. He and his wife have a 25-year-old son and a 21-year-old daughter, who live close by. They have a number of caged pets and two large dogs. Charles always enjoyed tinkering with his classic cars, taking the dogs for long walks and holidaying in their caravan. His wife is the main breadwinner and also carer for her mother-in-law. Their children are very supportive and visit regularly, looking after their grandmother while their parents are on holiday.

Charles presents with a number of medical conditions that have prevented him from working since the age of 35. He went into kidney failure and while awaiting a kidney transplant had dialysis three times a week. This resulted in a long period of depression, which was resolving when he had a successful kidney transplant at the age of 40, but he was then diagnosed with type II diabetes. As a result of the diabetes, Charles has peripheral neuropathy and a glaucoma in his left eye, as well as episodes of depression.

He had a right hemisphere stroke at the age of 43, with no rehabilitation follow-up on discharge from hospital, followed by a second left hemisphere stroke while at home. He was admitted to the acute stroke unit in his local hospital and is recovering well, but still presents with symptoms of fatigue, reduced fine motor dexterity, power and co-ordination and impaired balance and is again low in mood because of the frustrations of not being as active as he was following his successful transplant. Charles is also anxious that he will become depressed and lack motivation to engage in rehabilitation, delaying his discharge home. Charles is keen to return home to be able to work on his cars rather than instruct his wife in what to do, take the dogs for walks and be self-sufficient during the day when his wife is at work.

Planning and Preparing for Intervention

Aim.

- Using all available information, formulate an assessment of function and need and determine goals to be achieved.

Process.

- Using a semi-structured interview, explore occupational performance issues relevant to the individual.
- Consider self-care, productivity and leisure issues.
- Identify and document which issues are most important to the individual.
- Know the person's deficits.

The initial assessment meeting with the individual is crucial in setting the scene and establishing the parameters of the therapeutic encounter. Frequency, duration of sessions and the focus of occupational therapy are important parts of this phase. Once the person's problems have been identified, the next stage is to determine what goals need to be achieved. Once this has been agreed, the method of attaining them, the approach used and the individual responsibilities for specific aspects of intervention need to be confirmed. The person-centred approach may need explanation, as it may be unfamiliar to the individual who is used to a traditional model of encounter with medical staff. It is crucial that the individual understands the key issues of the working relationship you establish with them, as this will be built on throughout the encounter (Sumsion 1999).

This stage is all about exploration: what problems and issues need to be discussed, as well as how the individual wishes to see these changed. As the relationship with the person develops, the therapist should start to determine the individual's strengths and resources. During the assessment phase the therapist will help them understand how occupational therapy can support them and link this with an early understanding of the person's views of the problem.

Identification of problems and goal-setting are two of the most important elements of the rehabilitation process (Wressle et al 2002). Although goal-setting may be the domain of the therapist, an approach worth adopting that is more reflective of being person-centred is to formulate the intervention plan based on individual-identified issues (Parker 2013). This ensures intervention reflects individual needs, especially if issues are described in their own words. Therapists should be aware that time can be a barrier to the person-centred approach (Wilkins et al 2001, Maitra & Erway 2006), as it takes time to share information, develop the relationship and understand the outcome of the assessments before goals are agreed (Corring 1999).

Considerations

How do you introduce the assessment process with the person? Action:

- Use language that a person will understand when explaining how you are going to assess their skills and why.
- Be comfortable with your own words; if you are not, practice key phrases with peers or user focus groups.

Does the individual understand and agree with the reason for referral? Action:

- Check and note in the records an understanding of this.
- Use a consent form that they can sign, making sure they have a copy.
- An easy check is to note the actual way that the person expresses themselves.

Does the individual understand what the process of assessment means? Action:

- Explain clearly the steps of assessment and what is involved.
- Be aware that some people may view assessments as a test of their ability.
- Give reassurance that there is no one correct way of doing things.
- Respect the individual way an individual carries out activities.

Can the individual identify their own needs and problems? Action:

- In an unfamiliar environment, the person may require help to identify needs which relate to their home circumstances.
- Assist them by talking through their day, noting issues with which they may need support.
- Use this information to help the person formulate their own goals.
- Reflect back to them with an outline of their issues to ensure clarity.

Is there an issue of 'locus of control'? Action:

- Recognize the person's expert knowledge of their own condition and how it affects them.

- Listen to the way in which they explain their problems and articulate the issues of their life.
- Use a person-centred outcomes measure, like the COPM, to ensure that true person-centred intervention planning takes place.
- Encourage the individual in making choices and initiating ideas.

What happens if the individual is confused, cognitively impaired or lacking in capacity? Action:

- Clearly identify deficits through assessment.
- Explain these in simple terms to both the individual and carer together.
- Involve the person at all stages of intervention by not ignoring their changed mental state.
- Repeat instructions carefully and keep language simple.
- Use picture boards to remind or replicate complex directions.
- Balance risk identification and reduction to create a safe environment (Moats 2007).

Case Study: Part 2. Charles: planning and preparing for intervention.

The hospital occupational therapist met Charles on the ward and set about establishing his abilities and occupational performance issues. Charles told the occupational therapist that his key aim was to go home. The initial assessment and goal-setting enabled them to agree what support was required to enable him to go home and, because an initial date had been agreed for his discharge, a plan was mapped out.

Charles was eligible for a community service that supported an earlier discharge from hospital. This service was time limited and it was clear that there were long-term issues which needed addressing in the community on discharge from the hospital. Charles wanted to go home and be independent as well as carry on with his leisure interests.

Talking to Charles about his desire to go home as soon as possible, the occupational therapist helped him focus on what he needed to work on to be fit for discharge. Together they completed a COPM to help name and frame the occupational performance problems reflecting Charles's priorities. The following issues were identified and it was agreed that they would form the basis for the intervention plan:

- Self-care:
  - Managing to wash, shower and shave
  - Preparing hot drinks and cold lunch snacks
  - Managing self-medication
  - Mobilizing safely around his home
  - Ascending/descending steps and stairs.
- Productivity:
  - Being self-supporting during the day
  - Getting out and about.

- Leisure:
  - Regaining his ability to work on his classic cars
  - Wanting to feel safe when walking, to take the dogs for walks
  - Wanting to be able to go on holiday and enjoy the experience.

The five key issues he chose to concentrate on in hospital were

1. To be able to make hot drinks and sandwiches and look after himself during the day at home
2. To be able to manage his own medication
3. To be able to move around at home safely, without falling
4. To shower, dress and shave independently
5. To be able to tinker with his classic cars.

Implementing Intervention

Aim.

- To practice the skills necessary to achieve individual outcomes.

The intervention plan should set out how an individual's goals are to be met and in what time scale. It should be explicit about the approaches used, the activity to be carried out and the range of options available. Choices of where the intervention is to be carried out are also important. This may be at home, or in the community or therapy department; these choices may impact on performance. Intervention may not always be on a one-to-one basis; groups may provide a more suitable medium to achieve goals related to communication and social skills.

Process.

- Agree to a programme of intervention, negotiating time and duration.
- Be clear about what resources are and are not available.
- Provide feedback to the individual on their performance.
- Identify and explain risks and explore alternative actions.
- Listen to the person's opinions on progress and concerns.

Considerations

Does the individual understand how the intervention plan will address their issues?

Action:

- Explain the intervention plan to the person and check for understanding.
- Provide a copy for the individual to keep.
- Negotiate times within the constraints of everyday commitments and work pressures.
- Keep the person informed of changes to the plan that may have an impact on outcomes.

Does the individual understand that other agencies are involved in providing care and intervention?
Action:
- Gain consent to liaise with colleagues and carers.
- Carry out home visits and specialist interventions jointly, with the person, carers or community agencies present.
- Always ensure the individual's voice is heard amidst the professional ones.
- Review goals throughout the intervention stage to check against reality.

What happens if the individual changes their mind about what they want to achieve?
Action:
- Work in partnership with them—then you will understand the challenges they face.
- Listen to their views and concerns.
- Point out the risks of pursuing a particular course of action if there are concerns about risk or safety.
- Suggest alternative or safer options.
- Engage the person in active problem solving.
- Adjust the intervention plan to accommodate new goals.
- Use clinical reasoning to adjust and adapt intervention.
    Case Study: Part 3. Charles: implementing intervention.
The occupational therapist used the Canadian Model of Occupational Performance (CMOP) to provide the theoretical underpinning to her practice and selected the person-centred frame of reference to steer her practice. The intervention plan included assessment and practice using the shower (stepping in/out of the bath, transfers, standing and use of equipment), drink and snack preparation, fine motor dexterity, co-ordination and power (self-medication, shaving), mobility and falls management (in a variety of environments and terrains) and fatigue management strategies. The occupational therapist needed to be mindful of Charles's low mood and previous episodes of depression. Charles displayed his frustration when he did not see any significant improvements and the occupational therapist needed to ensure that objective measurements were taken, which demonstrated to Charles the improvements he had made in specific tasks and activities. This assisted to increase his mood and self-esteem and empowered him to engage in rehabilitation.

Evaluating Outcomes
Aim.
- To measure and evaluate intervention in relation to the plan agreed with the individual person.
Process.

- Evaluate performance.
- Carry out specific tests if indicated.
- Match performance with agreed outcomes.
- Agree on an action plan if there are deficits.
- Agree on referral to other agencies to meet further needs.

At an agreed point in the occupational therapy process, the therapist evaluates progress with the individual. This may be at frequent intervals throughout the therapeutic encounter, but ultimately the final evaluation of whether goals have been achieved will be made at the transition from one environment to another, usually at the point of discharge from a service. Evaluation is a means for determining continuation or change for both the therapist and the individual.

The evaluation of outcomes should take the form of a meeting between the therapist and service user to review goals and match intervention with progress. The most person-centred way of doing this is to use a person-centred outcomes measure, such as the COPM. This tool will ensure the individual is engaged in the occupational therapy process, as person-selected goals reflect prioritized issues of occupational performance, and change in a person's perception of their performance is measured during the course of occupational therapy (Law et al 1990) (see Chapter 7).

Considerations
What happens if the individual has not reached their goals or addressed their concerns? Action:
- Encourage realism throughout intervention by reminding them of the end goal or destination.
- Check that the person understands about any changes in role or environment.
- Clarify how satisfied the person is with progress.
- Use the COPM to match performance and satisfaction.
- Share outcome results with them.
    Case Study: Part 4. Charles: evaluating outcomes.
Once the discharge was agreed, Charles and the occupational therapist reviewed progress and Charles re-evaluated himself on the COPM with the change scores shown in Table 11.1.

This phase focused on his return home; however, because Charles had outstanding issues remaining, he was transferred to the earlier supported discharge team to carry on working on his identified goals with the occupational therapist, who worked with him to establish new goals, completing a new COPM and continuing intervention. These included kitchen skills practice with occupational therapy assistant support, attending a falls prevention group, carrying out a hand therapy programme at home (including specific exercises, functional related movements and tasks), support in fatigue management principles and adapting day-to-day activities, mobilizing within his local

TABLE 11.1   Canadian Occupational Performance Measure Scores for Charles at Discharge

Occupational Performance Problems	Performance 1	Satisfaction 1	Performance 2	Satisfaction 2
Unable to prepare own hot drinks and snacks	3	3	6	8
Reliant on wife to dispense and administer medication	1	1	7	8
Risk of falling within home environment	2	2	3	2
Difficulty carrying out personal care activities such as showering, dressing and shaving	3	3	8	8
Unable to work on his classic cars	1	1	3	3
Change in performance	3.4			
Change in satisfaction	3.8			

TABLE 11.2   Person-Centred Checklist

When I reflect on my practice do I:	Yes/no
Plan intervention around the needs of the person?	
Establish an empathic relationship with them?	
Respect and listen to what they say?	
Select therapeutic interventions to meet their needs?	
Offer choices and solutions?	
Naturally communicate with them in a genuine and honest manner?	
Cut down barriers to ensure they feel welcome in my service?	
Engage them actively in a partnership throughout the occupational therapy process?	
Negotiate with them about goals and outcomes?	
Treat them politely and equally?	
Respect them when they change their minds and re focus their goals?	
Ensure they understand about risks, safety issues and resource limitations?	
Demonstrate confidence in my practice?	
Am I person-centred?	

community without the dogs to get used to the environment and terrains. When Charles and the occupational therapist agreed that he had met his goals, she re-assessed his performance using the COPM and the change scores shown in Table 11.1 were calculated.

Satisfaction scores can usually be more significant with positive changes compared with performance scores. This is especially so for Charles, who has significant physical and mental health conditions, but his rehabilitation has enabled him to manage his activity limitations and participation restrictions in a different way, enabling him to meet his goals

The Individual's Perspective

This chapter has so far considered the person-centred frame of reference from a professional perspective, exploring values, practice and the process of delivering occupational therapy to our consumers. There remains limited exploration and understanding of the individual's views of person-centred care (Parker 2013), and so to successfully apply a person-centred frame of reference to practice, consider the issues Bibyk et al (1999) raised but which are still current:

- What does it feel like to be a person-centred therapist?
- What does a person-centred therapist act like?
- What does a person-centred practice look like?

The answers may help you reflect and apply a person-centred frame of reference to your own unique circumstances. To help you assess how person-centred you are, reflect on the questions listed in Table 11.2.

What Does a Person-Centred Therapist Feel Like?

- They respect each person as an individual.
- They are nonthreatening, nonauthoritarian and nonjudgemental.

- They actively listen to the individual and engage with them.
- Values are discussed but not imposed.
- Skilled communication is key to explore, discuss and evaluate progress.

What Does a Person-Centred Therapist Act Like?

- They are approachable and authentic.
- They treat each individual as an equal in the therapeutic partnership.
- They adopt a positive attitude in their relationship with each individual.
- They provide each individual with information to make choices.
- Ownership and direction for change remains with the individual.

What Does a Person-Centred Service Look Like?

- It provides a welcome.
- It pays attention to access, parking and other facilities.
- It provides information on services provided.
- It lacks physical barriers between the therapist and user.
- The environment does not make a person feel uncomfortable and powerless.

SUMMARY

This chapter has described a person-centred frame of reference, put it into context and explored its application in practice. At the heart of occupational therapy are the people for whom we train and educate each generation of occupational therapists: namely, our clients, patients and service users—all of whom are individuals. If we can harmonize our own values and beliefs, combining our clinical expertise and knowledge with each individual's needs

REFLECTIVE LEARNING

b0015

- What personal values are important to me as a therapist?
- Do I truly work in partnership with each individual, respecting their views?
- What role does person-centred practice have in my clinical reasoning?
- Which aspects of person-centred practice do I find easy? How can I maximize my use of these aspects?
- How can I encourage my peers in occupational therapy but also the wider multi-disciplinary/inter-disciplinary team to be person-centred?
- Which of the above items causes me the most challenges? What can I do to improve them?

and expectations in an environment that supports respect and partnership, in a way that provides us with a process of articulating and teaching this in the workplace, then we have achieved something worthwhile. Adopting the person-centred frame of reference should help you practice that, as it provides you with the opportunity to work together and achieve true partnership (Parker 2013).

REFERENCES

Banks, S., Crossman, D., Poel, D., & Stewart, M. (1997). Partnerships among health professionals and self help group members. *Canadian Journal of Occupational Therapy, 64*(3), 259–269.

Bibyk, B., Day, D. G., Morris, L., O'Brien, M., Rebeiro, K. L., & Seguin, P. (1999). Who's in charge here? The client's perspective on client-centred care. *Occupational Therapy Now, 1*(5), 11–12.

Blank, A. (2004). Clients' experience of partnership with occupational therapists in community mental health. *British Journal of Occupational Therapy, 67*(3), 118–124.

Brown, T. (2013). Person-centred occupational practice: Is it time for a change of terminology? *British Journal of Occupational Therapy, 76*(5), 207.

Canadian Association of Occupational Therapists. (2002). *Enabling occupation: An occupational therapy perspective.* Ottawa: CAOT Publications ACE.

Canadian Association of Occupational Therapists, Department of National Health and Welfare. (1983). *Occupational therapy guidelines for client-centred practice.* Toronto: CAOT.

Canadian Association of Occupational Therapists and Department of National Health and Welfare. (1991). *Occupational therapy guidelines for client-centred practice.* Toronto: CAOT Publications ACE.

Carpenter, L., Baker, G., & Tyldesley, B. (2001). The use of the Canadian Occupational Performance Measure as an outcome of a pain management programme. *Canadian Journal of Occupational Therapy, 68*(1), 16–22.

Chen, Y. H., Rodger, S., & Polatajko, H. (2002). Experiences with the COPM and client-centred practice in adult neuro rehabilitation in Taiwan. *Occupational Therapy International, 9*(3), 167–184.

Christiansen, C. (1991). Occupational therapy for life performance in occupational therapy. In C. Christiansen, & C. Baum (Eds.), *Overcoming human performance deficits.* Thorofare, NJ: Slack.

College of Occupational Therapists. (2015). *Code of ethics and professional conduct* (revised ed.). London: COT.

College of Occupational Therapists. (2017). *Professional standards for occupational therapy practice* (revised ed.). London: COT.

Conneeley, A. L. (2004). Interdisciplinary collaborative goal planning in a post-acute neurological setting: A qualitative study. *British Journal of Occupational Therapy, 67*(6), 248–255.

Corring, D. (1999). The missing perspective on client-centred care. *Occupational therapy now, 1,* 8–10.

Corring, D., & Cook, J. (1999). Client-centred care means that I am a valued human being. *Canadian Journal of Occupational Therapy, 66*(2), 71–82.

Creek, J. (2003). *Occupational therapy defined as a complex intervention.* London: College of Occupational Therapists.

Department for Constitutional Affairs. (2007). *Code of practice mental capacity act 2005.* London: Stationery Office.

Donnelly, C., & Carswell, A. (2002). Individualised outcome measures: A review of the literature. *Canadian Journal of Occupational Therapy, 69*(2), 84–94.

Falardeau, M., & Durand, M. J. (2002). Negotiation-centred versus client-centred: Which approach should be used? *Canadian Journal of Occupational Therapy, 69*(3), 135–142.

Foster, M. (2002). Theoretical frameworks in occupational therapy and physical dysfunction, principles, skills and practice. In A. Turner (Ed.), *Occupational therapy and physical dysfunction, principles, skills and practice* (5th ed.). Edinburgh: Churchill Livingstone.

Gan, C., Campbell, K., Snider, A., Cohen, S., & Hubbard, J. (2008). Giving Youth a Voice (GYV): A measure of youths' perceptions of the client-centredness of rehabilitation services. *Canadian Journal of Occupational Therapy, 75*(2), 96–104.

Hong, C. S., Pearce, S., & Withers, R. A. (2000). Occupational therapy assessments: How client-centred can they be? *British Journal of Occupational Therapy, 63*(7), 316–319.

Jamieson, M., Krupa, T., O'Riordan, A., et al. (2006). Developing empathy as a foundation of client-centred practice: evaluation of a university curriculum initiative. *Canadian Journal of Occupational Therapy, 73*(2), 76–85.

Lane, L. (2000). Client-centred practice: Is it compatible with early discharge hospital at home policies? *British Journal of Occupational Therapy, 63*(7), 310–315.

Law, M. (1998). *Client-centred Occupational Therapy.* Thorofare, NJ: Slack.

Law, M., Baptiste, S., McColl, M., et al. (1990). The Canadian Occupational Performance Measure: An outcome measure for occupational therapy. *Canadian Journal of Occupational Therapy, 57*(2), 81–87.

Law, M., Baptiste, S., & Mills, J. (1995). Client-centred practice: What does it mean and does it make a difference? *Canadian Journal of Occupational Therapy, 62*(5), 250–257.

Law, M., Polatajko, H., Baptiste, S., Opzoomer, A., Polatajko, H., & Pollock, N. (1997). Core concepts of occupational therapy. In E. Townsend, et al. (Ed.), *Enabling occupation: An occupational therapy perspective.* Ottawa: Canadian Association of Occupational Therapy Publications ACE.

Law, M., Baum, C., & Dunn, W. (2001). *Measuring occupational performance.* Thorofare, NJ: Slack.

Lewin, S. A., Skea, Z. C., Entwistle, V., Zwarenstein, M., & Dick, J. (2008). Interventions for providers to promote a patient-centred approach in clinical consultations (review). In *Cochrane collaboration.* John Wiley.

Lum, J. M., Williams, P. A. Rappolt, S. Landry, M. D. Deber, R. Verrier, M. (2004). Meeting the challenge of diversity: Results from the 2003 survey of occupational therapists in Ontario. *Occupational Therapy Now, 6*(4), 1–6.

Maitra, K., & Erway, F. (2006). Perception of client-centred practice in occupational therapists and their clients. *American Journal of Occupational Therapy, 60*(3), 298–310.

Mead, N., & Bower, P. (2000). Patient-centredness: A conceptual framework and review of the empirical literature. *Social Science & Medicine, 51,* 1087–1110.

Mew, M., & Fossey, E. (1996). Client-centred aspects of clinical reasoning during an initial assessment using the Canadian Occupational Performance Measure. *Australian Occupational Therapy Journal, 43,* 155–166.

Moats, G. (2007). Discharge decision-making, enabling occupations and client-centred practice. *Canadian Journal of Occupational Therapy, 74*(2), 91–101.

Moats, G., & Doble, S. (2006). Discharge planning with older adults: Towards a negotiated model of decision making. *Canadian Journal of Occupational Therapy, 73*(5), 303–311.

Morgan, S., & Yoder, L. H. (2012). A concept analysis of person centred care. *Journal of Holistic Nursing, 30*(1), 6–15.

Palmadottir, G. (2003). Client perspectives on occupational therapy in rehabilitation services. *Scandinavian Journal of Occupational Therapy, 10*(4), 157–166.

Parker, D. M. (2013). *An exploration of client-centred practice in occupational therapy: Perspectives and impact.* University of Birmingham. Unpublished PhD thesis.

Peloquin, S. M. (1997). Should we trade person-centred service for a consumer-based model? *American Journal of Occupational Therapy, 51*(7), 612–615.

Rebeiro, K. (2000a). Reconciling philosophy with daily practice: Future challenges to occupational therapy's client-centred practice. *Occupational Therapy Now, 2,* 4–12.

Rebeiro, K. L. (2000b). Client perspectives of occupational therapy practice: Are we truly client-centred? *Canadian Journal of Occupational Therapy, 67*(2), 7–14.

Rogers, C. R. (1939). *The clinical treatment of the problem child.* London: George Allen and Unwin Ltd.

Rogers, C. (1951). *Client-centred therapy.* New York: Houghton Mifflin.

Simon, C., & Daub, M. (1993). Human development across the lifespan. In H. Hopkins, & H. Smith (Eds.), *Willard and Spackman's occupational therapy* (8th ed.). Philadelphia: JB Lippincott.

Sumsion, T. (1997). Environmental challenges and opportunities of client-centred practice. *British Journal of Occupational Therapy, 60*(2), 53–56.

Sumsion, T. (1999). *Client-centred practice in occupational therapy: A guide to implementation.* Edinburgh: Churchill Livingstone.

Sumsion, T. (2000). A revised definition of client-centred practice. *British Journal of Occupational Therapy, 63*(7), 304–310.

Sumsion, T. (2006). *Client-centred practice in occupational therapy – a guide to implementation* (2nd ed.). Edinburgh: Churchill Livingstone Elsevier.

Sumsion, T., & Law, M. (2006). A review of evidence of the conceptual elements informing client-centered practice. *Canadian Journal of Occupational Therapy, 73(3)*, 153–162.

Sumsion, T., & Smyth, G. (2000). Barriers to client-centredness and their resolution. *Canadian Journal of Occupational Therapy, 67(1)*, 15–21.

The Health Foundation. (2016). *Person-centred care made simple. What everyone should know about person centred care.* London: The Health Foundation.

Townsend, E., Stanton, S., Law, M., et al. (1999). *Enabling occupation: An occupational therapy perspective.* Ottawa: Canadian Association of Occupational Therapy Publications ACE.

Turner, A. (2002). Theoretical frameworks. In A. Turner (Ed.), *Occupational therapy and physical dysfunction, principles, skills and practice* (5th ed.). Edinburgh: Churchill Livingstone.

Whalley Hammell, K. (2002). Informing client-centred practice through qualitative inquiry: Evaluating the quality of qualitative research. *British Journal of Occupational Therapy, 65(4)*, 175–185.

Wilkins, S., Pollock, N., Rochon, S., & Law, M. (2001). Implementing client-centred practice: Why is it so difficult to do? *Canadian Journal of Occupational Therapy, 68(2)*, 70–79.

Wressle, E., Eeg Olofsson, A., Marcusson, J., & Henriksson, C. (2002). Improved client participation in the rehabilitation process using a client-centred goal formulation structure. *Journal of Rehabilitation Medicine, 34*, 5–11.

12

The Cognitive–Behavioural Frame of Reference

Edward A.S. Duncan, Sarah Fletcher-Shaw

OVERVIEW

Cognitive–behavioural therapy (CBT) is a popular and evidence-based psychotherapeutic approach. Although its guiding principles are associated with ancient Greek thought, current developments emanate from the modern theoretical frameworks of behavioural therapy and cognitive therapy. Contemporary CBT represents a broad church of theoretical developments, interventions and professional groupings (Kennerley et al 2016, Swan & Sloan 2018). This chapter outlines the development and general principles of CBT. It continues by examining CBT's theoretical framework and general characteristics. Having provided an overview of CBT in general, the chapter explores the various uses of a cognitive–behavioural frame of reference in occupational therapy. In doing so, the criticisms that have been made of occupational therapists' use of CBT to date are acknowledged and proposals for ways in which the strengths of a cognitive–behavioural frame of reference can be integrated within occupationally focused practice are offered.

HIGHLIGHTS

This chapter
- provides an accessible overview of the historical development of CBT
- outlines a cognitive–behavioural frame of reference in occupational therapy
- presents criticisms of the use of CBT in occupational therapy
- illustrates how a cognitive–behavioural approach can be integrated within occupational therapy practice.

INTRODUCTION

'Cognitive Behavioural Therapy (CBT) is the term given to a specific psychological approach to conceptualizing and addressing clients' difficulties' (Duncan 2003a). Whilst CBT is frequently associated with the work of psychologists, it is more accurately described as a shared intervention by a variety of health professionals.

CBT's robust and developing evidence base has consistently drawn occupational therapists to use it in practice. However, in doing so, the potential to become a general mental health practitioner and not an occupational therapist has been noted. Considerable debate has taken place regarding the fact that occupational therapists may carry out CBT as a form of psychotherapy. The case for occupational therapists' use of their shared skills in this respect has been given elsewhere (Duncan 1999, 2003a, 2003b, Harrison 2003, Stewart 2003) and will not be repeated here. Distancing from the occupational therapy role is, however, not essential in order for a clinician to use a CBT approach in practice. In fact, the incorporation of a cognitive–behavioural frame of reference within occupational therapy is not only achievable but also highly desirable. Therefore, this chapter focuses on the use of a cognitive–behavioural frame of reference within an occupational therapy context.

WHAT IS COGNITIVE BEHAVIOURAL THERAPY?

Historical Development
CBT is a dynamic body of knowledge that has developed since the 1950s. It is strongly influenced by the theoretical and therapeutic traditions of behavioural therapy and

141

cognitive therapy. Behavioural therapy, in turn, has been significantly shaped by the evolutionary perspective of health. Its developmental roots stretch back to the beginning of the 20th century, when animal behaviour research was carried out and related to human beings (Hawton et al 1996). Cognitive therapy, whilst developing later than behavioural therapy, claims more historic roots. It cites the Roman emperor Epictetus, who wrote, 'Men are disturbed, not by things, but of the view they take of them', as an example of the early recognition of the power of thought on health (Beck et al 1979).

Behavioural Therapy

Two principles of animal learning theory have affected the development of behavioural therapy: classical conditioning and operant conditioning (Bernstein 2018). Both classical and operant conditioning are briefly outlined below; however, readers are encouraged to refer to other texts for a more comprehensive overview of these important theories.

Classical Conditioning

Ivan Pavlov, a Russian physiologist, developed the theory of classical conditioning at the turn of the 20th century. However, the original development of this theory could not have been further from its eventual applied role within behaviour therapy. Classical conditioning was discovered during an experiment into the digestive process of dogs, a study that would win Pavlov the Nobel Prize for physiology/medicine in 1904. In 1913, John Watson employed classical conditioning theory in the development of behaviourist theory. Watson's theory was popular, as it offered an objective and measurable basis for human behaviour, an approach that was in stark contrast to the other predominant psychological theories of the time (Hawton et al 1996, Duncan 2003a).

Operant Conditioning. The second influential learning theory in the development of behavioural theory was operant conditioning. This outlines 'the law of effect', whereby a behaviour that is rewarded will tend to be repeated, and behaviour that is punished will diminish (Hawton et al 1996).

Burrhus F. Skinner, an American psychologist, developed Pavlov's work by extending the principle of reinforcement. Previously, an action was considered to be reinforced if it increased or decreased behaviour. Skinner explored different types of reinforcers and consequences. It was observed that different types of reinforcers had different effects on behaviour, depending upon the nature of the action. Together, classical and operant conditioning provided the theoretical foundation for a variety of behaviour therapy interventions, mainly in mental health settings (Hawton et al 1996).

Although the benefits of behaviour therapy were widely recognized, the late 1960s and early 1970s witnessed a developing disillusionment with behaviour therapy as the theoretical shortcomings and practical failures associated with the approach came into focus. Such disillusionment, at least amongst some, supported the birth of another related form of therapy known as cognitive therapy.

Cognitive Therapy

The original attribution of a cognitive approach to therapy is given to Meichenbaum (1975). However, it is the work of Aaron T. Beck, an American psychiatrist, that has become synonymous with the term *cognitive therapy*. Aaron Beck (b. 1921) developed cognitive therapy through an examination of the links between the environment, the person and his/her emotion and motivation. Surprisingly, Beck, a medical doctor, did not come from a foundation in behaviourism. Instead, Beck's theoretical roots were found in the psychoanalytical perspective (Duncan 2003a). Beck's career commenced in psychiatry, and he trained in psychoanalytical theory and practice. Despite initially questioning the nature of psychoanalytical theory, he embraced the approach, even undertaking research aimed at proving the efficacy of the approach in relation to depression. However, this study reignited his initial doubts about psychoanalytical theory and in doing so led to the development of cognitive therapy. Subsequently, Beck has published extensively on the theory and practice of cognitive therapy. For those who are interested in finding out more about Aaron Beck, a biography of his life and work has been published (Weishaar 1993). Cognitive therapy and behaviour therapy, whilst taking significantly different views about the causal factors of a disorder (i.e., that it has a cognitive or behavioural root), have many commonalities. It was perhaps inevitable, therefore, that both theories became combined into the generally accepted framework of CBT.

Conditions in Which Cognitive Behavioural Therapy Is Commonly Used. Owing to its strong evidence base in a variety of contexts (e.g., anxiety, depression and psychosis) (Hofman et al 2012) and support in a range of clinical guidelines from both the National Institute of Health and Clinical Excellence (NICE) and the Scottish Intercollegiate Guidelines Network (SIGN), CBT has become an increasingly popular method of intervention and has swiftly developed over the last 20 years. As well as having a strong evidence base for practice in the forenamed conditions, CBT is often associated with interventions to address alcohol abuse (e.g., Longabaugh & Morgenstern 1999), personality disorders (e.g., Rafaeli et al 2010,

Davidson et al 2006), family therapy (e.g., Epstein 2003) and drug abuse (e.g., Beck et al 1993, Waldron & Kaminer 2004). As well as conditions traditionally found within the mental health spectrum of interventions, CBT has also been positively associated with various other conditions, including chronic pain (Strong 1998, McCracken & Turk 2002, Vlaeyen & Morley 2005), chronic fatigue syndrome (Prins et al 2001, Price et al 2008) and knee osteoarthritis (Murphy et al 2018).

An Introduction to the Theoretical Framework of Cognitive Behavioural Therapy. CBT takes a problem-focused perspective of life difficulties and focuses on five aspects of life experience:

- thoughts
- behaviours
- emotion/mood
- physiological responses
- the environment (Greenberger et al 2016).

Each aspect of life experience is influenced by the social and physical environment in which they are placed (Fig. 12.1). CBT suggests that changes in any factor can lead to an improvement or deterioration in the other factors. For example, if we exercise (behaviour), we feel better (mood); if we feel nervous (mood), we may experience an increased heart rate or sweat more (physiological reaction); if we find large social gatherings difficult (social environment), we may avoid them (behaviour).

The way in which CBT is delivered depends on the training of the therapist and the needs of the client. In practice, the majority of clinicians using these approaches draw from its richness of technique and theory. However, therapists' training and personal preferences can lead to a greater emphasis on a cognitive or behavioural approach:

- Cognitive therapy places an emphasis on rapid and automatic interpretations of events and the importance of underlying beliefs and values.
- Behaviour therapy emphasizes our automatic learned responses to stimuli and the way in which our behaviour is shaped by its consequences.

One of the key theoretical components to understanding the theoretical basis of CBT is its postulated levels of cognition.

Levels of Cognition. Cognitions are the way in which we know, sense or perceive reality (Chambers 1994; Box 12.1). Beck et al (1979), in their seminal text *Cognitive Therapy of Depression*, outlined three levels of cognition that are amenable to therapeutic intervention. Key to this conceptualization is the idea that, unlike other psychotherapeutic approaches (e.g., psychodynamic psychotherapy), each of these levels is accessible by the client. The levels are hierarchical in nature, with automatic thoughts being the most frequently occurring and easily accessible, beliefs being more constant and core schema representing the building blocks of thought processes and being more challenging to shift.

Automatic Thoughts. Automatic thoughts are habitual and plausible. They are the uninvited thoughts that pop into your head (e.g., 'I'll sound stupid if I ask a question in this class') Everyone has automatic thoughts and it is likely that you will have some while reading this chapter (e.g., What am I having for tea? Is this going to help me with my

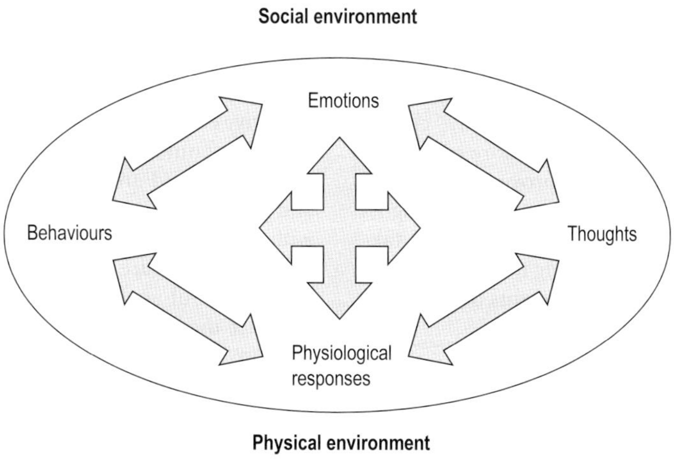

Fig. 12.1 The influence of the social and physical environment on aspects of life experience. (Reproduced with the permission of Kathlyn L. Reed.)

Imagine you are asleep in bed ... Suddenly you are awakened by a loud crashing sound from downstairs. How would you feel?
- How would you feel if you knew there had been a spate of violent burglaries in your neighbourhood?
- How would you feel if you had just bought a new kitten that has been knocking over everything in sight?

The nature of feelings is largely determined by the way we think.

assignment? When am I seeing my next client?). However, for clients, more often than not automatic thoughts will be negative in nature. Another characteristic of automatic thoughts is that they can be situation-specific—a client may be plagued by unhelpful automatic thoughts whilst in a stressful work situation and find it difficult to cope, whilst appearing to function without difficulty when in the home environment.

It is useful to understand the automatic thoughts a client is having, as these can have a direct impact on their presentation in sessions and their ability to carry out day-to-day life activities. Several techniques can be used to elicit automatic thoughts:
- *Direct questioning.* What is (was) going through your mind just now?
- *Inductive questioning.* Use a series of open questions and reflexive statements to help a client recall an emotional situation (e.g., What happened next? What did you do?).
- *Re-enacting/recreating a situation.* Use imagery, role play and in vivo experiments.
- *Recording thoughts.* Use thought diaries and so on.

Where thoughts are recognized as being unhelpful, the therapist and clinician can work together to help the client to change the nature of their thinking—in the knowledge that this will help their behaviour. Importantly, changing thoughts is not the same as thinking more positively, which is unlikely in itself to lead to improved functioning (Greenberger et al 2016). Challenging automatic thoughts is about gaining a sense of perspective on a situation, taking alternative perspectives and exploring new perspectives and solutions. Methods to challenge thoughts include
- Looking at the evidence:
  - What do I know about this situation?
  - How well do my thoughts fit the facts?
  - Do I have experiences that suggest my thoughts are not completely true?
  - Would my thoughts be accepted as correct by other people?

- Looking at other possible interpretations:
  - Are there other interpretations that fit the facts just as well?
  - How might a friend think of this situation?
  - How will I think about this in 6 months or a year?
- Looking at the helpfulness of thinking this way:
  - If the facts are bleak, does my way of thinking help?
  - Is this type of thinking likely to make me feel worse?
  - Am I brooding over questions with no clear-cut answers?
  - Am I behaving in ways that may make the situation worse?

Beliefs. These are conditional beliefs that we hold about ourselves. They may be unhelpful in nature (e.g., 'I always make a fool of myself when I meet my friends in the pub'). Although automatic thoughts are often easily accessible, beliefs tend to be slightly less obvious. They can sometimes be inferred from individuals' actions. If beliefs are to be put into words, then they often take the form of 'if ... then ...' sentences (e.g., *If* I cannot do my job to perfection, *then* everyone will think I am a failure') or of statements that contain 'should' (e.g., I *should* be the life and soul of a party) (Greenberger et al 2016). Conditional beliefs lie beneath and shape the automatic thoughts that pop into our head; they can be viewed as guiding principles that affect our daily life experiences. All lives are governed by beliefs to a certain extent and these in turn govern our behaviour. Some people, however, develop unhelpful beliefs about a range of issues and these can often significantly affect the way in which they lead their lives.

Although unhelpful beliefs can be varied in nature, there are several categories in which the most common beliefs can be placed. It is often helpful to discuss these categories with clients to see if any of them resonate with their experience (Box 12.2).

Core Schemas. Schemas are the most stable of the three cognitive constructs. These are absolute core beliefs that we hold about ourselves. Schemas are formed during the early years of life and are influenced by childhood experiences and genetic composition. Often when working with clients with mental health difficulties, schemas are found to be unhelpful in nature, for example, 'I am worthless' or 'I am bad'. A useful analogy to understand core schemas is to consider them as the building blocks of cognition. From the core schemas develop the beliefs, and from the beliefs come our automatic thoughts. Core schemas are not as immediately accessible as automatic thoughts or beliefs; however, through specialist CBT it is possible for a client to become aware of these processes (Rafaeli et al 2010). Changing a client's schemas is, however, very difficult,

BOX 12.2   Typical Forms of Unhelpful Beliefs

Overgeneralization
- Making sweeping judgements on the basis of single instances. *'Everything I do goes wrong'*

Selective Abstraction
- Attending only to negative aspects of experience. *'Not one good thing happened today'*

Dichotomous Reasoning
- Thinking in extremes, also known as black and white thinking. *'If I can't get it right, there's no point in doing it at all'*

Personalization
- Taking responsibility for things that have little or nothing to do with oneself. *'I must have done something to offend him'*

Arbitrary Influence
- Jumping to conclusions without enough evidence. *'This course is rubbish'* (when you have only just started it!).

because these processes are deeply ingrained within each person. This is a specialist skill and should be left to individuals with specialist cognitive–behavioural training. Interestingly, however, significant differences can be made to a person's life using cognitive and behavioural principles, without ever exploring the issue of core schemas.

General Characteristics of Cognitive Behavioural Therapy.
CBT can be distinguished from other psychotherapeutic approaches by its general characteristics.

Present-focused. Whereas historic information (e.g., about a client's childhood and family relationships) can provide helpful information to give a context to a client's difficulties, this information is not the focus of traditional CBT. Therapists using CBT are much more interested in exploring what a client's current difficulties are and examining ways in which these can be directly addressed.

Time-limited. CBT is a time-limited procedure. The guiding principle here, however, is not predetermining the length of the intervention, but that an agreement is made between the therapist and client regarding the approximate length of intervention and agreed time-points for evaluation of therapy.

Collaborative. Beck et al (1979) describe the relationship between a therapist and a client as one of 'collaborative empiricism', in which both parties work together and develop a shared understanding of a client's problem.

Problem-focused. Cognitive–behavioural therapists take a problem-focused approach. Frequently, the first form of collaboration between the therapist and client is the development of a 'problem list'. Together, the therapist and client then decide upon the priorities for intervention, and the focus of interventions is consequently developed.

Assessment and formulation. Assessment is an ongoing process within CBT. Initial assessment focuses on information-gathering and appraisal of a client's problems. This is achieved through a variety of methods including interviews, questionnaires, observational techniques and self-monitoring (Wells 1997). Information gathered from these assessments is then considered in the development of an individual case formulation. A case formulation is a conceptualization of the therapist's understanding of the client's problems. It takes into account the effects of the client's thinking, behaviour, physiological responses, emotions and environment, as well as other related information. This formulation is shared with the client by the therapist as a method of explaining their perspective of the client's problems. Crucially, the therapist should introduce the formulation and ask the client for their feedback on their perception of its accuracy. In doing so, the formulation becomes a collaborative effort to understand a client's difficulties. This document often becomes a key component of the intervention and can be referred to and refined throughout the course of therapy (Duncan 2003a).

Socialization. Socialization is the term given to the education of clients about the theoretical basis of CBT. This education enables clients to understand the rationale for therapy and empowers them as collaborators in the therapeutic process. Educating clients about the theoretical background to CBT can occur in a variety of manners, including verbal explanations and the provision of written or audio-visual material as well as providing examples and demonstrations of the links between cognition, behaviour and emotion.

Intervention. CBT interventions are very varied. Whereas cognitive–behavioural therapists frequently engage clients in didactic (one-to-one) interaction, they are also found out of such settings *doing* therapy whilst engaged in specific *activities* (e.g., shopping, using public transport, etc.). Such an active engagement in therapy can bear close resemblance to occupational therapy and, again, gives an indication of why so many occupational therapists are attracted to this frame of reference.

Concluding therapy. One of a cognitive–behavioural therapist's key objectives is to assist a client to become their own therapist. This is again an empowering process. It involves educating a client about the triggers that have initiated their problems and the development of effective strategies for dealing with them in the future. Through this process, known as 'relapse prevention', the chances of future difficulties are decreased.

Each of these characteristics resonates with the guiding principles of occupational therapy practice today. Indeed, many of the interventions even appear to be similar to occupational therapy in practice. Perhaps it is these factors, together with CBT's impressive evidence base, that attracts so many occupational therapists to embrace CBT in practice.

The Cognitive–Behavioural Frame of Reference in Occupational Therapy

CBT describes a range of approaches developed under a shared theoretical umbrella. Indeed, CBT is so vast in its development and application that the professional body that represents CBT in the United Kingdom has asked, 'What is CBT?'

Within occupational therapy, the practice of CBT is complicated. Occupational therapists can describe using cognitive–behavioural theory or practice within an occupational therapy framework but refer to it as CBT (Duncan 2003a). To avoid confusion, it is important to clarify terminology. It is proposed that all forms of primarily didactic psychotherapy that use a CBT approach are referred to as CBT, whereas the use of cognitive–behavioural theory or practice within core skill occupational therapy is referred to as employing a cognitive–behavioural frame of reference.

History of Cognitive Behavioural Therapy and the Cognitive–Behavioural Frame of Reference in Occupational Therapy.
Cognitive–behavioural interventions within occupational therapy can be traced back as far as 1969 (Braund & Moore 1969). Later, the basic concepts of behaviour therapy were summarized and their use in the practice of occupational therapy outlined. Behaviour therapy was viewed as 'particularly relevant to occupational therapists' work because it concentrates on the behavioural repertoire of the patient and his interaction with the environment rather than on his internal state' (Jodrell & Sanson-Fisher 1975).

Despite an apparent lack of integration of CBT into occupational therapy, it continued to be used in practice. Taylor (1988) rationalized the use of cognitive–behavioural techniques in the following manner:

To function in everyday life, a person must be able to perform skills that enable him or her to engage in a variety of adaptive behaviors. If anger regularly interferes with an individual's ability to perform adaptive behaviors, it is the responsibility of the occupational therapist to assist such a person in the management of anger.

Taylor (1988) also attempted to ground the cognitive–behavioural approach within an occupational performance context and highlighted the benefits to occupational therapists as follows:

- The approach is based on theories already familiar to occupational therapists and readily incorporated into practice.
- The methods of assessment are also familiar to therapists.
- The flexibility of the approach is attractive to the client group with whom occupational therapists often work.
- The approach lends itself to scientific investigation.

Taylor (1988) justifies the use of CBT within occupational therapy by illustrating the impact that such interventions have on occupation. However, the nature of the therapy Taylor (1988) describes is essentially a CBT intervention, not occupational therapy. Several other publications support occupational therapists' embracement of CBT as a method of skill enhancement (O'Neil 1989, Gilbert & Strong 1994, Keable 1997, Prior 1998a, 1998b).

Although some colleagues from other disciplines have expressed surprise at occupational therapists' use of CBT (Stewart 2003), occupational therapists' continued use of cognitive–behavioural techniques, especially within mental health settings, appears to be generally well accepted. Meeson (1998) found that anxiety management and problem-solving techniques (both cognitive–behavioural approaches) contributed towards 28% of intervention choices in a survey of British occupational therapists working in community mental health teams.

Recently, in an initial attempt to articulate a cognitive–behavioural frame of reference within occupational therapy, Duncan (2003a) highlighted the shared areas of concern and practice of CBT and occupational therapy, illustrating the overlap that existed in several areas of practice (Fig. 12.2). This articulation of the potential role of a cognitive–behavioural frame of reference in occupational therapy was in response to the growing criticism of its use. However, it was only a partial explanation of cognitive–behavioural theory's relevance to occupational therapy.

Criticisms of the Use of Cognitive Behavioural Therapy in Occupational Therapy.
Acceptance of CBT without a direct occupation focus has been criticized as leading to role blurring and dilution of therapeutic expertise (e.g., Kaur et al 1996). Another concern is that occupational therapists' use of CBT is a response to dissatisfaction about the perceived effectiveness of occupational therapy and a desire for enhanced professional respect (Mocellin 1996, Harrison 2003). These concerns appear to be supported by Harrison and Hill (2003), who outline 'personal interest' and the 'impact of the intervention' as decisive factors in the use of CBT by a group of occupational therapists in mental health.

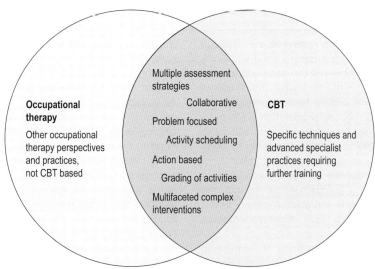

Fig. 12.2 The relationship between cognitive–behavioural therapy and occupational therapy. *CBT,* Cognitive–behavioural therapy. (From Everett, T., Donaghy, M., Fearver, S. (Eds.), (2003). *Interventions for mental health: an evidence based approach*, Butterworth Heinemann, reprinted with permission of Elsevier Ltd.)

Integrating a Cognitive–Behavioural Approach Within Occupational Therapy

Using Cognitive–Behavioural Techniques in Occupational Therapy. One method in which occupational therapists can effectively use a cognitive–behavioural frame of reference is to integrate cognitive–behavioural techniques appropriately into their occupational therapy-focused interventions. Indeed, the use of cognitive–behavioural techniques in occupational therapy has, at times, been deemed a research priority (Fowler et al 2000). Such techniques include the use of anxiety management strategies (e.g., deep breathing exercises, relaxation, thought-challenging, diary-keeping, etc.) and techniques used for assisting people with phobias (e.g., systematic desensitization) or chronic fatigue (e.g., graded activity scheduling). An example of how cognitive–behavioural techniques can be used appropriately within occupational therapy practice is outlined next.

CASE VIGNETTE

Katie works as an occupational therapist in a cardiovascular rehabilitation team in the community. She receives a referral for a gentleman named Sol. He is 45 years old and had a myocardial infarction resulting in a cardiac arrest 4 months ago while at work. He has been attending the rehabilitation classes and progressing well but is expressing fears and concerns about returning to his hobbies and work.

Katie carried out an initial assessment with Sol after the rehabilitation class at the hospital. During the assessment Sol is very tearful and reports he feels 'my life is over' because he is too anxious to return to his previous hobby of singing in a band and to return to work. He describes physical symptoms of his mouth going dry, his heart racing and his becoming breathless when thinking about these two occupations (anxiety symptoms). Katie uses Socratic questioning to explore this further with Sol and he discloses he is fearful of having another heart attack whilst at work or whilst performing (negative automatic thoughts). Katie takes a psychoeducation approach with Sol during the initial assessment and helps him understand the symptoms he is experiencing when thinking about work and singing from a cognitive–behavioural perspective (environmental triggers–thoughts–feelings–behaviour).

Katie further assesses Sol's identified issues by utilizing a Likert scale (1–10) to measure how important these occupations are to Sol and how anxious he feels about engaging in them. Sol rates both occupations as a 10 for importance and he rates the anxiety level of returning

Continued

CASE VIGNETTE—cont'd

to work as a 9 and returning to singing as a 7. Through collaborative discussion using a goal-focused approach, Sol and Katie agree that goals will be set to address Sol returning to singing, as it is the occupation which scores lower on the Likert scale and he feels returning to the place where he had his myocardial infarction is too overwhelming at present. Sol feels if he can sing again this will improve his confidence to address returning to work. Katie agrees with him and they set long- and short-term goals using a graded activity scheduling approach. A graded activity scheduling approach helps Sol increase his activity tolerance in a safe and gradual manner whilst also reducing his anxiety as a result of graded exposure resulting in habituation.

Katie also recognizes the importance of addressing the distressing anxiety symptoms Sol is experiencing and increasing his coping strategies which help him succeed in his graded activity plan. Sol identifies the breathlessness as the most distressing symptom so Katie suggested they work on breathing techniques as an intervention in sessions together which can then be used during the graded activity plan and whenever Sol feels they will be of benefit to him. Katie and Sol work together to agree a graded activity plan, using a Likert scale of perceived anxiety to inform them. This approach is also used to adapt the plan in vivo as needed. They agree the following stages: (1) Katie and Sol to discuss his singing (score 5, when reduced to a 3 they will move to next step), (2) Katie and Sol to sing together at the rehabilitation unit (score 6, when reduced to a 3 they will move to the next step), (3) Katie and Sol to visit his singing venue (score 7, when reduced to a 3 they will move to the next step), (4) Sol to sing with Katie present at his singing venue (score 7, when reduced to a 3 they will move to the next step), (5) Sol to sing with his band at his singing venue with no audience (score 7, when reduced to a 3 Sol will then return to singing in public). Sol also practises the breathing techniques at home twice a week, so he can utilize these to help manage his symptoms to increase the likelihood of successful engagement in his occupations. Once Sol completed the fourth steps of the singing plan he felt ready to take the same approach to return to work, with Katie's support. This took place over a 12-week period and on the final session Katie concluded therapy with a final assessment, reviewing his goals and utilized the Likert scales to measure Sol's anxiety and his confidence in sustaining his goals. Sol gradually returned to his meaningful and purposeful occupations as his activity levels and tolerance increased whilst his anxiety level reduced.

Socratic questioning (a technique that uses guided questions to get clients to reconsider how they view unhelpful thoughts) and *graded activity scheduling* (that involves the therapist and client agreeing an increasing schedule of meaningful activities for the client to undertake) are only two of the cognitive–behavioural techniques that are used by occupational therapists in practice. There are numerous cognitive–behavioural techniques and their appropriate use is outlined in a variety of specialist cognitive–behavioural textbooks (e.g., Beck et al 1979, Greenberger et al 2016, Hawton et al 1996, Wilding 2015).

Cognitive–behavioural techniques are undoubtedly useful tools for occupational therapists to have as part of their therapeutic repertoire. However, these should not be employed lightly, as they can appear to be deceptively simple. Careless employment of such techniques without consideration being given to the broader conceptualization of a client from a cognitive–behavioural frame of reference can result in a therapist becoming 'gimmick orientated' (Beck et al 1979).

Theory of Mind

A 'theory of mind' is an understanding of the inner psychological workings of a person (Wellman & Lagattuta 2004). There are numerous conceptualizations of how people understand each others' interactions, behaviours, relationships and lives in general. Daily, we form opinions about the rationale of other people's actions, a process that has become known as 'folk psychology' (Wellman & Lagattuta 2004). Some theories of mind are formalized (e.g., the person-centred frame of reference discussed in Chapter 11 and the cognitive–behavioural frame of reference discussed in the current chapter). Rather than relying on idiosyncratic folk psychology to guide a clinician in their interactions and conceptualization of clients, I propose that clinicians should develop the ability to use an evidence-based theory of mind. The cognitive–behavioural approach has undergone rigorous research to underpin its theoretical basis. We contend that the evidence base and pragmatic here-and-now philosophy of the cognitive–behavioural frame of reference mean that it lends itself to being the theory of mind of choice for occupational therapists in practice. The benefit of using a cognitive–behavioural frame of reference as a theory of mind is outlined in the case vignette below.

CASE VIGNETTE

Helen works as an occupational therapist in a medium-secure forensic unit. She has been qualified for 8 months. One afternoon she enters a ward day room to gather together a group of clients due to attend their regular kitchen session. Two of the clients willingly get up and prepare for the group; however, the third (Jack) shouts from a distance saying that 'she can stuff her group!' Helen approaches Jack and suggests that she is surprised that he does not want to attend, because he had appeared to be getting a lot of satisfaction from previous sessions. In response, Jack launches into a verbally aggressive discourse about his feelings about the unit and several of the staff. He concludes by stating that he wants nothing more to do with her, occupational therapy or any of the other staff. Clients and staff watch to see how Helen will react. Initially, she feels like walking away—after all, he has made his position very clear! However, taking a cognitive–behavioural theory of mind, Helen is aware that the real issue for Jack may not be being verbalized at present and in fact his current behaviour is likely to be a consequence of other issues. Helen sits down near Jack (but mindful of her own safety). She acknowledges Jack's anger and states that she respects his right to make decisions about his care. Jack appears a little surprised at this and states, 'nobody cares about my side of things'. Helen recognizes this as a verbalization of an unhelpful automatic thought and asks Jack what he means. Jack continues by explaining (in an angry but less aggressive manner) that he has just found out that his request for an unescorted leave of absence from the unit has been rejected. Continuing to use the cognitive–behavioural approach as her guiding theory of mind, Helen understands that Jack's outburst at her (emotion) and refusal to attend his occupational therapy session (behaviour) were a result of a recent decision by the clinical team (social environment). Helen acknowledges Jack's disappointment and asks if she can return later to chat to him some more. Jack replies that he still does not want to go to the group today but would be happy for Helen to return later. He appears more settled now and is talking at an appropriate rate and in an appropriate tone. Helen leaves, having a greater understanding of Jack's problem and with an invitation from Jack to continue the conversation.

There can be many occasions when it is useful to use a theory of mind when engaging with clients. Had Helen not used a cognitive–behavioural theory of mind, she may well have left the day room without engaging any further with Jack, or alternatively responded in a way that would not have been constructive. Conscious use of an evidence-based theory of mind enhances a clinician's ability to reason about clinical situations and lessens the potential for them to be influenced by their own biases and feelings.

The Cognitive–Behavioural Frame of Reference and Conceptual Models of Practice

The cognitive–behavioural frame of reference does not enable an occupational therapist to have a detailed understanding of a client's occupational performance and identity needs. However, it can support a clinician's guiding occupation-focused conceptual model of practice. Conversely, occupation-focused conceptual models of practice provide excellent means for an occupational therapist to conceptualize the occupational challenges facing a client but do not contain all the theoretical basis required for an occupational therapist to practice effectively. The cognitive–behavioural frame of reference assists occupational therapists to understand their clients more comprehensively and work collaboratively with them to address their occupational performance challenges. However, the cognitive–behavioural frame of reference in an occupational therapy context is not as straightforward as cutting and pasting from CBT literature. It requires an explicit use of a cognitive–behavioural frame of mind and judicious use of cognitive–behavioural techniques in practice, in clear conjunction with the therapist's occupation-focused conceptual model of practice.

SUMMARY

This chapter explored the historical basis, theoretical framework and broad evidence base of CBT. The guiding principles of CBT (problem-focused, working in the here and now, collaborative and time-limited) were recognized as principles that resonated with occupational therapy theory and practice. It is suggested, therefore, that the principles of CBT should be integral to occupational therapy practice. This proposal would certainly resonate with Aaron Beck, who stated (cited in Salkovskis 1996),

I hope in 10 years it no longer exists as a school of therapy … what we call cognitive therapy … will be taken for granted as the basics of all good therapy, just as Carl Rogers's principles of warmth, empathy and genuine regard for patient were adopted as necessary basics for all therapy relationships.

Although the principles and characteristics of CBT are congruent with occupational therapy, the method of their integration into practice has drawn criticism. Critics suggest that the use of CBT in occupational therapy practice has led to a loss of professional confidence and identity. To address these criticisms, this chapter has explored methods by which occupational therapists can effectively use a cognitive–behavioural frame of reference while remaining true to their professional role and identity. It is proposed that the cognitive–behavioural frame of reference, when used in conjunction with an occupation-focused conceptual model of practice, enhances a clinician's therapeutic potential by increasing their understanding of a client and allowing appropriate and judicious use of cognitive–behavioural techniques within an occupational context.

✳ REFLECTIVE LEARNING

- Can you explain to a friend who is not a health professional what CBT is? Try to use everyday language, but give as in-depth a description as you can.
- What differentiates between an occupational therapist using CBT and an occupational therapist taking a cognitive–behavioural frame of reference?
- Recall a practice setting in which you have had a placement or worked. How could a cognitive–behavioural frame of reference been applied in this setting?
- What differentiates the cognitive–behavioural frame of reference from other psychological frames of reference presented in this text?
- What are the similarities between the cognitive–behavioural frame of reference with other psychological frames of reference presented in this text?

REFERENCES

Beck, A. T., Rush, A. J., Shaw, B. F., et al. (1979). *Cognitive therapy of depression*. New York: Guilford.

Beck, A. T., Wright, F. D., Newman, C. F., et al. (1993). *Cognitive therapy of substance abuse*. New York: Guilford.

Bernstein, D. (2018). *Essentials of psychology*. Cengage Learning.

Braund, J. L., & Moore, R. J. (1969). The use of behaviour therapy in occupational therapy with psychiatric patients. *Australian Occupational Therapy Journal*, Boston. *16*(3), 27–32.

Chambers. (1994). *The Chambers dictionary*. Edinburgh: Chambers.

Davidson, K., Norrie, J., Tyrer, P., et al. (2006). The effectiveness of cognitive behavior therapy for borderline personality disorder: Results from the Borderline Personality Disorder Study of Cognitive Therapy (BOSCOT) Trial. *Journal of Personality Disorders, 20*(5), 450–465.

Duncan, E. A. S. (1999). Occupational therapy in mental health: It is time to recognise that it has come of age. *British Journal of Occupational Therapy, 62*(11), 521–522.

Duncan, E. A. S. (2003a). Cognitive-behavioural therapy in physiotherapy and occupational therapy. In T. Everett, M. Donaghy, & S. Feaver (Eds.), *Interventions for mental health: An evidence based approach*. Edinburgh: Butterworth–Heinemann.

Duncan, E. A. S. (2003b). Cognitive behaviour therapy: Seeking a common understanding. *British Journal of Occupational Therapy, 66*(5), 231.

Epstein, N. (2003). Cognitive-behavioral therapies for couples and families. In L. L. Hecker, & J. L. Wetchler (Eds.), *An introduction to marriage and family therapy*. Binghamton, NY: Haworth Clinical Practice Press.

Fowler-Davis, S., & Bannigan, K. (2000). Priorities in mental health research: The results of a live research project. *British Journal of Occupational Therapy, 63*(3), 98–104.

Gilbert, J., & Strong, J. (1994). Dysfunctional attitudes in patients with depression: A study of patients admitted to a private psychiatric hospital. *British Journal of Occupational Therapy, 57*(1), 15–19.

Greenberger, D., Padesky, C. A., & Beck, A. T. (2016). *Mind over mood: Change how you feel by changing the way you think* (2nd ed.). New York, NY: Guilford Press.

Harrison, D. (2003). The case for generic work in community mental health occupational therapy. *British Journal of Occupational Therapy, 66*(3), 110–112.

Harrison, D., & Hill, S. (2003). Mental health occupational therapy and cognitive behaviour therapy. *Mental Health Occupational Therapy, 8*(3), 101–105.

Hawton, K., Salkovskis, P., Kirk, J., et al. (Eds.). (1996). *Cognitive behaviour therapy for psychiatric problems: A practical guide*. Oxford: Oxford University Press.

Hofmann, S. G., Asnaani, A., Vonk, I. J., Sawyer, A. T., & Fang, A. (2012). The efficacy of cognitive behavioral therapy: A review of meta-analyses. *Cognitive Therapy and Research, 36*(5), 427–440.

Jodrell, R. D., & Sanson-Fisher, R. (1975). An experiment involving adolescent girls. *American Journal of Occupational Therapy, 29*(10), 620–624.

Kaur, D., Seager, M., & Orrell, M. (1996). Occupation or therapy? The attitudes of mental health professionals. *British Journal of Occupational Therapy, 59*(7), 319–322.

Keable, D. (1997). *The management of anxiety: A guide for therapists*. Edinburgh: Churchill Livingstone.

Kennerley, H., Kirk, J., & Westbrook, D. (2016). *An introduction to cognitive behaviour therapy: Skills and applications*. Los Angeles: Sage.

Longabaugh, R., & Morgenstern, J. (1999). Cognitive-behavioral coping-skills therapy for alcohol dependence: Current status and future directions. *Alcohol Research and Health, 23*(2), 78–86.

McCracken, L., & Turk, D. (2002). Behavioral and cognitive-behavioral treatment for chronic pain: Outcome, predictors of outcome, and treatment process. *Spine, 27*(22), 2564–2573.

Meichenbaum, D. (1975). A self-instructional approach to stress management: A proposal for stress inoculation training. In C. Spielberger, & I. Sarason (Eds.), *Stress and anxiety in modern life*. New York: Winston.

Meeson, B. (1998). Occupational therapy in community mental health, part 1: Intervention choice. *British Journal of Occupational Therapy*, *61*(1), 7–12.

Mocellin, G. (1996). Occupational therapy: A critical overview, part 2. *British Journal of Occupational Therapy*, *59*(1), 11–16.

Murphy, S. L., Janevic, M. R., Lee, P., & Williams, D. A. (2018). Occupational therapist–delivered cognitive–behavioral therapy for knee osteoarthritis: A randomized pilot study. *American Journal of Occupational Therapy*, *72*(5) 7205205040p1–7205205040p9.

O'Neil, H. (1989). *Managing anger*. London: Whurr.

Price, J. R., Mitchel, E., Tidy, E., et al. (2008). Cognitive behaviour therapy for chronic fatigue syndrome in adults. *Cochrane Database of Systematic Reviews*, *16*(3), CD001027.

Prins, J. B., Bleijenberg, G., Bazelmans, E., et al. (2001). Cognitive behaviour therapy for chronic fatigue syndrome: A multicentre randomised controlled trial. *Lancet*, *357*, 841–847.

Prior, S. (1998a). Determining the effectiveness of a short-term anxiety management course. *British Journal of Occupational Therapy*, *61*(5), 207–213.

Prior, S. (1998b). Anxiety management: Results of a follow up study. *British Journal of Occupational Therapy*, *61*(6), 284–285.

Rafaeli, E., Bernstein, D. P., & Young, J. (2010). *Schema therapy: Distinctive features*. Hove: Routledge.

Salkovskis, P. M. (Ed.). (1996). *Frontiers of cognitive therapy*. New York: Guilford.

Stewart, A. (2003). The case for generic working in mental health. *British Journal of Occupational Therapy*, *66*(4), 180.

Strong, J. (1998). Incorporating cognitive-behavioural therapy with occupational therapy: A comparative study with patients with low back pain. *Journal of Occupational Rehabilitation*, *8*(1), 61–71.

Swan, J., & Sloan, G. (2018). An introduction to the art and science of cognitive behavioural psychotherapy. In *European psychiatric/mental health nursing in the 21st century* (pp. 59–73). Cham: Springer.

Taylor, E. (1988). Anger intervention. *American Journal of Occupational Therapy*, *42*(3), 147–155.

Vlaeyen, J. W. S., & Morley, S. (2005). Cognitive-behavioral treatments for chronic pain: What works for whom? *Clinical Journal of Pain*, *21*(1), 1–8.

Waldron, H. B., & Kaminer, Y. (2004). On the learning curve: The emerging evidence supporting cognitive-behavioral therapies for adolescent substance abuse. *Addiction*, *99*(Suppl. 2), 93–105.

Weishaar, M. (1993). *Aaron T*. London: Beck. Sage.

Wellman, H. M., & Lagattuta, K. H. (2004). Theory of mind for learning and teaching: The nature and role of explanation. *Cognitive Development*, *19*, 479–497.

Wells, A. (1997). *Cognitive therapy for anxiety disorders: A practical manual and conceptual guide*. Chichester: Wiley.

Wilding, C. (2015). Cognitive Behavioural Therapy (CBT): Evidence-based, goal-oriented self-help techniques: A practical CBT primer and self help classic. *Teach Yourself*, London.

13

The Biomechanical Frame of Reference

Ian R. McMillan

OVERVIEW

This chapter explains why implementing a biomechanical frame of reference within occupational therapy continues to be relevant in practice. Occupational therapists are concerned with the relationship between people's occupations and their health, and assess people's disengagement from their occupations, provide ways for them to re-engage in their occupations, or suggest alternatives so that people's quality of life may improve. Core values and beliefs about the importance of occupation to humans constitutes a paradigm of occupation. This is seen in daily practice; occupational role issues that individuals may experience can be appreciated by referring to conceptual models of practice using a 'top-down' approach. Examples of such models of practice are the Canadian Model of Occupational Performance (CMOP; Townsend & Polatajko 2007) and the Model of Human Occupation (MOHO; Taylor 2017). Such models provide the knowledge, skills and attitudes necessary to understand how we analyze, intervene and evaluate individuals in relation to their roles and efficacy of occupational performances, for example, in self-care, work and leisure. However, to understand the individual's specific occupational performance problems, it is also necessary to analyze and understand their 'performance capacities' in more detail. Performance capacities refer to cognition, behaviour, neural development, personal and social interactions and, most importantly for this chapter, movement. The biomechanical frame of reference deals exclusively with the capacity for movement, whereas other frames of reference deal with other capacities, for example, the cognitive–behavioural frame of reference deals with cognition and behaviour. A biomechanical frame of reference is useful in assessment, intervention and evaluation with people who have occupational performance problems, created primarily by disease, injury or life events that impinge on their voluntary movement, muscle strength, endurance or, usually, a combination of all three. The loss of one or more of these capacities will interfere to some degree with an individual's ability to perform their occupations to their satisfaction. The biomechanical frame of reference assists in understanding the assessment, intervention and evaluation strategies associated with changing physical performance capacities (and/or modifying the environment) to help individuals re-engage in their occupations.

INTRODUCTION

The 'biomechanical frame of reference', in its original form, was not constructed for occupational therapy practice today and therefore some translation of the original frame of reference (from a professional perspective) is necessary to ensure a 'fit' with the philosophy of occupational therapy. This chapter describes and articulates a biomechanical frame of reference from an occupational therapist's perspective.

The biomechanical frame of reference used in occupational therapy has a long tradition and at different points in history has been termed Baldwin's reconstruction approach (1919), Taylor's orthopaedic approach (1934), and Licht's kinetic approach (1957) (Curtin et al 2017). This frame of reference continues to be widely

---

HIGHLIGHTS

This chapter

- explores the evolution and use of the biomechanical frame of reference in occupational therapy.
- asserts the biomechanical frame of reference can be located within a 'top-down' approach to occupational therapy.
- explains how the biomechanical frame of reference helps you deal with a person's problems related to their capacity for movement in their daily occupations.
- presents why the biomechanical frame of reference can be used to shape assessment, intervention and evaluation strategies, to assist individuals to re-engage in their occupations.

used today in practice thinking (whether occupational therapists realize it or not), and occupational therapists are continuing to present this frame of reference in different ways, for example, Trombly Latham appears to have incorporated a biomechanical frame of reference into the Occupational Functioning Model (Radomski & Trombly Latham 2013).

Reflecting on the biomechanical frame of reference (encompassing a variety of knowledge, skills and attitudes) broadens your knowledge and provides more insight into practice experiences with individuals and an understanding of how practice can inform theory-building and vice versa.

CONCEPTUAL MODELS OF PRACTICE

Occupation (Taylor 2017, Polatajko & Townsend 2007), within the context of occupational therapy, is part of the human condition, necessary to society and culture, required for physical and psychological well-being, entails underlying performance components and is a determinant and product of human development. Further, the intrinsic values of occupational therapy as a practice grounded in humanism affirm the dignity and worth of individuals, the participation in occupation, self-determination, freedom and independence, latent capacity, caring and the interpersonal elements of therapy, human uniqueness and subjectivity, and mutual cooperation in the therapeutic process. Occupational performance is usually expressed in terms of self-care/daily living tasks, work/productivity and leisure/play, depending on which conceptual model is being employed (Taylor 2017, Townsend & Polatjko 2007).

Studying and considering human occupation has to be paramount and is the core business of being an occupational therapist. When necessary, occupation can be analyzed (e.g., the biological, psychosocial, environmental, etc.) in terms of its content and meaning for the individual, to determine what has gone wrong or what performance is missing because of disease and injury.

Occupational therapists who can expertly analyze occupations are able to perceive the meaning for that person and assist them in regaining the necessary skills (or compensate for their permanent loss) through the medium of occupation and/or by modifying the environment or the attitudes of others in society.

If an individual has temporarily or permanently lost an occupational role (e.g., worker) because of occupational performance problems primarily concerning movement, the biomechanical frame of reference is key to informing the therapist and assisting the overall therapeutic process.

Ultimately, the majority of individuals seen by an occupational therapist will have problems of 'body and mind' (irrespective of diagnostic labels), which can only be discerned within the context of that individual's environment, perspectives and value systems. This requires adopting a top-down approach to practice (Kramer et al 2003, Brown & Chien 2010) by using an occupational therapy conceptual model of practice to appreciate the significance of an individual's occupational performance problems and then using one or more frames of reference (in this case, the biomechanical frame of reference) and others to appreciate the performance component issues.

Top-Down Approach to Practice

The values and beliefs inherent in an occupation paradigm imply that occupational therapists first need to view their clients as occupational beings. We need to choose conceptual models of practice that focus on describing the occupational nature of the client. There are a number of unique occupational therapy models of practice available to choose from, such as the MOHO (Taylor 2017), the CMOP (Townsend & Polatajko 2007) and the Person–Environment–Occupation Model (Law et al 1996, Strong et al 1999). Practice is further supported with other frames of reference when required (e.g., the biomechanical frame of reference), so occupational performance issues relative to movement in occupations can be specifically analyzed and managed.

Figure. 13.1 implies the occupation paradigm influences every aspect of an occupational therapist's thinking and practice. The use of knowledge located in a biomechanical frame of reference needs to be altered or filtered by the occupational therapist's values (the occupation filter) that are located within the occupation paradigm. This filter ensures the focus of interventions remains occupational in nature. The focus of the biomechanical frame of reference is the musculoskeletal capacity to create movement (range of motion), strength and endurance to carry out meaningful occupations. Movement, strength and endurance can be assessed within the context of a person completing their occupations, and occupations will be used therapeutically to restore, maintain or compensate for lack of movement, strength and endurance.

OCCUPATION FILTER

The following points constitute the notion of the occupation filter, and occupational therapists ought to reflect on these statements when using the biomechanical frame of reference (or any other frame of reference) to enrich

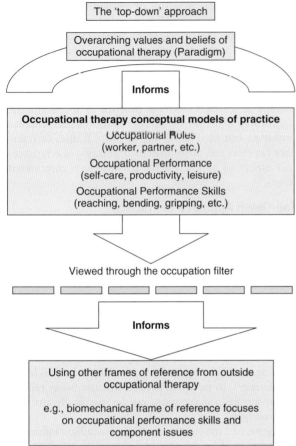

The 'top-down' approach

Overarching values and beliefs of
occupational therapy (Paradigm)

Informs

Occupational therapy conceptual models of practice

Occupational Roles
(worker, partner, etc.)

Occupational Performance
(self-care, productivity, leisure)

Occupational Performance Skills
(reaching, bending, gripping, etc.)

Viewed through the occupation filter

Informs

Using other frames of reference from outside
occupational therapy

e.g., biomechanical frame of reference focuses
on occupational performance skills and
component issues

Fig. 13.1 The 'top-down, approach. (Modified by McMillan (2018) from Forsyth and McMillan, personal communication (2001).)

practice (Mallinson & Forsyth, personal communication 2000). These points are

- A person's occupational performance. The primary concern here is understanding how movement, strength and endurance influence the person's performance of their occupational roles.
- Assess through occupation. Analyze and assess movement, strength and endurance within the context of the person's performance of their occupational roles.
- Occupation restores/maintains/compensates. This reinforces the person's performance of occupational roles during the restoration and/or maintenance and/or compensation of movement, strength and endurance.
- The outcome of occupational therapy is satisfying. Meaningful performance in occupations. Occupational therapists ought to view the satisfying, meaningful

performance of occupation as the primary outcome of therapy.

Using the top-down approach implies that a biomechanical frame of reference used by an occupational therapist will be different from a biomechanical frame of reference used by other health professionals. Understanding the use of this frame of reference in our professional practice means that occupation and occupational performance incorporating movement and its potential restoration are key. Movement for the sake of movement divorced from the individual's occupations is more likely to be the aim of other professionals, reflecting a more traditional 'bottom-up approach' (Kramer et al 2003, Brown & Chien 2010).

DETAILS OF THE BIOMECHANICAL FRAME OF REFERENCE

This frame of reference is primarily concerned with an individual's movements during occupations. Movement in this context can be understood in more detail as the capacity for movement, muscle strength and endurance (the ability to resist fatigue).

An individual's quality of movement may be compromised as they carry out their occupations because of the effects of disease or injury. These effects may compromise specific body systems and structures (e.g., bones and joints) that create movement seen during occupational performance. Additionally, an individual's quality of movement has to be viewed in the context of the environment that may facilitate or inhibit their movement when executing their occupations.

Aim and Objectives

The biomechanical frame of reference aims to address the quality of movement in occupations. Specific objectives are to

- prevent deterioration and maintain existing movement for occupational performance
- restore movement for occupational performance, if possible
- compensate/adapt for permanent loss of movement in occupational performance.

Compensation and *adaptation* are terms that have often been associated with 'rehabilitation' or the 'rehabilitative model' in the past. Some practitioners believe the biomechanical frame of reference deals comprehensively with the topic of compensation and some believe that a rehabilitation model deals with compensation. This author believes that rehabilitation may be viewed as an 'aim' and that compensation is more comprehensively addressed within the biomechanical frame of reference.

Whom Would You Use the Biomechanical Frame of Reference With?

This frame of reference is principally used with individuals who experience the following problems in their daily occupations:

Limitations in Movement During Occupations

This describes the capacity of the person to use their muscles in conjunction with bones and joints to move freely when engaging in occupations. This is usually attributed to one or more of the following problems:

- contracture (shortening) of soft tissues, that is, muscle tissue, muscle connective tissues, tendons, ligaments, fibrous capsules and skin
- the presence of inflammation, oedema or haematoma
- localized destruction of bone (e.g., rheumatoid arthritis, osteoarthrosis)
- amputation
- congenital issues
- acute and persistent/chronic pain
- maladaptive environmental conditions.

Inadequate Muscle Strength for Use in Occupations

This describes the capacity of the person to initiate and maintain muscle strength during their occupations (e.g., using the forearm muscle groups to facilitate gripping an object effectively in the hand). Inability to do this may be attributed to one or more of the following problems:

- limitations in movement
- disuse or atrophy of muscle (e.g., postfracture immobilization)
- primary muscle pathology (e.g., muscular dystrophy)
- spinal (anterior horn cell) pathology (e.g., motor neurone disease)
- peripheral neuropathy (e.g., diabetes)
- peripheral nerve damage (e.g., mononeuropathy of the median nerve)
- acute and persistent/chronic pain
- maladaptive environmental conditions.

Loss of Endurance in Occupations

This describes the ability of the person to resist subjective fatigue and therefore sustain their occupations over time and distance to their satisfaction. Issues in this area are usually attributed to one or more of the following problems:

- limitations in movement
- inadequate muscle strength
- compromised cardiovascular and/or respiratory function
- acute and persistent/chronic pain
- maladaptive environmental factors.

Biomedical Conditions

People who experience limitations in movement, inadequate muscle strength and loss of endurance while engaging in their occupations usually have a diagnosis of one or more of the following biomedical conditions:

- rheumatoid arthritis, osteoarthrosis or a combination of the two, or the individual may have experienced surgical arthroplasty
- amputations, burns and other soft-tissue damage frequently seen in hand and limb injuries
- fractures and various orthopaedic conditions
- Guillain–Barré syndrome, muscular dystrophy, motor neurone disease and the long-term effects of poliomyelitis (post-polio syndrome)
- peripheral neuropathy, mononeuropathy, brachial plexus lesions
- cardiac problems in the form of ischaemic heart disease (angina, myocardial infarction), cardiac failure or the effects of bypass surgery
- respiratory problems in the form of various obstructive airways diseases
- persistent/chronic pain as a result of occupational overuse syndrome (OOS), back injuries, neck injuries, fibromyalgia or pain associated with any of the conditions outlined above.

To appreciate the application of the biomechanical frame of reference implies an understanding of the biomedical conditions outlined above but also of the anatomical and physiological details of certain body systems and structures, which are outlined below:

- the musculoskeletal system, which comprises muscles, tendons, ligaments, bone and related tissues, and synovial joints (fibrous capsules, synovial tissues)
- the peripheral nervous system, comprising neural and connective tissues
- the integumentary system (skin), comprising the epidermis, dermis, blood vessels, hair follicles, sebaceous glands and sweat glands
- the cardiorespiratory system, comprising the heart, blood vessels and lungs.

It should be understood that the biomechanical frame of reference principally concerns the capacity to execute purposeful movement in everyday occupations; however, it is important to understand other factors that underpin this concept.

Other Factors

Understanding the biomechanical basis of movement includes understanding the musculoskeletal system (how bones and joints perform together, especially in relation to the appendicular skeleton), active and passive joint range of movement (a.ROM and p.ROM), the function of skeletal muscle, types of muscle work (concentric and eccentric, isotonic and isometric contraction), muscle architecture and role, the peripheral nervous system (motor, sensory and autonomic) and the relationship between the peripheral nervous system (synaptic transmission and innervation) and muscle action (sliding filament theory).

In addition, the biomechanical basis of movement includes understanding concepts of force, gravity, friction, resistance, leverage, stability and equilibrium, and how these elements interact to affect the nature of motion in human beings (Spaulding 2005), for example, when standing up from the seated position, and so on.

The relationship between occupational performance and the biomechanical frame of reference also requires understanding locomotion, the stance and swing phases of the gait cycle, prehension and the prehensile patterns of hand grips (power and precision), skeletal muscle and cardiovascular endurance, and the effects of fatigue on human occupations, all of which have to be considered for the execution of purposeful movement. McMillan and Carin-Levy (2012) provide a detailed explanation of all of the above, and this text is recommended as further reading to understand these factors in greater detail.

In summary, the capacity for occupational performance and movement is a synthesis of forces (the capabilities of the musculoskeletal system and the nervous system co-ordinating the work of groups of muscles to produce movement and stabilize joints) acting on the body. Endurance (the ability to sustain occupational performance) is predominantly a function of muscle physiology and the ability of the body systems to transport the required material towards, and waste materials away from, the muscle tissues.

Individuals' occupational performance problems that can be addressed through the biomechanical frame of reference *should* have an intact, fully matured central nervous system (CNS). In other words, no evidence of biomedical conditions or pathology that might affect the following body systems should be evident:

- motor control systems (cortex/basal ganglia/cerebellum)
- sensory discrimination (cortex/thalamus/cerebellum)
- perceptual qualities (association areas of the cortex and parietal lobe functions)
- cognition (localization of function)
- behaviour (localization of function).

This is because an individual with movement problems described in the biomechanical frame of reference still has the capacity in their CNS to initiate the wilful production of smooth, controlled isolated movements (Boyt Schell & Gillan 2018). This is in sharp contrast to individuals with CNS damage who would have different types of motor problem and therefore a different frame of reference would have to be considered, that is,

the theoretical approaches to motor control and cognitive–perceptual function (see this book for further information). However, it is also apparent that occupational therapists do use the biomechanical frame of reference at certain times with selected individuals who do have CNS damage in the form of stroke, multiple sclerosis, Parkinson disease and persistent/chronic pain. This is because, inevitably, some individuals do sustain permanent loss of the control of movement in various parts of their body and, in the long-term, compensating for this loss of movement in occupational performance is not only necessary but desirable.

The next part of this chapter concentrates on the assessment of movement seen in occupational performance.

PRINCIPLES OF ASSESSMENT AND MEASUREMENT

Rationale for Assessment

Occupational therapists ought to be concerned with the principles of assessment and measurement in their practice to facilitate collaborative goals, build intervention plans and document measures of outcomes. This process of assessment can be undertaken through client-driven assessment, therapist observation and the use of standardized and nonstandardized instruments.

Assessment facilitates the collection of quantitative and qualitative data, which when analyzed permits the interpretation of the effectiveness of an intervention by both the client and the therapist. This interpretative process, in relation to hard and soft data, assists in monitoring and implementing change, helps in building goals, facilitates decision-making and produces evidence that is readily understood, for the benefit of clients and other health professional and managerial colleagues.

General Aims of Assessment

The aims of occupational therapy assessment are generally to

- decide whether occupational therapy is appropriate or necessary
- establish roles, occupational performance, abilities, disabilities and the effects of the environment on an individual's occupations
- formulate a package of information (data collection) to plan collaborative goals
- formulate a baseline to compare progress and/or regress over time
- assist decision-making regarding the modification of intervention plans
- involve (through collaboration), inform, educate and motivate the individual

- establish the efficacy (and evidence base) of occupational therapy intervention
- assist resource decision-making regarding demands on service provision
- produce tangible outcomes/evidence for the benefit of the individual, healthcare and management colleagues.

Methods of Assessment

In the context of the biomechanical frame of reference these may consist of
- observation of occupational performance
- interviews (informal/unstructured through to formal/structured)
- questionnaires (open and closed questions)
- checklists (paper, computer and application based)
- rating scales (paper, computer and application based)
- performance evaluations (specific tasks, electrical, mechanical and computer equipment).

Framework for Assessment and Occupation

Assessments frequently reflect the theoretical perspectives of certain conceptual models of practice or frames of reference. It is important to reflect on which theoretical perspectives have informed the construction of assessments administered in your practice. Although occupational therapists use a wide range of assessments, Mathiowetz (1993), Kielhofner (2009) and Fisher (1998), all occupational therapists, assert that in concert with the values and philosophy of the profession, assessment ought to be focused on occupation, with a view to re-engaging the person in their occupations, and be as comprehensive as possible within the constraints of time. Because different assessments have arisen from different conceptual models of practice and frames of references, it is important to be able to discriminate between assessments constructed by occupational therapists and assessments constructed by other professionals. These differences reflect varying professional philosophies and need to be understood, so that it is clear when to use multiple assessments from conceptual models and frames of reference appropriately.

Molineux (2004) believes that a hierarchical order ought to be imposed on assessment, with occupational role and occupational performance being more important than the assessment of performance components. Mathiowetz (1993) previously advocated this approach because he believed occupational therapists ought to be primarily concerned with the daily effects of loss of occupational performance, thus reflecting the importance of the link between individuals and occupations. Specific occupation-focused assessments ought to be used in the first instance reflecting the top-down approach, for example, the Worker Role Interview (Braveman et al 2005) and the COPM (Law et al

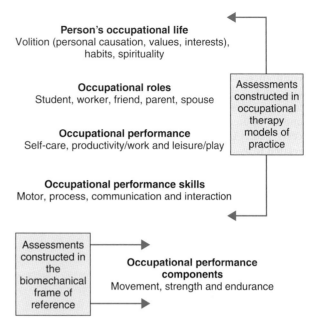

Fig. 13.2 Assessment and occupation. (From McMillan and Forsyth (2001). Personal communication

1990, Law et al 2014), would capture occupational performance as described above. However, Wilby (2007) also believes that performance components ought to be recognized in occupational therapy practice and that specific assessments may be required in specialist areas of practice that are drawn from other frames of reference. This would help inform therapists about specific performance component issues that are the building blocks of occupational performance; that is, an occupational therapist would assess loss of movement, which influences occupational performances.

In summary, assessments are drawn from occupational therapy models first and then more detailed observations/data about movement, strength and endurance (performance components) could also be collected using specific instruments to provide a comprehensive picture of the individual or this information could be made available by other professionals to meet the same end. Figure. 13.2 reflects this approach.

Assessment of Performance Components for Occupation

As previously mentioned, an area of expertise within the biomechanical frame of reference is to collect data from individuals, which provides greater detailed evidence to understand an individual's specific occupational performance problems. Because of the nature of the biomechanical frame of reference, assessments mostly relate to movement. There are various methods (mostly quantitative) available to assess occupational performance components in terms of movement, strength and endurance. The majority of these are readily available and can be easily applied with some practice. During the last few years there has been an increase in electronic and computer technology to assist the assessment process. Table 13.1 identifies specific testing procedures related to assessing the capacity for movement, strength and endurance. This table also details other factors, such as sensation (including pain) and other tests, which may fall within the remit of the biomechanical frame of reference.

Assessment of Specific Performance Components

Occupational therapists frequently use tests of 'function', although the exact meaning of this term is debatable. These tests tend to examine performance skills and components related to the upper limb and especially power

TABLE 13.1 Assessment of performance components	
Movement	
Range of motion (ROM) in joints	
Observation	Radomski & Trombly Latham (2013)
Goniometry	McHugh Pendleton & Schultz-Krohn (2016)
Odstock method	Roberts (1989)
Strength	
Muscle power	
Oxford rating scale	Radomski & Trombly Latham (2013)
Other scales	McHugh Pendleton & Schultz-Krohn (2016)
Grip strength in the hand	
Dynamometer	Radomski & Trombly Latham (2013)
	McHugh Pendleton & Schultz-Krohn (2016)
Pinch strength in the fingers	
Pinch meter	Radomski & Trombly Latham (2013)
Muscle bulk	
Observation	Radomski & Trombly Latham (2013)
Tape measure	Radomski & Trombly Latham (2013)
Presence of swelling in limbs	
Observation	McHugh Pendleton & Schultz-Krohn (2016)
Tape measure	McHugh Pendleton & Schultz-Krohn (2016)
Volumeter	McHugh Pendleton & Schultz-Krohn (2016)
Endurance	
Observation	McHugh Pendleton & Schultz-Krohn (2016)
Cardiorespiratory	McHugh Pendleton & Schultz-Krohn (2016)
Functional	McHugh Pendleton & Schultz-Krohn (2016)
Sensation	
Light touch and pressure	Radomski & Trombly Latham (2013)
Weinstein monofilament	Radomski & Trombly Latham (2013)
Thermal sensation	Radomski & Trombly Latham (2013)
Pain[a]	Radomski & Trombly Latham (2013)

[a]The management of pain as part of the biomechanical frame of reference is a contentious issue. Pain is a perception (not merely a sensation) formulated in the cerebrum and is therefore within the remit of a different frame of reference; however, pain can be apparent in a multitude of conditions that fall within the remit of the biomechanical frame of reference and affect the occupational performance of individuals.

and precision grips of the hand (see Fig. 13.2). Examples of these include (Curtin et al 2017):

- Bennett Hand Tool Test
- Jebsen–Taylor Hand Function Test
- Moberg Pick Up Test
- Valpar Work Samples.

PRINCIPLES OF INTERVENTION

The principles of intervention located in a biomechanical frame of reference should reflect the philosophy and values of our profession. This implies filtering the knowledge associated with the biomechanical frame of reference through the occupation filter, as described earlier. The philosophy and values of occupation provide the rationale for coherent principles, skills and techniques that are applied to meet the needs of individuals, regarding occupational performance problems and movement.

Occupation in Therapeutic Intervention

Occupational therapy intervention varies considerably in terms of contact time with individuals. This may range from performing an assessment and discharge planning service (<1 day) to constructing programmes where the individual may be seen by you for longer periods of time (especially on an outpatient basis). This helps distinguish, to some extent, different practices that attempt to restore, maintain or compensate for 'lost' (temporarily or permanently) occupational performance. The use of meaningful occupation energizes intervention and defines the unique philosophy of occupational therapy (Trombly 1995, Ferguson & Trombly 1997, Fisher 1998, Perrin 2001, Pollard & Ikiugu 2015). In summary, principles related to meaningful occupation, the quality of movement and intervention techniques are blended together to manage the problems the individual experiences. This usually relates to restoring (or compensating) an individual's physical performance in terms of movement, strength and endurance to carry out tasks in self-care, work and leisure in different contexts of practice.

Practice Settings

Occupational therapists tend to be employed in different practice settings, and usually these are denoted by specialized areas of expertise. The application of theory and techniques associated with the biomechanical frame of reference is usually experienced with people in the following areas of practice:

- amputation and amputee problems
- assistive technology (wheelchairs, orthotics and other devices for home and personal use)
- burns and plastic surgery

- cardiac rehabilitation
- general medical problems
- hand therapy
- housing (ergonomic) modifications in the community
- older people (usually problems with falls, stability and mobility)
- orthopaedics
- orthotics and prosthetics
- pain management
- spinal cord injury
- work rehabilitation
- worksite ergonomic modification.

All of these may take place in specialized units, hospital or community-based settings.

To link the theory described in this chapter clearly with practice, the next section will illustrate the use of the biomechanical frame of reference with a hypothetical case study of a person who has difficulties in her daily life with occupational performances.

Case Vignette: Alison

Anne Alison is a 50-year-old woman who currently lives independently in her own apartment, with a very supportive partner. She has a 10-year history of rheumatoid arthritis (RA) and reports the main effects of her condition on her occupational lifestyle are fatigue at work and some experience of pain in her hands.

Anne Alison is employed full-time in an office as an administration assistant, mainly using a computer for multiple tasks in her worker role.

She still pursues leisure interests including socializing with friends, reading and listening to music, but has given up skiing, cycling and generally keeping fit. However, attempts are being made to reintroduce these occupational performances.

Anne appears to manage (in her own words) her occupational roles; however, during an initial interview with the occupational therapist, she does report having some minor difficulties.

ASSESSMENT

The occupational therapist could use various rigorous assessments drawn from MOHO (Taylor 2017) or use the COPM (Law et al 2014) to collect self-report data regarding occupations. Assessments related to movement, strength and endurance could then be administered to collect objective data on specific performance component issues. Based on the client's perceived problems (from the selected occupational therapy conceptual model of practice assessments) and objective assessments from the biomechanical frame of reference, the following are apparent:

- Occupational roles—no major concerns expressed at this time in terms of fulfilling her role expectations of being a partner, daughter, worker and friend.
- Occupational performance—no self-care problems evident except in relation to heavy housework (lack of endurance). Work and productivity (especially using a computer keyboard) provoke more anxiety in terms of future capability. Leisure is not reported as being problematic.
- Occupational performance skills—problems at times in terms of mobility, reaching, bending, gripping, manipulating objects and endurance in her occupations.
- Occupational performance components—objective findings related to loss of muscle bulk, strength, hand grip and overall endurance.
- Environment—problems with work environment, especially the work desk and other people's attitudes towards her productivity, and minor problems in her home environment.

INTERVENTION

The aim of the biomechanical frame of reference in this case vignette is to address the quality of movement in Ms A's occupations. General objectives relative to Alison are to

- prevent further deterioration and maintain existing movement for occupational performance (computer usage at work, joint protection techniques and acknowledging/managing pain)
- restore movement for occupational performance, if possible (by improving muscle strength)
- compensate/adapt for loss of movement in occupational performance (energy conservation techniques and using assistive technology).

It should be noted that, although individual objectives are documented, all three objectives are probably being addressed simultaneously when Ms A engages in any occupation in a therapeutic manner.

Using Computers at Work

Alison uses a computer at her work every day, and therefore the topic of ergonomics is relevant to her situation. Ergonomics is the application of scientific information concerning human beings to the design of objects, systems and environments for human use (Jacobs 2007).

This subject is principally associated with the design of everyday objects in the environment, and, in this case, analyzing the computer work station at the point of interaction with Alison, to prevent OOS, postural deformity, excessive fatigue and pain, whilst also ensuring safety.

In relation to occupational performance in its widest context, occupational therapists should be concerned with biological efficiency, health and safety in the home and workplace, and the comfort and ease of use of objects (Hignett 2000). The United Kingdom Royal College of Occupational Therapists has a vocational rehabilitation strategy (RCOT 2008), and this document would provide more information on this important role for an occupational therapist intervening with Alison.

OOS is defined as those disorders that are caused, precipitated or aggravated by repeated exertions or movements of the human body. It involves a number of similar conditions arising from overuse of soft tissues (tendons, muscles, nerves, vascular structures), usually of the upper limb, and is caused by repeated 'micro trauma' rather than sudden instant injury (McNaughton 1997). Alison may be at risk of developing OOS because of repetitive or prolonged keyboard use, awkward postures as a result of poorly designed chairs, localized contact stress on her forearms and hands as a result of the table edge and poorly designed workstations in general. Alison may complain of stiffness, discomfort, pain, alteration in sensation and clumsiness because of OOS, in addition to the problems associated with RA. In response, intervention may be delivered in terms of altering the ergonomics of her computer workstation and specifically the following:

Chair

Ensure that Alison uses the correct chair, which should have a five-spoked base with castors and an adjustable backrest. The backrest angle should be adjusted to 110 degrees, and ought to support her lumbar region up to the inferior aspect of her scapulae. Adjust her chair for height; when her fingers are placed on the keyboard, her forearms ought to be roughly parallel with the floor. Ensure that her feet are firmly placed on the floor with her knee angle at roughly 90 to 110 degrees. If her feet are not touching the floor, use a footrest. Some space between the top of the thighs and the underside of the desk ought to exist.

Workstation

Adjust the position of Alison's monitor by ensuring that her feet are flat on the floor and her head is in the midline; when she is looking straight ahead, the top of the screen should be at or just below eye level height. The monitor should be at least 18 to 30 inches from her eyes (arm's length). The posture of her hands on the keyboard is important. Preferably, the hands and wrists should be neutral relative to the forearm (no excessive flexion, extension, or radial or ulnar deviation). Instruct her to hold the mouse loosely and to avoid resting the forearm or wrist on the edge of the desk. Discourage hyperextending the little finger and advise her to use a light touch when clicking the mouse. Use workstation devices, for example, a copy stand or document holder, a gel wrist rest at the front of the keyboard, a gel mouse mat, a lumbar roll if necessary, and a footrest and telephone headset if appropriate. Check her arc of reach on the desk when seated and place important objects to hand to prevent overstretch (Jacobs & Bettencourt 1995, Jacobs 2007).

Lighting

Try to reduce glare on the computer screen by placing the monitor at right angles to a window (light source), if possible, using blinds on windows if these are fitted. Tilt the monitor slightly so that overhead lighting does not create screen glare. Use the brightness, colour and contrast controls on the monitor to compensate for glare.

Adaptive Posture

Encourage Alison to take frequent breaks from keyboarding, by varying her routines and walking about to perform other tasks, for example, a 30-second break every 10 minutes. A 'standing desk' would be of benefit so Alison can alternate sitting and standing when working.

The same advice would be applied to Alison if she also uses a computer at home for work or leisure. You should consult Holmes (2007) or Langman (2011) for further information on vocational rehabilitation.

Joint Protection and Occupational Performance

Joint protection is principally an educational and training programme used in conjunction with connective tissue diseases and has historically been utilized in the management of rheumatoid disease in the upper limb. The principles are designed to teach Alison about the inflammatory process and potential deformities seen in RA (Hammond 2013). Instruction in joint protection techniques addresses the following points:

- reducing joint stress
- decreasing pain
- preserving joint structure
- maximizing occupational performance and conserving energy.

Alison will require careful instruction, so that joint protection techniques can be consistently employed in all of her occupations to maintain maximal capacity for motion and to prevent damage and long-term deformity.

Seven principles of joint protection are outlined below in title only, and further research is recommended to understand fully the detail required for implementing each of these principles before instructing Alison in their application. The detail regarding these principles can be found in most occupational therapy textbooks on physical dysfunction (e.g., McHugh Pendleton & Schultz-Krohn 2016):

- Respect pain at all times.
- Maintain muscle strength and joint range of movement.
- Avoid positions of deformity and deforming stress.
- Use each joint in its most stable, anatomical and functional position.
- Use the strongest joints available for the activity.
- Avoid using muscles or holding joints in one position for any undue length of time.
- Never begin an activity that cannot be stopped immediately.

The success of these techniques with Alison depends on the need for education teaching her about preventing deterioration or maintaining her present occupational performance. Occupational therapists are constantly required to reinforce existing knowledge or impart new skills, which may alter habits in some way to facilitate change. In relation to Alison, the key to learning (and teaching) involves using the techniques in conjunction with her occupational performances in self-care, work and leisure that she has identified as problematic. Effective learning methods also imply planning ahead, imparting information at the correct level, providing clear instructions, eliciting feedback, evaluating learning, promoting the highest level of learning and using different methods to impart new information (French et al 1994, Boyt Schell & Gillen 2018). Techniques drawn from the cognitive–behavioural frame of reference (see Chapter 12) are important here.

Alison may also have a problem with persistent/chronic pain. Although it is beyond the remit of this chapter to deal with the extensive information about the management of chronic pain, attention to computer usage, joint protection techniques and pacing during occupations may help to change the perception of chronic pain. McMillan and Carin-Levy (2012) give further information on the occupational therapist's role in the management of pain and presents a related case study.

Improving Muscle Strength

Muscle strength is the amount of force that can be exerted by a single muscle or groups of muscles in a voluntary contraction. Muscle strength can be seen in isometric and isotonic activity, both of which are required for occupational performance. There is a relationship between the recruitment of motor units and the production of maximum muscle tension in response to external loads on muscle groups. Periods of muscular inactivity as a result of disease or trauma may lead to muscle atrophy (decreased strength), the inability to sustain performance and a loss of co-ordination during occupational performances.

To increase muscle strength, stress (demand) has to be applied to a muscle through the use of occupational performances so that all the motor units are recruited to maintain and restore the muscle. This activity will ensure maximum (or near-maximum) contraction of the muscle, thus hypertrophying muscle fibres by influencing changes in the amount of contractile proteins. An increase in the amount of proteins and cross-bridges improves muscle cross-sectional size and therefore strength (Radomski & Trombly Latham 2013).

Hypothetically, muscle tension needs to reach 50% to 67% of the maximum potential capability of that muscle or group of muscles, and an increase in strength will result. This implies that, as the muscle increases in strength, the amount of stress placed upon it should also be increased over time to increase strength further. This is termed the *overload principle* and requires grading of stress through occupations placed on the client's affected muscle groups over time. Overloading is a positive stressor and will improve adaptation to the demands placed on Alison when carrying out her self-care, work and leisure performances. Radomski & Trombly Latham (2013) argue that *occupation as a means* of therapeutic change and *occupation as an end result* have to be apparent to the individual for muscle strengthening to fall within the remit of an occupational therapist.

Muscle strengthening (through overloading) involves the analysis and grading of occupation and is dependent on the following factors, all of which can be graded:
- type of occupation (self-care, work/productivity and leisure)
- intensity (resistance of muscles against the performance)
- duration (time taken to complete the occupation)
- speed (of the limbs and so on during the occupation)
- frequency (how often the occupation is undertaken).

Occupations should be motivating and have meaning for Alison in relation to her occupational performances. The most important factor other than the occupation itself is the intensity, which concerns the muscle groups being resisted whilst attempting to produce motion for occupation. Resistance can be altered by changing the position of Alison relative to the occupation, changing the length of lever arms, changing the materials used, increasing the difficulty of the occupation, using different tools, and changing the weight of any objects used for the occupation.

Engaging in occupational performance is usually aimed at restoring muscle strength and improving motion in one area of the body, for example, the upper limbs. However, to carry out her desired occupations in a sustained fashion, Alison's muscular (whole-body) endurance also has to be improved. For example, this could be attained by looking at the weight of the clothes that she loads into her washing machine and gradually increasing that load over time. The 'reserve' of the cardiorespiratory system in resisting fatigue is then considered as part of the occupation. McHugh Pendleton & Schultz-Krohn (2016) provides further detail on increasing cardiorespiratory reserve.

Energy Conservation

Energy conservation techniques are generally used in the management of chronic pathological conditions in which strength and particularly endurance are compromised. This implies compensation on a temporary or permanent basis. The aims of the techniques are to eliminate wasted body motion to preserve physical and psychological energy resources. This is especially the case when Ms A perceives a relapse in the course of her condition of RA.

Alison could be instructed to reduce energy expenditure (physical and psychological) by planning ahead, organizing storage in the home and at work, sitting to perform kitchen work instead of standing where possible, reducing the weight of briefcases, bags of shopping and so on, and ensuring good working conditions with respect to lighting, ventilation and heating.

She could also use alternative sources of energy (human resources and assistive technology devices) by asking her partner, immediate family and relatives to undertake certain tasks for her at times (shopping, laundry, vacuuming). In the longer term, if her condition did deteriorate, then volunteer and 'home care' services (ironing, laundry, etc.) would be worth considering.

Assistive Technology and Occupational Performance

This section describes technology that can help an individual maintain, restore or compensate for loss of occupational performance.

Assistive technology can be used over short or long periods of time, depending on the client's potential for restoration or compensation. Assistive technology in its simplest form includes personal and domestic devices, for example, adapted cutlery, plates, easy chairs, dressing devices, communication devices, bath boards, kitchen devices and manual wheelchairs. Some of these simpler devices may be appropriate for Alison at certain times. On a more complex level, static and dynamic orthoses, prostheses, burn pressure garments, electric wheelchairs, stair lifts, adapted vehicles and environmental control systems can also be viewed as assistive technology (Cook & Polgar 2015).

One aspect of assistive technology that may assist Alison temporarily is the use of a wrist–hand orthosis or splint. Orthotics (or splinting) involves the design, manufacture and application of thermoplastic material to manage individuals' biomechanical problems. Although thermoplastic orthoses can potentially be applied to any area of the body, occupational therapists most often apply orthoses to the prehensile structures (i.e., the hand and upper limb), and locomotor structures (i.e., the foot and lower limb).

In general, orthoses are biomechanical in design and are used to manage problems associated with limitations resulting from problems of the musculoskeletal system, peripheral nervous system and integumentary system. Despite the different designs (static and dynamic orthoses) and materials, orthoses are generally used to meet the following aims, dependent on the individual's problems:

- to achieve an optimal anatomical position and physiological state, therefore maximizing functional ability
- to provide pain relief (especially during sleep)
- to facilitate correct anatomical healing
- to prevent and correct soft-tissue deformity
- to maintain the function of unaffected parts
- to maintain the improvements achieved by other forms of treatment
- to restore or maintain joint alignment and stabilization
- to assist the function of weak muscles and prevent overstretch
- to provide a substitution for absent muscle power
- to protect vulnerable anatomical structures.

In addition to the skill of manufacture and application, comprehensive assessment procedures and specific knowledge about the musculoskeletal structures necessary for motion are necessary. Effective management of problems by the application of orthoses depends as much on efficient manufacture as the clients' attitudes to wearing the device. Individuals like Alison have to understand why wearing any orthosis is important; this can be achieved through educational principles, which are the key to successful management and treatment. See Coppard and Lohman (2015) for further information about orthoses.

SUMMARY

Some occupational therapists have argued that a biomechanical frame of reference is essentially reductionist and narrow in its focus, because it is based on a biomedical view of the world (Molineux 2004) and may have no place in current practice. However, thinking about only using one frame of reference reflects a 'bottom-up' approach to practice, and occupational therapists who attempt to use the biomechanical frame of reference in isolation from occupational therapy conceptual models of practice will certainly find its use limiting. Recently Burley et al (2018) undertook a scoping review of hand therapy and the use

of the biomechanical model that appears to highlight the shortcomings of using this model disconnected from occupation-focused models (a bottom-up approach). Ultimately, it is not necessarily the theoretical base of a specific frame of reference that makes it narrow in application, but one's view of the world as an occupational therapist and how different conceptual models of practice/frames of reference are used to address the multiple needs of an individual. In isolation, the biomechanical frame of reference is not universally applicable; however, the management of any individual (e.g., Alison) will always require a blend of conceptual models of practice and frames of reference viewed through the occupation filter. For example, the successful management of Alison will require knowledge about occupational therapy conceptual models of practice, the biomechanical frame of reference and the cognitive–behavioural frame of reference (see Chapter 12) to address her problems of occupational performance created by conditions that affect mind and body.

✷ REFLECTIVE LEARNING

- What features make the biomechanical frame of reference different from other frames of reference in this book?
- Which areas of human performance does a biomechanical frame of reference help you understand as an occupational therapy student?
- In what ways could a biomechanical frame of reference inform you how to assess and intervene with people who have issues in their daily occupations?
- What would be the consequences of assuming that a biomechanical frame of reference could be applied in isolation from models and other frames of reference in occupational therapy?
- Reflecting on your most recent practice experiences, in what ways could you have enriched the interventions that you undertook with individuals with movement problems in their daily occupations?

REFERENCES

Braveman, B., Robson, M., & Velozo, C. (2005). *The worker role interview (Version 10).* Chicago: University of Illinois, Department of Occupational Therapy, Model of Human Occupation Clearinghouse.

Brown, T., & Chien, W. (2010). Top-down or bottom-up occupational therapy assessment: Which way do we go? *British Journal of Occupational Therapy, 73*(3), 95.

Boyt Schell, B. A., & Gillen, G. (2018). *Willard and Spackman's occupational therapy* (13th ed.). Baltimore: Walters Kluwer .

Burley, S., Di Tommaso, A., Cox, R., & Molineux, M. (2018). An occupational perspective in hand therapy: A scoping review. *The British Journal of Occupational Therapy*, *81*(6), 299–318.

Coppard, B. M., & Lohman, H. (2015). *Introduction to splinting: A clinical reasoning and problem-solving approach* (4th ed.). St Louis: Elsevier.

Cook, A., & Polgar, J. M. (2015). *Assistive technologies: Principles and practice* (4th ed.). St Louis: Elsevier.

Curtin, M., Adams, J., & Egan, M. (2017). *Occupational therapy for people experiencing illness, injury or impairment: Promoting occupation and participation*. Edinburgh: Elsevier.

Ferguson, J. M., & Trombly, C. A. (1997). The effect of added-purpose and meaningful occupation on motor learning. *American Journal of Occupational Therapy*, *51*(7), 508–515.

Fisher, A. G. (1998). Uniting practice and theory in an occupational framework. *British Journal of Occupational Therapy*, *52*(7), 509–521.

French, S., Neville, S., & Laing, J. (1994). *Teaching and learning: A guide for therapists*. Oxford: Butterworth–Heinemann.

Hammond, A. (2013). Chapter 8: Joint Protection. In L. Goodacre, & M. MacArthur (Eds.), *Rheumatology practice in occupational therapy: Lifestyle management* (1st ed) (pp. 111–132). Chichester: Wiley-Blackwell.

Hignett, S. (2000). Occupational therapy and ergonomics: Two professions exploring their identities. *British Journal of Occupational Therapy*, *63*(3), 137–139.

Holmes, J. (2007). *Vocational rehabilitation*. Oxford: Blackwell.

Jacobs, K., & Bettencourt, C. M. (1995). *Ergonomics for therapists*. Boston: Butterworth–Heinemann.

Jacobs, K. (2007). *Ergonomics for therapists* (3rd ed.). St Louis, Missouri: Mosby Elsevier.

Kielhofner, G. (2009). *Conceptual foundations of occupational therapy* (4th ed.). Philadelphia: FA Davis.

Kramer, P., Hinojosa, J., & Brasic Royeen, C. (2003). *Perspectives in human occupation: Participation in life*. Philadelphia: Lippincott Williams & Wilkins.

Langman, C. (2011). *Introduction to vocational rehabilitation*. Oxon: Routledge.

Law, M., Cooper, B., Strong, S., Stewart, D., Rigby, P., & Letts, L. (1996). The Person–Environment–Occupation Model: A transactive approach to occupational performance. *Canadian Journal of Occupational Therapy*, *63*(1), 9–23.

Law, M., Baptiste, S., Carswell, A., McCall, M. A., Polatajko, H., & Pollock, N. (2014). *Canadian Occupational Performance Measure* (5th ed.). Toronto: Canadian Association of Occupational Therapists.

Law, M., Baptiste, S., Opzoomer, A., Polatajko, H., & Pollock, N. (1990). Canadian Occupational Performance Measure. *Canadian Journal of Occupational Therapy*, *57*(2), 82–87.

Mathiowetz, V. (1993). Role of physical performance component evaluations in occupational therapy functional assessments. *British Journal of Occupational Therapy*, *47*(3), 225–230.

McHugh Pendleton, H., & Schultz-Krohn, W. (2016). *Pedretti's occupational therapy: Practice skills for physical dysfunction* (8th ed.). St Louis, Missouri: Elsevier.

McMillan, I. R., & Carin-Levy, G. (2012). *Tyldesley & Grieves' muscles, nerves and movement in human occupation* (4th ed.). Oxford: Wiley Blackwell.

McMillan, I. (2001). Assumptions underpinning a biomechanical frame of reference. In Duncan EAS (Ed) (2001) Foundations for Practice in Occupational Therapy. Edinburgh: Elsevier.

McNaughton, A. (1997). Occupational overuse syndrome/repetitive strain injury: The occupational therapist's role. *British Journal of Occupational Therapy*, *60*(2), 69–72.

Molineux, M. (2004). *Occupation for occupational therapists*. Oxford: Blackwell.

Perrin, T. (2001). Don't despise the fluffy bunny: A reflection from practice. *British Journal of Occupational Therapy*, *64*(3), 129–134.

Pollard, N., & Ikiugu, M. N. (2015). *Meaningful living across the lifespan: Occupation-based intervention strategies for occupational therapists and scientists (Occupational Therapy for a Changing World)*. London: Whiting & Birch.

Radomski, M. V., & Trombly Latham, C. A. (2013). *Occupational therapy for physical dysfunction* (7th ed.). Philadelphia: Walters Kluwer, Lippincott Williams & Wilkins.

Roberts, C. (1989). The Odstock hand assessment. *British Journal of Occupational Therapy*, *52*(7), 256–261.

Royal College of Occupational Therapists. (2008). *Vocational rehabilitation strategy*. London: Royal College of Occupational Therapists.

Spaulding, S. J. (2005). *Meaningful motion: Biomechanics for occupational therapists*. Edinburgh: Churchill Livingstone.

Strong, S., Rigby, P., Stewart, D., et al. (1999). Application of the Person–Environment–Occupation Model: A practical tool. *Canadian Journal of Occupational Therapy*, *66*(3), 122–133.

Taylor, R. R. (2017). *Kielhofner's model of human occupation: Theory and application* (5th ed.). Philadelphia: Walters Kluwer.

Townsend, E., & Polatajko, H. (2007). *Enabling occupation ii: Advancing an occupational therapy vision for health, well-being, & justice through occupation*. Ottawa: CAOT Publishers.

Trombly, C. A. (1995). Occupation: Purposefulness and meaningfulness as therapeutic mechanisms. *British Journal of Occupational Therapy*, *49*(11), 960–972.

Wilby, H. J. (2007). The importance of maintaining a focus on performance components in occupational therapy practice. *British Journal of Occupational Therapy*, *70*(3), 129–132.

14

Application of Theoretical Approaches to Movement and Cognitive–Perceptual Dysfunction Within Occupation-Focused Practice

Leisle Ezekiel, Sally Feaver

◎ HIGHLIGHTS

- Occupational therapy practice is moving from an impairment focus to an occupation focus within neurological practice.
- The motor control frame of reference and acquisitional frame of reference enable therapists to use current theories about motor learning and skill acquisition to support their clinical reasoning and practice.
- The occupational task-oriented approach, dynamic interactional approach and neurofunctional approach all help therapists to integrate theory and research evidence within occupation-focused practice.

OVERVIEW

Movement, cognitive and perceptual deficits are common in neurological disorders and are key foci of occupational therapy interventions, as these deficits may result in significant occupational dysfunction.

The contemporary paradigm in occupational therapy is occupation-focused and recognizes the importance of occupation for long-term health and well-being (Kielhofner 2009). This paradigm shift is reflected in the development of occupation-focused approaches in neurological practice. Occupational therapists use a variety of approaches to aid their planning of interventions for people with neurological disability with the aim of maximizing occupational engagement and social participation.

This chapter focuses on two frames of reference that inform occupational therapy practice. Firstly, the motor control frame of reference is explored. This frame of reference is exemplified using the task-oriented approach and principles of motor learning. Next, the acquisitional frame of reference is discussed. The acquisitional frame of reference brings together theories of learning, cognitive neuroscience and activity analysis to guide occupational therapy interventions for clients with cognitive and perceptual dysfunction (Luebben & Royeen 2010). The acquisitional frame of reference is centred around therapists, use of teaching and learning strategies to support occupational performance (Greber et al 2007).

A brief summary of key theories will be discussed along with approaches to assessment and intervention planning for each frame of reference. A synopsis of the evidence base supporting intervention approaches will be given along with vignettes to illustrate the integration of theory into practice.

INTRODUCTION

Acquired brain injury is an umbrella term that includes both traumatic and nontraumatic causes of brain injury (stroke, for example). It is a leading cause of death and disability globally (Dewan et al 2018, Feigin et al 2014). Acquired brain injury results in diverse impairments which cause physical, cognitive and perceptual dysfunction and has long-term consequences for occupational engagement, participation and quality of life (Ezekiel et al 2018, Larsson et al 2013).

With the profession's focus on occupation, occupational therapists are well placed to address the long-term impacts of acquired brain injury. In recent years, occupational therapy interventions in stroke and brain injury rehabilitation have moved from being impairment-focused to activity-focused, reflecting the biopsychosocial model of health, disability and function (Gillen et al 2015, Radomski et al 2018). As a result, therapists take an occupational focus to intervention planning and enable clients to perform occupations with the motor and cognitive deficits they have, whilst recognizing that practicing everyday activities takes advantage of activity-dependent neuroplasticity and supports recovery (Sabari 2016).

There are now several intervention approaches that address the occupational performance challenges arising from motor, cognitive or perceptual dysfunction. These intervention approaches are supported by a growing body of evidence, but integrating evidence and theory into occupation-focused practice can be challenging (Radomski et al 2018). Consequently, this chapter aims to explore the main approaches currently used to plan occupation-focused interventions for people experiencing motor dysfunction and cognitive–perceptual dysfunction, as well as discuss their theoretical basis and available evidence.

THE MOTOR CONTROL FRAME OF REFERENCE

Motor control is defined as 'the ability to regulate or direct the mechanisms essential to movement' (Shumway-Cook and Woollacott 2017).

Systems Theory

Our understanding of motor control has shifted from being of a reflex and hierarchical nature to a systems theory of motor control (Shumway-Cook & Woollacott 2017). Systems theory suggests that motor control is distributed across several interconnected subsystems of the central nervous system acting in parallel. Thus movement is thought to emerge from multiple systems (neuromuscular, sensory, cognitive and perceptual) working together to solve motor problems (Muratori et al 2013).

A key feature of systems theory is Bernstein's problem of the elimination of redundant degrees of freedom (Latash 2012). Bernstein viewed the body as a mechanical system and he theorized how the body co-ordinates movement with so many different ways of configuring movement across multiple joints. Bernstein suggested that groups of muscles are constrained together to act as a unit (synergy) and thereby reduce the available degrees of freedom. Viewing the body as a mechanical system means understanding how external forces and the musculoskeletal system contribute to movement, along with the central nervous system (Bernstein, cited in Whiting 1984).

In more recent years, Latash (2012) revisited these concepts and suggested that redundant degrees of freedom are useful and help the system to cope with the unexpected.

Rather than eliminate redundant degrees of freedom, synergies ensure flexibility in task performance. The implications of this theory on clinical practice have not yet been established (Piscitelli 2016). However, Latash et al (2007) suggest that therapeutic interventions should explore flexibility rather than develop fixed solutions to motor performance problems.

Dynamic systems theory (DST) was developed from systems theory and explains the significance of the environment and tasks for motor control. DST suggests that movement emerges not only from the interactions of multiple systems (as described above) but also from interactions with the task and the environment (Shumway-Cook & Woollacott 2017).

Gibson's ecological theory of perception and action (Gibson 1966, cited in Shumway-Cook & Woollacott 2017) also explains the significance of the environment on movement. When we interact with objects within a task, we need to perceive the object, have accurate spatial awareness of the object and successfully integrate sensory and motor systems (Yamani et al 2015). Gibson proposed that environments and objects offer possibilities for action (object affordances) and these object affordances elicit particular movements, for example, a cup offers the action of reaching and grasping and thus affects the pattern of movement of the hand and arm (Mon-Williams & Bingham 2011).

Current practice reflects these theories and thus embraces a contextual approach to motor control and motor behaviour (McHugh et al 2013). The main features of the motor control frame of reference can be summarized as follows:

- Movement arises from the interaction of motor, sensory, cognitive and perceptual systems (Shumway-Cook & Woollacott 2017).
- The central nervous system is part of a complex system responsible for skilled movement. Different movement patterns emerge if other parts of the system change (Muratori et al 2013).
- Task demands and environmental factors affect the neural organization of movement (Teasell & Hussein 2018).

Motor control theories explain how motor behaviour emerges but to address the impact of motor dysfunction on occupational performance, therapists need to understand how motor behaviour is learnt. Hence contemporary approaches to motor dysfunction are also underpinned by theories of motor learning.

Motor Learning

Motor learning is defined as 'the acquisition or modification of skilled action' (Shumway-Cook & Woollacott 2017). It is beyond the remit of this chapter to offer a detailed discussion of motor learning theories but we will introduce key theories and summarize their implications for practice.

Skill Acquisition. Skilled and purposeful movement needs to be consistent, flexible and efficient (Muratori et al 2013). However, the learning process is not linear and it is important for therapists to understand where their patient is in terms of learning or relearning a motor skill.

Gentile (1998) described two stages to skill acquisition. In the initial stage, the learner explores basic movement patterns and identifies key environmental components relevant to the task. Patterns of movement during this stage are variable as the learner explores different movement strategies. This stage can be summarized as learning what movements are necessary (Muratori et al 2013) and involves cognitive processes such as problem solving.

Once a successful movement pattern has been discovered, the learner begins to refine their movement, learning how to move more efficiently. This stage is process of consolidation.

Gentile also suggested that motor learning involved explicit and implicit learning processes that occur in parallel. Explicit learning occurs as the learner consciously attends to the goal of the movement and uses feedback from the task and the environment to refine and improve movement. Gentile proposed that verbal instruction, demonstration and structuring the environment could be used to support explicit learning processes (Gentile 1998).

Implicit learning, however, involves the ability to predict the external forces affecting movement (for example, moving against gravity) and refine internal force dynamics accordingly. Internal force dynamics arise from muscle contractions and co-contractions. Implicit learning processes are not conscious processes and cannot be accessed by the therapist in the same way as explicit learning processes. Gentile suggested that implicit learning occurs when the learner engages in tasks that elicit the appropriate production of force. The therapist manipulates the tasks and the environment to provide the 'just-right' challenge. The implications of motor learning principles for therapists can be summarized as follows:

- Learning involves the acquisition, retention and transfer of skills (Muratori et al 2013).
- Motor learning involves sensory, perceptual and cognitive processes.
- Motor learning is contextual to the person, task and environment.
- As motor skills are learnt, movement patterns may be initially variable and unstable (Gentile 1998).

- Practice is an essential part of motor learning and can be structured to facilitate motor skill acquisition (Gentile 1998).

An occupational therapist using the motor control frame of reference would seek to explain motor function and dysfunction by analyzing the interactions between cognitive, perceptual, sensory and motor systems, the demands of the task, and the environment in which the task is performed. The therapist would focus on optimizing motor performance within meaningful tasks, using principles of motor learning. This involves providing opportunities for whole task practice in real life or simulated environments, enabling exploration of movement strategies and developing a practice schedule that supports the retention and transfer of learning (Mathiowetz 2016).

There are several approaches that integrate the motor control frame of reference and motor learning principles, including motor relearning (Carr & Shepherd 2003) and task-oriented approaches (Shumway-Cook & Woollacott 2017). Task-oriented approaches in particular have been recommended to form the basis of interventions for motor deficits after stroke (Nilsen et al 2015, Cotoi et al 2018). However, these approaches are not specific to occupational therapy and the therapist needs to translate the approach to retain an occupation focus.

Mathiowetz (2016) developed the occupational therapy task-oriented approach, which successfully integrates the task-oriented approach into the occupational therapy process.

OCCUPATIONAL THERAPY TASK-ORIENTED APPROACH

The occupational therapy task-oriented approach is an occupation-focused approach based on systems theory of motor control and motor learning (Mathiowetz 2016). It embeds these theories into occupational therapy practice and provides a structure for assessing the impact of motor deficits on occupational performance. The approach was developed for use in stroke rehabilitation but more recently has expanded to other patient populations (Muratori et al 2013). In this chapter, we will summarize how occupational therapists understand and optimize motor behaviour and occupational performance, using the motor control frame of reference and motor learning principles within the occupational therapy task-oriented approach.

Principles of Assessment

The task-orientated approach uses a top down approach to occupational therapy assessment by initially exploring the patient's roles, interests and needs (Mathiowetz 2016). The next step is to identify which areas of occupation are affected and to select tasks for further assessment. Therapists use observational assessments of everyday tasks to determine how performance is affected by sensory, motor, cognitive or perceptual difficulties and where performance breaks down. Task analysis of observed performance is a key aspect of the therapist's assessment (Preissner 2010). However, the therapist uses multiple assessment methods to determine the critical factors affecting occupational performance.

During task analysis, the therapist also assesses the impact of environmental factors on task performance to determine how to grade and adapt the task to provide the just-right challenge. The therapist observes the strategies used to accomplish the task and develops hypotheses about the underlying sensory, motor, cognitive and perceptual difficulties experienced and how these interact to affect the person's performance (Shumway-Cook & Woollacott 2017). The therapist needs to determine which of the factors affecting motor performance are critical and therefore need to be addressed.

Principles of Intervention Planning

Mathiowetz (2016) describes five key treatment principles in the occupational therapy task-oriented approach, outlined here:

1. Help clients adjust to role limitations.
2. Create environments that provide typical challenges of everyday life.
3. Practice functional tasks or close simulations.
4. Provide opportunities for practice outside of therapy.
5. Minimize ineffective and inefficient movement patterns:
   - Use motor learning principles in training or retraining skills.
   - Remediate critical factors affecting performance, if possible.
   - Adapt the environment and/task to optimize performance.
   - Constrain the degrees of freedom of movement.
   - Use constraint-induced movement therapy for those with learned nonuse.

The following vignette focuses on step 4. The scenario takes a narrow focus to allow demonstration of the approach.

CASE VIGNETTE

Miriam is a 55-year-old woman who experienced a stroke affecting the right side of her body. She is now several weeks post stroke and is being seen by the community stroke team at home. Miriam is independent in personal care tasks such as dressing and washing but mostly uses one-handed techniques. She has some movement in her right hand and arm but struggles to incorporate this into her everyday tasks. Using the Canadian Occupational Performance Measure (Law et al 1998), the occupational therapist determined Miriam's priorities for intervention. One of Miriam's goals was to go out for a meal with her husband and be able to cut up her own food. She had difficulty grasping objects with her right hand. The therapist initially assessed Miriam's motor skills whilst Miriam was eating, noting where her task performance broke down. The first area of task breakdown was Miriam's ability to form a secure grasp on the knife. The second area was in placing the knife on the plate and co-ordinating a smooth sawing motion. Miriam used lateral trunk flexion to place her hand on the plate but was unable to maintain her hand position against gravity. Miriam did not have any sensory, cognitive or perceptual deficits affecting her task performance. However, the therapist noted that Miriam had reduced grip strength, which also affected her ability to keep hold of the knife. Critical control parameters were identified by the therapist as grip strength and maintaining shoulder flexion against gravity.

The therapist and Miriam explored her movement during task performance, trying out different strategies until Miriam was able to perform the task with a degree of success. Examples were trying different hand positions to grip the knife, varying the size of the knife handle, reducing the degrees of freedom by increasing proximal support, therapist demonstration of movement and provision of verbal cues. The therapist encouraged Miriam to explore her movement by analyzing the task and problem-solving potential solutions. The therapist then devised a practice schedule with Miriam that includes both task practice and hand-strengthening exercises (to remediate the critical control parameter of grip strength). Task practice was organized around graded tasks that challenged Miriam's forward reach and grasp. As Miriam's movement with the task became more efficient and effective, the task difficulty increased (for example, reducing proximal support and reducing the size of the knife handle).

Evidence Base

There is moderate-quality evidence for the efficacy of the broader task-oriented approach in improving hand and arm function after stroke (French et al 2016, Pollock et al 2014). However, there is insufficient evidence to recommend one approach over another and further research is needed to establish the optimum dose of therapy (Pollock et al 2014). Variation in intervention protocols across research studies also hinders the translation of research into practice (Cotoi et al 2018).

Although there is evidence supporting elements of the occupational therapy task-oriented approach, as yet there have been no large randomized controlled trials to establish its efficacy. However, the approach offers an occupation focus to intervention planning while using theories of motor control and motor relearning.

ACQUISITIONAL FRAME OF REFERENCE

A range of different interventions are described in the research literature that address cognitive and perceptual impairments. These include training in the use of internal compensatory strategies, external compensatory strategies, metacognitive strategy training, remedial activities (for example, computer programmes) and errorless learning (Cicerone et al 2011).

These interventions are often categorized as remedial or compensatory approaches (Stephens & Williamson 2015) but this more traditional way of thinking about cognitive rehabilitation is potentially unhelpful for therapists and inaccurate, as it creates false dichotomies (Sohlberg & Turkstra 2011). For example, Thickpenny-Davis and Barker-Collo (2007) found that memory strategy training (considered compensatory) both reduced the behavioural impact of memory impairment and improved performance on neuropsychological memory assessments. Katz (2011) and Katz et al (2011) suggest that approaches within cognitive rehabilitation should be viewed on a continuum rather than as discrete categories.

There has also been a shift in occupational therapy practice away from an impairment or neuropsychological focus of cognition and perception to an occupation focus. Occupational therapists are now concerned with how to optimize occupational performance and engagement for people experiencing cognitive and perceptual dysfunction (Gillen 2008).

When it comes to frames of reference guiding occupational therapy practice in cognitive and perceptual rehabilitation, there continues to be a lack of consensus on a clearly defined frame of reference. Furthermore, the terms *frame of reference*, *approach* and *model*, while clearly defined within this textbook, are used interchangeably within occupational therapy literature in general For example, Toglia's dynamic interactional approach is described as an approach (Toglia 2005), a model (Josman 2005) and a frame of reference (Nash & Mitchell 2017). Selecting and using relevant frames of reference is vital to ensure therapists integrate theory into practice and hence support clinical reasoning (Dirette 2013).

An important part of reasoning with frame of reference is understanding the target of therapeutic change. In Toglia's dynamic approach, the target area of change for therapists is enabling clients to learn and use strategies that

optimize occupational performance. This target is shared by other approaches, for example, the cognitive orientation to occupational performance (CO-OP) (Missiuna et al 2001) and the perceive, recall, plan, perform system of task analysis (Nott et al 2009). Approaches such as the neurofunctional approach also identify learning as a key therapeutic focus (Clark-Wilson et al 2014).

The acquisitional frame of reference is primarily concerned with restoring or developing skills necessary for occupational performance and engagement. It explains the function–dysfunction continuum simply as being able to perform occupations or unable to perform occupations (Luebben and Royeen 2010). Although this frame of reference is mostly used within paediatric occupational therapy, within adult rehabilitation it supports occupation-focused practice as exemplified by the neurofunctional approach (Giles 2011).

The acquisitional frame of reference guides the therapist to take a teaching and learning orientation to therapeutic intervention, whilst recognizing that the personal factors that affect occupational performance also affect learning (Greber et al 2007). As such, the acquisitional frame of reference does not focus on cognitive and perceptual impairment but focuses on learning of necessary skills to support performance. These skills include the effective selection and use of cognitive strategies. The acquisitional frame of reference captures the centrality of teaching and learning in current approaches to cognitive and perceptual dysfunction, as it explains how learning arises from the interactions between the person, the task being learnt and the environment (Luebben and Royeen 2010).

Key Theories

The acquisitional frame of reference is underpinned by learning and behavioural theories as well as cognitive neuroscience. Here we will discuss key theories relevant to learning.

Vygotsky's Zone of Proximal Development. Lev Vygotsky was a developmental psychologist who proposed the social development theory of cognition. Vygotsky stressed the importance of social contexts and teacher–learner relationships in supporting cognitive development, leading to a collaborative approach to teaching and learning (Greber et al 2007).

Vygotsky defined the zone of proximal development (ZPD) as 'the distance between the actual development level as determined by independent problem-solving and the level of potential development as determined through problem-solving under adult guidance or in collaboration with more capable peer' (Vygotsky 1978, p.86). For the occupational therapist, the ZPD is the difference between how an individual performs without any support compared with their performance with therapist's support. Support strategies are described as 'the psychological tools or prompts designed to supplement inadequate cognitive resources' (Greber et al 2007). The process of applying support strategies is known as scaffolding. As the learner progresses through their zone of proximal development, they move from other-regulation to self-regulation. The therapist facilitates this by gradually withdrawing support until the person performs the task independently. Further generalization of learning to other tasks and situations requires metacognitive skills such as self-awareness (Greer et al 2007). Vygostky's ZPD is a key principle of dynamic assessment—a process where the therapist seeks to understand the person's occupational performance and identify interventions that enable them to move to the next level of competence (Lidz 1995). Although the ZPD was originally used to describe learning and cognitive development in children, it has been suggested that the ZPD has applications in brain injury rehabilitation as it represents the restoration potential of clients with acquired brain injury (Toglia 2011).

Cognitive Information Processing. An information-processing approach to understanding cognition comprises a number of different theories. One key theory is Atkinson and Shiffrin's (1968) stage theory of memory where information is processed and stored in three stages: sensory register, short-term (working) memory and long-term memory (Atkinson & Shiffrin 1968). For information to move from the sensory register to the short-term memory and then to long term, we first must attend to the information. Any information not processed in these first two stages is lost. Within long-term memory, information is organized as declarative memory (for example, episodic memory) or nondeclarative memory (e.g., procedural memory) (Squire & Dede 2015). Declarative and nondeclarative memory have been summarized as 'knowing what' and 'knowing how' (Roediger et al 2008).

Information processing theories suggest that we have limited capacity to process information and there are bottlenecks in the system. For example, short-term memory stores hold limited information for up to twenty seconds, unless the information is repeated. Information flow is also two directional as we use information from the environment and from our memory to make sense of our experiences (Huitt 2003).

Baddeley (2001) suggested a concept of working memory where information is processed and manipulated in three different storage components: phonological loop (auditory and written verbal information), visual–spatial sketchpad and the episodic buffer. The episodic buffer allows manipulation of information from the long-term memory store (Roediger et al 2008). A control mechanism is also necessary to oversee processing, storage and retrieval

of information. The control mechanism (executive function) also uses the processing capability of the system. New and complex tasks in new environments require greater executive control and hence are more taxing on the information processing system (Huitt 2003).

These theories have implications for understanding occupational performance and the acquisition of skills across all areas of occupational therapy practice. However, they are particularly pertinent when working with people with acquired brain injury because the deficits arising from acquired brain injury affect the learning process. Therapists need to understand how to structure learning experiences for clients and optimize their occupational performance in accordance with the severity and nature of the patient's cognitive dysfunction.

Two occupational therapy approaches that focus on the acquisition of skills for occupational performance for clients with cognitive or perceptual dysfunction are the dynamic interactional approach (Toglia 2005) and the neurofunctional approach (Clark-Wilson et al 2014).

The Dynamic Interactional Model of Cognition

In Toglia's dynamic interactional model, cognition is defined as 'an ongoing product of the dynamic interaction of the person, activity and environment' (Toglia 2005, p.30). Toglia suggests that optimum occupational performance depends on the person's self-awareness of their cognitive strengths and limitations, their selection of processing strategies, their personal contexts, activity demands and environmental factors. Using this approach, the therapist uses dynamic assessment principles to investigate the contextual factors and processing strategies that influence a patient's occupational performance (Toglia 2011). Processing strategies are defined as mental tools used when learning a new task or dealing with complex information and are considered part of normal cognitive functioning (Toglia et al 2012).

Occupational dysfunction occurs when the patient has difficulty selecting and using efficient processing strategies, limited anticipation and monitoring of performance, limited use of previous experience and knowledge to guide performance, and insufficient flexibility to apply knowledge and skills in different tasks and environments (Toglia 2011). The patient may have limited awareness of their cognitive functioning (metacognitive skills) and be unable to select processing strategies to meet the demands of the task within a given environment (Toglia 2000).

The aim of occupational therapy intervention is to initially facilitate the patient's self-awareness of their performance difficulties and promote the selection of effective processing strategies. Therapeutic interventions later aim to optimize the patient's performance as the patient learns to apply processing strategies flexibly across different tasks and environments.

Principles of Assessment

1. The dynamic interactional approach takes a top-down approach to assessment and starts by the therapist understanding their patient's personal contexts, goals and occupational challenges.
2. The therapist also needs to assess the individual's self-awareness of their performance. Self-awareness is predominately assessed as part of occupational performance by the therapist investigating a patient's self-perceptions before, during and after a task.
3. Dynamic assessment of occupational performance to determine the patient's cognitive modifiability. The therapist determines the client's zone of proximal development and notes how cues, task adaptations and feedback support optimal occupational performance (Toglia 2011).

Intervention Principles

1. Build self-awareness through engaging clients in structured learning experiences. The therapist guides the client to anticipate their performance, to review their performance and any challenges during the task, and to reflect back on their performance after the task. Therapists use feedback, questionnaires and discussion to promote the client's self-awareness of their performance difficulties (Zlotnik et al 2009).
2. Generate processing strategies with the client. The therapist explores the client's ideas of strategies that might support their performance in the task or may suggest strategies if the client is unable to think of any. Single or multiple strategies might be suggested by the therapist. Using multiple strategies better reflects how strategies are used within occupations (Toglia 2011).
3. Train in strategy use. As the client learns to predict their performance and anticipate difficulties, they practice identifying potential strategies to use within a task, and reflect on how using the strategy affected their task performance. Single or multiple strategies might be practiced according to the client's needs. Some example strategies are mental rehearsal, time pressure management and self-talk (verbalizing the steps of the task).
4. Develop a practice schedule to generalize learning; the client practices strategy use across a continuum of tasks and environments.

Case Vignette 2

Peter is in his early thirties and is recovering from a moderate brain injury following a road traffic collision. He previously worked in an information technology department for a local business and is hoping for a graded return to work. However, he has noticed that he struggles to concentrate, particularly when attempting paperwork and administration tasks.

After interviewing Peter and establishing his needs, challenges and goals, the therapist agreed a task with Peter for an observational dynamic assessment; observing how he reviews and answers recent emails on his laptop.

The therapist saw Peter at home and asked him to approach the task of checking emails on he computer as he usually would. Before starting the task, the therapist asked Peter to rate how difficult he anticipated the task to be and to identify any potential challenges. Then the therapist observed Peter completing the task.

The therapist noted that Peter was disorganized in his approach and distracted by notifications on his laptop and his phone. He would lose track of what he was doing, often having several applications and emails open at the same time. During the task Peter noticed that he couldn't make sense of some emails as there was too much information on the screen for him to take in. He reported feeling mentally tired and increasingly frustrated. During the assessment, the therapist redirected Peter when he became distracted and prompted him to close unnecessary windows and programmes. The therapist suggested increasing the size of the email window so that Peter could only see one or two emails at a time.

Through discussion and reflection on his performance, Peter started to identify key areas of task difficulty. He recognized that his laptop screen was overcrowded at times and that he found multi-tasking extremely difficult. He had not noticed how distracting his phone was, or that he struggled to return to the task after being distracted.

The therapist used 'understanding my attention' worksheets to help Peter understand how the environment affected his ability to stay focused on a task (Fish et al 2017). Peter decided to create a quiet workspace in his flat to minimize distraction and put his phone in a different room when working on the computer. He chose to use a simple checklist to help him to work systematically through his emails. He also reduced the amount of information displayed on his laptop. Peter then discussed how these strategies affected his task performance and identified other similar tasks that he struggled with. The therapist worked with Peter to devise a graded practice schedule that entailed effectively applying his chosen processing strategies in different tasks and environments. Peter also increased his awareness of optimum conditions necessary for him to tackle cognitively demanding tasks.

Evidence Base

There are a number of case studies that support the use of the dynamic interactional approach in people with acquired brain injury (Zlotnik et al 2009, Toglia et al 2010, Toglia et al 2011).

The evidence for the components of the approach is more robust. Metacognitive training and strategy training have been shown to be effective in addressing attention, memory and executive dysfunction for people with mild to moderate acquired brain injury (Cicerone et al 2011). Gillen et al (2015) also identified performance-based interventions, strategy training and compensatory techniques as common features of more effective interventions for cognitive dysfunction after stroke. There is also evidence to support the use of feedback for increasing self-awareness after acquired brain injury but further research is needed to clarify how feedback is best delivered (Schmidt et al 2011). Dymowski et al (2015) also found that the person-centred and individualized approach involved in strategy training was preferred by participants to impairment-focused approaches.

NEUROFUNCTIONAL APPROACH

The neurofunctional approach has been described as an occupation-focused approach that targets patients' occupational performance rather than cognitive impairments. It was designed for people experiencing severe occupational dysfunction following traumatic brain injury but is used in other neurological conditions (such as stroke) (Clark-Wilson et al 2014, Rotenberg-Shpigelman et al 2012). The approach is characterized by developing routines and real-world skills, and by using environmental supports for occupational performance (Giles 2011). The approach is client-centred and the creation of a positive therapeutic alliance between therapist and client is essential to success (Clark-Wilson et al 2014). Therapists focus on understanding the person–occupation–environment interactions that affect performance and develop a structured skill retraining programme using meaningful everyday activities. The retraining programme is designed to support the generalization of skills to each client's everyday life (Giles 2011).

Principles of Assessment

1. Assessment starts with developing an understanding of client's goals, context, motivation and needs.
2. The therapist then establishes the client's occupational performance through observational assessments in naturalistic environments.
3. The therapist uses standardized assessments if needed to understand the client's occupational dysfunction.
4. The therapist analyzes her/his assessment results (considering the person, environment, occupation interactions) and identifies the client's strengths and needs, as

well as any impairments that need to be accommodated in intervention planning.
5. Task analysis is used to define key steps of the task, identify areas where the task is likely to break down and to inform the therapist's use of cues.

Intervention Principles

Practice and repetition is key to this approach. The therapist should use errorless learning if clients have severe impairment in declarative memory and poor self-awareness of deficits. Intervention plans should include whole task practice, use blocked and random practice as necessary, and promote intensity of practice and a high number of repetitions (Clark-Wilson et al 2014).

The therapist uses teaching and learning strategies to engage the patient and improve performance, for example, fading of cues and prompts as performance of the task improves; forwards or backwards chaining; feedback; and reinforcement strategies to increase patient engagement and self-efficacy such as positive reinforcement, collaboration and problem-solving with the patient (Giles 2011).

Case Vignette 3

Edward is a 77-year-old man who experienced a stroke resulting in severe motor and cognitive dysfunction. He required assistance with all aspects of personal care and presented with left-sided visual neglect. Edward did not seem to be aware of his neglect. He had good communication skills and was motivated to be more independent but his occupational performance was severely limited. After gathering information from Edward and his wife about Edward's interests and goals, the therapist observed Edward in self-care tasks such as eating and drinking, washing his face and upper body, and upper body dressing. During observational assessments, the therapist noted where Edward's task performance broke down and how he responded to cues. The therapist didn't provide immediate assistance during the assessment but observed Edward's performance, whether he noticed difficulties in task performance and how he adapted to meet the demands of the task. The therapist analyzed the task, person and environment interactions that affected Edward's occupational performance.

The therapist also completed the Oxford Cognitive Screen (OCS) (Demeyere et al 2015) to understand the nature and severity of Edward's cognitive impairments. Edwards, scores on the OCS confirmed neglect of objects presented to his left (known as egocentric neglect) and impaired memory and executive functions.

Starting with the task of washing his hands and face in the ward bathroom, the therapist adapted the task for

Edward to wash himself using one hand. This included optimizing his position and seating for the task. The therapist then broke the task into component parts and developed a schedule of verbal cues and visual prompts to guide Edward. The therapist cued him to progress from one aspect of the task to the next, and used cueing and visual prompts for him to turn his head to his left and scan the left side of his space.

Evidence Base

The evidence base to support the neurofunctional approach is limited, but promising. There is high-quality randomized controlled trial evidence that this approach had a long-term positive effect on independent living status for a subsection of research participants (those who were over 30 years old and not employed) (Vanderploeg et al 2008). Parish and Oddy (2007) suggested the approach benefits occupational performance and quality of life of people with severe brain injury. However, the study was small, with only four participants. Elements of the approach are also supported by evidence. For example, a review by Cicerone et al (2011) of cognitive rehabilitation literature recommended errorless learning or the use of external compensation in daily activities for people with severe memory impairment after acquired brain injury. Further research is needed to establish the effectiveness of this approach in improving occupational performance and engagement for people with acquired brain injury, specifically large-scale pragmatic trials of the neurofunctional approach.

SUMMARY

There is a growing evidence base to support a range of interventions for addressing movement, cognitive and perceptual dysfunction after acquired brain injury. However, occupational therapy practice is increasingly occupation-focused within neurorehabilitation and there is currently a lack of research into the efficacy of occupation-focused approaches. Therapists currently need to integrate research evidence within the contemporary paradigm and occupation-focused practice.

The motor control frame of reference, motor learning and the acquisitional frame of reference are underpinned by theories that explain how person, occupation and environment factors interact to effect occupational performance. These theories inform intervention approaches that enable therapists to integrate research evidence with occupation-focused practice. Using these frames of reference, the therapist designs structured experiences of meaningful everyday tasks to optimize occupational performance and maximize practice opportunities.

REFLECTIVE LEARNING

- What are the challenges to implementing occupation-focused practice within rehabilitation?
- How does your practice context influence your choice and application of the task-orientated, dynamic interactional or neurofunctional approach?
- How would you maximize practice opportunities sufficiently to enable learning and change in your client group?
- What factors would you consider when choosing an approach to address cognitive dysfunction after acquired brain injury?

REFERENCES

Atkinson, R. C., & Shiffrin, R. M. (1968). Human memory: A proposed system and its control processes. *Psychology of Learning, 2,* 89–195.

Baddeley, P. (2001). Is working memory still working? *The American Psychologist, 56,* 849–864.

Carr, J. H., & Shepherd, R. B. (2003). *Neurological rehabilitation: Optimizing motor performance.* Butterworth-Heinemann, Oxford.

Cicerone, K. D., Langenbahn, D. M., Braden, C., et al. (2011). Evidence-based cognitive rehabilitation: Updated review of the literature from 2003 through 2008. *Archives of Physical Medicine and Rehabilitation, 92,* 519–530.

Clark-Wilson, J., Giles, G., & Baxter, D. (2014). Revisiting the neurofunctional approach: Conceptualizing the core components for the rehabilitation of everyday living skills. *Brain Injury, 28,* 1646–1656.

Demeyere, N., Riddoch, M. J., Slavkova, E. D., Bickerton, W. L., & Humphreys, G. W. (2015). The Oxford Cognitive Screen (OCS): Validation of a stroke-specific short cognitive screening tool. *Psychological Assessment, 27,* 883–894.

Dewan, M. C., Rattani, A., Gupta, S., et al. (2018). Estimating the global incidence of traumatic brain injury. *Journal of Neurosurgery,* 1–18.

Dirette, D. P. (2013). Letter from the Editor: The importance of frames of reference. *The Open Journal of Occupational Therapy, 1.*

Dymowski, A. R., Ponsford, J. L., & Willmott, C. (2016). Cognitive training approaches to remediate attention and executive dysfunction after traumatic brain injury: A single-case series. *Neuropsychological rehabilitation, 26,* 866–894.

Ezekiel, L., Collett, J., Mayo, N. E., Pang, L., Field, L., & Dawes, H. (2018). Factors associated with participation in life situations for adults with stroke: A systematic review. *Archives of Physical Medicine and Rehabilitation, 100,* 945–955.

Feigin, V. L., Forouzanfar, M. H., Krishnamurthi, R., et al. (2014). Global and regional burden of stroke during 1990–2010: Findings from the global burden of disease study 2010. *Lancet, 383,* 245–254.

Fish, J., Hicks, K., & Brentnall, S. (2017). Attention. 2017. In A. Winson, B. A. Wilson, & A. Bateman (Eds.), *The brain injury rehabilitation workbook* (pp. 36–67). The Guildford Press. New York.

French, B., Thomas, L. H., Coupe, J., et al. (2016). Repetitive task training for improving functional ability after stroke. *Cochrane Database of Systematic Reviews.*

Gentile, A. M. (1998). Movement science: Implicit and explicit processes during acquisition of functional skills. Scandinavian Journal of Occupational Therapy, 5, 7–16.

Giles, G. (2011). *A neurofunctional approach to rehabilitation following brain injury. Cognition, occupation and participation across the life span.* Bethesda: AOTA Press.

Gillen, G. (2008). *Cognitive and perceptual rehabilitation.* Elsevier. Edinburgh.

Gillen, G., Nilsen, D. M., Attridge, J., et al. (2015). Effectiveness of interventions to improve occupational performance of people with cognitive impairments after stroke: An evidence-based review. *American Journal of Occupational Therapy, 69,* 1–9.

Greber, C., Ziviani, J., & Rodger, S. (2007). The four-quadrant model of facilitated learning (Part 1): Using teaching–learning approaches in occupational therapy. *Australian Occupational Therapy Journal, 54,* S31–S39d.

Huitt, W. (2003). The information processing approach to cognition. Educational psychology interactive, 3(2), 53.

Josman, N. (2005). The dynamic interactional model in schizophrenia. In N. Katz (Ed.), *Cognition across the lifespan: Models for intervention in occupational therapy* (2nd ed.). AOTA Press. Bethesda.

Katz, N. (2011). *Cognition, occupation, and participation across the life span: Neuroscience, neurorehabilitation, and models of intervention in occupational therapy.* AOTA Press. Bethesda.

Katz, N., Baum, C. M., & Maeir, A. (2011). Introduction to cognitive intervention and cognitive functional evaluation. In N. Katz (Ed.), *Cognition, occupation, and participation across the lifespan: Neuroscience, neurorehabilitation, and models of intervention in occupational therapy* (3rd ed.). AOTA Press. Bethesda.

Kielhofner, G. (2009). *Conceptual foundations of occupational therapy practice.* F.A. Davis Company. Philadelphia.

Larsson, J., Björkdahl, A., Esbjörnsson, E., & Sunnerhagen, K. (2013). Factors affecting participation after traumatic brain injury. *Journal of Rehabilitation Medicine, 45,* 765–770.

Latash, M. L. (2012). The bliss of motor abundance. *Experimental Brain Research, 217,* 1–5.

Latash, M. L., Scholz, J. P., & Schoner, G. (2007). Toward a new theory of motor synergies. *Motor Control, 11,* 276–308.

Law, M. C., Baptiste, S., Carswell, A., McColl, M. A., Polatajko, H., & Pollock, N. (1998). *Canadian Occupational Performance Measure: COPM.* CAOT Publ. ACE. Ottawa.

Lidz, C. S. (1995). Dynamic assessment and the legacy of L.S.Vygotsky. *School Psychology International, 16,* 143–153.

Luebben, A. L., & Royeen, C. B. (2010). An acquisitional frame of reference. In P. Kramer, & J. Hinojosa (Eds.), *Pediatric occupational therapy* (3rd ed.). Philadelphia.

Mathiowetz, V. (2016). Task oriented approach to stroke rehabilitation. In G. Gillen (Ed.), *Stroke rehabiliation: A function based approach* (4th ed.). New York: Elsevier.

Mchugh, G., Swain, I., & Jenkinson, D. (2013). Treatment components for upper limb rehabilitation after stroke: A survey of UK national practice. *Disability and Rehabilitation, 36,* 925–931.

Missiuna, C., Mandich, A. D., Polatajko, H. J., & Malloy-Miller, T. (2001). Cognitive orientation to daily occupational performance (CO-OP): Part I – theoretical foundations. *Physical and Occupational Therapy in Pediatrics, 20,* 69–81.

Mon-Williams, M., & Bingham, G. P. (2011). Discovering affordances that determine the spatial structure of reach-to-grasp movements. *Experimental Brain Research, 211,* 145–160.

Muratori, L. M., Lamberg, E. M., Quinn, L., & Duff, S. V. (2013). Applying principles of motor learning and control to upper extremity rehabilitation. *Journal of Hand Therapy, 26,* 94–103.

Nash, B. H., & Mitchell, A. W. (2017). Longitudinal study of changes in occupational therapy students' perspectives on frames of reference. *American Journal of Occupational Therapy, 71,* 7.

Nilsen, D., Gillen, G., Geller, D., Hreha, K., Osei, E., & Saleem, G. (2015). Effectiveness of interventions to improve occupational performance of people with motor impairments after stroke: An evidence-based review. *American Journal of Occupational Therapy, 69,* 6901180030 1–9.

Nott, M. C., Chapparo, C., & Heard, R. (2009). Reliability of the perceive, recall, plan and perform system of task analysis: A criterion–referenced assessment. *Australian Occupational Therapy Journal, 56,* 307–314.

Parish, L., & Oddy, M. (2007). Efficacy of rehabilitation for functional skills more than 10 years after extremely severe brain injury. *Neuropsychological Rehabilitation, 17,* 230–243.

Piscitelli, D. (2016). Motor rehabilitation should be based on knowledge of motor control. *Archives of Physiotherapy, 6,* 5.

Pollock, A., Farmer, S. E., Brady, M. C.Langhorne, P. E., Mead, G. E., Mehrholz, J. , & van Wijck, F. (2014). Interventions for improving upper limb function after stroke. *Cochrane Database of Systematic Reviews,* (11).

Preissner, K. (2010). The motor performance of a patient with cognitive limitations. *American Journal of Occupational Therapy, 64,* 727–734.

Radomski, M. V., Anheluk, M., Arulanantham, C., Finkelstein, M., & Flinn, N. (2018). Implementing evidence-based practice: A context analysis to examine use of task-based approaches to upper-limb rehabilitation. *British Journal of Occupational Therapy, 81*(5), 285–289.

Roediger III, H.L., Zaromb, F.M., Lin, W. (2017) A Typology of Memory Terms. In:Menzel, R. (ed.), Learning Theory and Behavior, Vol. 1 of Learning and Memory: A Comprehensive Reference, 2nd edition, Byrne, J.H. (ed.). pp. 7–19.

Rotenberg-Shpigelman, S., Erez, A. B., Nahaloni, I., & Maeir, A. (2012). Neurofunctional treatment targeting participation among chronic stroke survivors: A pilot randomised controlled study. *Neuropsychological Rehabilitation, 22,* 532–549.

Sabari, J. C. (2016). Activity based intervention in stroke rehabilitation. In G. Gillen (Ed.), *Stroke rehabilitation: A function based approach* (4th ed.). London: Elsevier.

Schmidt, J., Lannin, N., Fleming, J., & Ownsworth, T. (2011). Feedback interventions for impaired self-awareness following brain injury: A systematic review. *Journal of Rehabilitation Medicine, 43*, 673–680.

Shumway-Cook, A., & Woollacott, M. (2017). *Motor control: Translating research into clinical practice.* Philadelphia: Wolters Kluwer.

Sohlberg, M. M., & Turkstra, L. S. (2011). *Optimizing cognitive rehabilitation: Effective instructional methods.* Guilford Press. New York.

Squire, L. R., & Dede, A. J. (2015). Conscious and unconscious memory systems. *Cold Spring Harbor Perspectives in Biology, 7.*

Stephens, J. A., & Williamson, K. N. C. (2015). Cognitive rehabilitation after traumatic brain injury: A reference for occupational therapists. *OTJR: Occupation, Participation and Health, 35*, 5–22.

Teasell, R., & Hussein, N. (2018). Background Concepts in Stroke Rehabilitation. Available: http://www.ebrsr.com/sites/default/files/v18-SREBR-CH3-NET.pdf. Accessed 22/11/18.

Thickpenny-Davis, K. L., & Barker-Collo, S. L. (2007). Evaluation of a structured group format memory rehabilitation program for adults following brain injury. *Journal of Head Trauma Rehabilitation, 22*, 303–313.

Toglia, J. (2000). Understanding awareness deficits following brain injury. *Neurorehabilitation, 15*, 57–70.

Toglia, J. (2011). The dynamic interactional model of cognition in cognitive rehabilitation. In N. Katz (Ed.), *Cognition, occupation, and participation across the lifespan: Neuroscience, neurorehabiliation, and models of intervention in occupational therapy* (3rd ed.). Bethesda: AOTA Press.

Toglia, J., Goverover, Y., Johnston, M. V., & Dain, B. (2011). Application of the multicontextual approach in promoting learning and transfer of strategy use in an individual with TBI and executive dysfunction. *OTJR (Thorofare N J), 31*, S53–S60.

Toglia, J., Johnston, M. V., Goverover, Y., & Dain, B. (2010). A multicontext approach to promoting transfer of strategy use and self regulation after brain injury: An exploratory study. *Brain Injury, 24*, 664–677.

Toglia, J. P. (2005). A dynamic interactional approach to cognitive rehabilitation. In N. Katz (Ed.), *Cognition & occupation across the lifespan: Models for intervention in occupational therapy* (2nd ed.). Bethesda: AOTA Press.

Toglia, J. P., Rodger, S. A., & Polatajko, H. J. (2012). Anatomy of cognitive strategies: A therapist's primer for enabling occupational performance. *Canadian Journal of Occupational Therapy, 79*, 225–236.

Vanderploeg, R. D., Schwab, K., Walker, W. C., et al. (2008). Rehabilitation of traumatic brain injury in active duty military personnel and veterans: Defense and veterans brain injury center randomized controlled trial of two rehabilitation approaches. *Archives of Physical Medical Rehabilitation, 89*, 2227–2238.

Vygotsky, L. S. (1978). *Mind in society: The development of higher psychological processes.* Cambridge, MA: Harvard University Press.

Whiting, H. T. A. (1984). *Human motor actions: Bernstein reassessed.* Amsterdam: Elsevier.

Yamani, Y., Ariga, A., & Yamada, Y. (2015). Object affordances potentiate responses but do not guide attentional prioritization. *Frontiers in Integrated Neuroscience, 9*, 74.

Zlotnik, S., Sachs, D., Rosenblum, S., Shpasser, R., & Josman, N. (2009). Use of the dynamic interactional model in self-care and motor intervention after traumatic brain injury: Explanatory case studies. *American Journal of Occupational Therapy, 63*, 549–558.

Evolving Areas of Knowledge

15

The Evolving Theory of Clinical Reasoning

Carolyn A. Unsworth

OVERVIEW

This chapter explores clinical reasoning in occupational therapy. It provides an overview of the development of clinical reasoning in occupational therapy and definitions of the different types of clinical reasoning and associated constructs and explains how acquisition of expertise is promoted through clinical reasoning. A structured approach to using clinical reasoning when engaging with an occupational therapy model for practice is then presented to assist novices bridge the theory-to-practice gap. An overview of clinical reasoning research over the past 38 years is then presented. Although it has long been established that clinical reasoning enables therapists to integrate theory into practice, the final section of the chapter examines the process of theory development and maps this against developments and research growth in the area of clinical reasoning in occupational therapy. Hence, this chapter builds an argument that clinical reasoning is developing into a theory.

◎ HIGHLIGHTS

- Clinical reasoning has been studied by occupational therapy researchers since 1982. Clinical reasoning is distinct from clinical decision making, and is referred to using a variety of terms, including *professional reasoning*.
- Many types or modes of clinical reasoning have been identified and described, including narrative, procedural, interactive, conditional, ethical and pragmatic reasoning.
- One of the hallmarks of expertise is the therapist's ability to reason rapidly and intuitively. The clinical reasoning of an expert is deeply internalized, and the therapist can draw appropriately on relevant ideas, solutions or information from an extensive knowledge bank and range of experiences.
- There have been over 155 journal articles discussing and investigating the clinical reasoning of occupational therapists. Qualitative and quantitative findings from this research are slowly building a picture of clinical reasoning in occupational therapy.
- Clinical reasoning is evolving into a theory in its own right. Research evidence to support the evolving theory of clinical reasoning is slowly assembling. Further studies that build on existing work organizing this phenomenon into a conceptual framework and empirically testing this framework are required to refine and test this theory.

INTRODUCTION

In 1983, Schön (p.42) penned the following analogy:

In the varied topography of professional practice, there is a high hard ground in which practitioners can make effective use of the research-based theory and technique. Moreover, there is the swampy lowland in which situations are confusing 'messes' incapable of technical solution. The difficulty is that the problems of the high hard ground, however great their technical interest, are often relatively unimportant to clients or to the larger society, whereas in the swamp, the problems of greatest human concern are found.

This chapter welcomes you to the swamp!

The way we think and reason, in essence, makes us who we are as individuals. Furthermore, groups of people who come together for specific purposes often share patterns, modes and constellations of thinking and reasoning. As a professional group, occupational therapists share a mode of thinking and reasoning that is quite particular and quite different from that of other health professionals. Of course, many elements and aspects of this thinking are shared with other clinicians, but it is the way the thinking is constructed and how this reasoning enables our theories of human occupation to be practiced that is unique. Writing about clinical reasoning in occupational therapy today is commonplace, and all the introductory texts and compendia in the profession include material on clinical reasoning. Furthermore, I would guess that all occupational therapy education programmes internationally include some training or exposure to the idea of clinical reasoning, particularly to assist students bridge the theory-to-practice gap before or during professional practice experiences. However, clinical reasoning has only been described in our profession over the past 32 years or so. Although the idea was first brought to the attention of therapists by Rogers (1982) and Rogers and Masagatani (1982), and Rogers' Eleanor Clarke Slagle lectureship the following year (1983), it was not until the *American Journal of Occupational Therapy* released its special edition on clinical reasoning in November 1991, and Mattingly and Fleming published their text *Clinical Reasoning: Forms of Inquiry in a Therapeutic Practice* in 1994, that the idea of clinical reasoning entered mainstream practice and became the buzz word of the early 1990s. News of this concept spread rapidly around the occupational therapy world, and there was an 'ah-ha' moment as the profession collectively recognized clinical reasoning as a way of naming and explaining all the hidden elements of practice that were so essential in the art (as opposed to the science) of occupational therapy practice. Early scholarly activities investigating clinical reasoning revealed that our thinking was indeed special and unique, and construction of a language to describe the tacit as well as overt elements of practice commenced. But what exactly is clinical reasoning? How does a therapist do it? What can make a therapist better at it? Some ideas to answer these questions are provided in this chapter, commencing with the first section, which provides an overview of what clinical reasoning is.

WHAT IS CLINICAL REASONING?

Issues in Arriving at a Definition

It is not easy to put forth a simple definition of clinical reasoning, because this is quite a complex construct.

To start, we must acknowledge that clinical reasoning is also described in the occupational therapy literature as *therapeutic reasoning* (Kielhofner & Forsyth 2002), *professional reasoning* (Schell & Schell 2018) and *occupational reasoning* (Rogers 2010). All of these are also excellent terms. The terms *professional reasoning* and *therapeutic reasoning* acknowledge that occupational therapy practice is not confined to the clinic. Using the term *occupational reasoning* ensures that our thinking is targeted to the 'systematic method of thinking about the occupational engagement of humans that supports the occupational therapy process' (Rogers 2010, p.57). But renaming the clinical reasoning rose does not make it smell any sweeter. Therefore, although this chapter adopts the traditional term that is so easily recognized, the reader is asked to consider that other terms can also be used.

The second issue to raise, before a definition is offered, concerns the intertwined nature of clinical reasoning and clinical decision making. In discussing reasoning and decision making in occupational therapy practice, Harries and Duncan (2009) observed that in the occupational therapy literature clinical reasoning tends to be used to cover all the thinking processes that involve reasoning, problem-solving judgement and decision making. These authors go on to present material on two theories of judgement and decision making from cognitive psychology: cognitive continuum theory (Hammond & Brehmer 1973) and dual-processing theory (Stanovich & West 2000), and show how these theories can further our understanding of occupational therapy practice. Harries and Duncan describe how, within dual-processing theory, two thinking systems are outlined that have been shown to be neurologically different (Goel et al 2000). The S1 system, as it is called, is a fast, automatic form of processing. Through the S1 system, judgements are largely tacit. However, the slower and more deliberate S2 system is more analytical, focuses on one task at a time and considers the outcome of different decisions from a more objective basis. The S1 system is more focused on the art of clinical reasoning and the S2 on the science of objective decision making. Ideally, we need both these elements in a successful clinical practice, and we need to explore both literatures to gain an understanding of what these approaches offer us. However, it is beyond the size and introductory nature of this chapter to explore both these concepts. This chapter focuses on the more context-dependent, phenomenologically grounded clinical reasoning. Texts that delve deeper into clinical reasoning in the allied health literature include those by Schell and Schell (2018) and Higgs et al (2008). In addition, a recent text by Cronin and Graebe (2018) presents clinical reasoning as a five-step process and then applies this across a range of theoretical approaches used in occupational therapy such as motor learning. This chapter will refer to decision making, but not describe it in any detail. To gain an appreciation of the full complexity of the science of judgement and decision making, the reader is referred to Dowie and Elstein (1988), Hardman (2009) or Sox et al (2013).

Definition of Clinical Reasoning

It is hard to be succinct when defining clinical reasoning. The *Oxford Dictionary* defines reasoning as 'the intellectual faculty by which conclusions are drawn from premises … [and] to reach conclusions by connected thought' (Thompson 1995, p.1144). But this definition does not convey the scope or complexity of clinical reasoning in occupational therapy. Higgs and Jones (2000, p.11)define clinical reasoning as 'a process in which the clinician, interacting with significant others (client, caregivers, healthcare team members), structures meaning, goals and health management strategies based on clinical data, client choices, and professional judgment and knowledge'. In occupational therapy, clinical reasoning can be defined as the reflexive thinking associated with engaging in a client-centred professional practice. This includes the thinking when planning to be with the client (and their caregivers and other health professionals), when the therapist is with the client and afterwards when reflecting on time with the client. Clinical reasoning draws on empathy, intuition, judgement and common sense. Clinical reasoning is constantly changing in response to a multitude of hidden and overt influences and contextual factors, which may be inhibitory or enabling. Clinical reasoning plays out in the occupational therapist's mind in narratives and images (adapted from Unsworth 1999). Within the clinical reasoning construct, many modes or types of reasoning have been identified. These are described in the next section of the chapter.

A LANGUAGE TO DESCRIBE THE MODES OF CLINICAL REASONING

Cheryl Mattingly (a medical anthropologist) and Maureen Fleming (an occupational therapist) worked with a large team of experts, including Gilette, Schön and Cohen, to conduct the first large-scale enquiry into the clinical reasoning of occupational therapists. The American Occupational Therapy Foundation funded a study between and 1986 and 1988 involving 14 therapists at a 900-bed acute care facility in a large city in the United States of America. The two major findings of the study were an understanding of the practice cultures that occupational therapists work within and the beginnings of a language to describe the modes of reasoning used by occupational therapists (Mattingly & Fleming 1994). Many refinements and additions have been made to this framework, but the fundamental ideas laid out in Mattingly and Fleming's text provide the foundation for understanding clinical reasoning in occupational therapy. The language that has now developed in occupational therapy in the field of clinical reasoning has been drawn from medicine, philosophy, anthropology and sociology.

An overview of these different modes of clinical reasoning and related terminology used in the field are provided below. Table 15.1 provides explanations of the different terms commonly used in clinical reasoning and is arranged in the same format as the model of clinical reasoning used in this chapter as presented in Figure 15.1. Table 15.2 then provides the remaining definitions of terms related to clinical reasoning, and the second column of Table 15.2 provides an example of how all the terms from Tables 15.1 and 15.2 might be used in clinical practice in the narrative (first-person) form. The use of narrative examples to illustrate how therapists reason is now quite popular in occupational therapy texts. Mattingly and Fleming's text came to life through the use of these narratives, and the first occupational therapy writers to adopt this approach to illustrate texts with both what and how a therapist thinks included Unsworth (1999) and Kielhofner (2008). This approach helps students and novice therapists to learn both what a particular therapy technique is and, very importantly, what a therapist thinks as they engage in practice.

Narrative Reasoning and Chart Talk

Mattingly documented how occupational therapy was a profession that sat comfortably between two practice cultures, and therefore described occupational therapy as a 'two body practice' (1994, p.37). This interpretation still holds true over 26 years later. On the one hand, occupational therapists work within a biomedical framework. Even when therapists do not work in a medical setting, our profession is primarily concerned about the relationship between health, occupation and well-being. Therefore, our concern with health connects us to medicine and a biomechanical understanding. Occupational therapists also have their own professional practice culture, which operates in the social, cultural and psychological sphere that is concerned with the client's experience of the illness and the meaning of the illness (Mattingly 1994). Usually, a biomechanical or scientific approach (the body as a machine) does not sit well alongside the more phenomenological sphere (the lived body). However, in occupational therapy, these two seem to make perfect sense (Shell & Schell 2018). As Mattingly

TABLE 15.1   Commonly Used Terms in Clinical Reasoning

Worldview:
Global outlook on the world, and underlying assumptions about life and reality. Worldview is not a type of reasoning, but influences all professional reasoning and therefore is at the top of the hierarchy in the model. Worldview encompasses a therapist's ethics, values, beliefs, faith and spirituality.

Ethical Reasoning:
The thinking that accompanies analysis of a moral dilemma where one moral conviction or action conflicts with another, and then generating possible solutions and selecting action to be taken.

Scientific Reasoning:	**Narrative Reasoning:**
Draws on a biomedical approach. When reasoning scientifically, therapists use the language of 'chart talk'. The process of hypothesis generation and testing that generally is referred to as hypothetico-deductive reasoning.	Draws on a phenomenological approach to understanding the person and involves storytelling and story creation. The emphasis is on understanding the meaning of the person's illness and illness experience

Diagnostic Reasoning:	**Procedural Reasoning:**	**Interactive Reasoning:**	**Conditional Reasoning:**
Used to identify underlying impairments or occupational performance issues, define desired outcomes, set goals, develop interventions/solutions. Provides a basis for procedural reasoning.	These are the reasoning processes associated with the evaluations and interventions to be used with a person. This reasoning refers to all the 'procedures' of therapy. Procedural reasoning includes systematic data collection, hypothesis formation and testing, as well as the reasoning that underpins interventions.	Used when communicating, both verbally and nonverbally. Interactive reasoning is used to engage the person in therapy, consider the best approach to communicate with the person, to understand who the person is and the problems from the person's point of view, individualize therapy, convey a sense of acceptance/trust/hope, break tension through the use of humour, build a shared language of actions and meanings, and monitor how the treatment session is going. Referred to as the underground practice because therapists often describe what they do with the person, but generally not their interactions.	One of the more complex models to understand, and has several components. A therapist is reasoning conditionally when thinking about the person's condition, and how change is conditional upon participation in the therapeutic process. The therapist is reasoning conditionally when thinking temporally about the person's past, present and future to understand what the person's life was like before the therapy encounter, what it is like now, and what it could be in the future. Hence, this type of reasoning is used when trying to understand what is meaningful to the person in their social and cultural world.

Pragmatic Reasoning:
Reasoning related to personal, organizational, political and economic contexts. Hence, this thinking is about how therapy can operate given resource and financial considerations such as who is funding therapy. Personal context includes the reasoning surrounding the therapist's own motivation, negotiation skills, repertoire of therapy skills and life knowledge and assumptions.

(1994) notes, occupational therapists seemed to have the ability to shift rapidly and easily between thinking about the client and the disease process and resulting occupational performance issues (for example), developing an understanding of the person and the client's experience of the illness.

When therapists are thinking and working in a biomechanical sphere, they use chart talk to present information on the client and discuss evaluation and intervention issues. Hence, chart talk is generally used when the occupational therapist is talking about the client's medical problem or writing case notes using brief

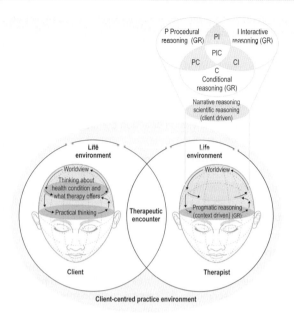

Fig. 15.1 The Occupational Therapy Model of Clinical Reasoning (also referred to as a hierarchical model of clinical reasoning). This model is based on an earlier version (Unsworth 2004a) and attempts to draw in elements from the other models to work towards building a conceptual framework. GR, generalisation reasoning.

and factual language. This kind of communication fits well in the biomedical world. However, when working in the more phenomenological practice sphere, occupational therapists use narrative reasoning to tell the story of therapy (Mattingly 1994, Unsworth 2004a). Storytelling is never static. Stories can be told of the past and of the present and created for the future. Stories can be rewritten and changed mid-stream. Hence, thinking in narratives fits perfectly with the ever-changing therapy environment.

The Therapist with the Three-Track Mind

Although narrative reasoning may be described as a core form of reasoning, Fleming (1994) went on to develop the idea of 'the therapist with the three-track mind' (p.119). The therapist with the three-track mind describes three dominant modes of reasoning found in the clinical reasoning study and confirmed in subsequent research (Alnervik & Sviden 1996, Unsworth 2004a). Fleming argued that therapists use these different kinds of reasoning when working in the different practice spheres. Therefore, procedural reasoning, which is similar to the problem-solving or hypothetico-deductive approach used in medical enquiry, fits well in the

biomechanical sphere. The other forms of reasoning described by Fleming, interactive reasoning and conditional reasoning, fit more readily in the phenomenological or meaning-making practice sphere (Fleming 1994). These forms of reasoning are all defined and described in Table 15.1. However, it is important to note how intertwined these are throughout the therapy process. Mattingly and Fleming (1994) described how the perspective gained from reasoning in one track might inform reasoning in another. This idea, that the different forms of reasoning interact and overlap, has been supported in clinical reasoning research (Unsworth 2004a).

Other Modes of Clinical Reasoning and Related Terms

Early clinical reasoning researchers, such as Rogers and Masagatani (1982) and Barris (1987), as well as researchers following in the footsteps of Mattingly and Fleming, have also contributed terms to describe modes of clinical reasoning, or to describe constructs that fit with clinical reasoning. Some of these terms, such as *ethical, scientific, pragmatic, generalization* and *diagnostic reasoning,* and related constructs such as intuition, embodiment, worldview and reflection, are defined and illustrated in Tables 15.1 and 15.2. It is important to note that some of these terms, such as *procedural, interactive, conditional* and *pragmatic reasoning,* fit better within an S1 or reasoning approach to understanding thinking processes. Other terms, such as *scientific* and *diagnostic reasoning,* fit better with an S2 approach.

CLINICAL REASONING AND EXPERTISE

Differences Between the Clinical Reasoning of Novice and Expert Therapists

Research in occupational therapy on novice–expert differences has often portrayed this construct as a dichotomy. However, as described by Dreyfus and Dreyfus (1980) in their seminal work on chess players and airline pilots, and then adapted for use in the health sciences by nursing researcher Benner (1984), expertise occurs on a continuum. It is now widely accepted that there are five phases one passes through on the journey from novice to expert, and these are novice, advanced beginner, competent, proficient and expert. It is also widely documented that increasing years of experience do not always equate with increasing expertise; some therapists never reach expert status but remain stuck at the level of competent or proficient practice (Benner et al 1996, Gibson et al 2000, Unsworth 2001). There have been several occupational

TABLE 15.2 Types/Modes of Clinical Reasoning in Occupational Therapy and Other Related Constructs

Mode of thinking. Researchers who coined/use this term. Description provided (if not in Table 15.1)	Clinical example
Narrative reasoning (Mattingly & Fleming 1994)	Robyn enters the hospital's allied health staff lunchroom and flops into a chair. Her colleagues, Dana, Matty and Pip are already there. Pip observes that Robyn looks exhausted. Robyn replies: 'I've just been working with the new lad. He's only four, but he spent the whole session wailing for his mum. The puppets caught his attention for a few minutes, and I made a start but that was about it. His leg muscles are so tight, but I'm sure the [tendon release] surgery will make a huge difference in the long run … I just need to find what will turn on the light and get him interested and motivated. I'm going to try and call his mum later and get some more information from her …'
Scientific reasoning (Schell & Cervero 1993)	Saran reports on her initial assessment of 73-year-old Peter at the team meeting. 'I assessed the new client, Peter, yesterday in terms of ability to complete personal ADLs. I found him to be independent with verbal supervision for all tasks such as toileting, showering, dressing and grooming. He plans to return to his home without any support and use public transport to get to the shops, visit his doctor and do his banking. Given what I observed yesterday, I doubt he will be independent in all these activities by next week. I will commence an IADL assessment today, and intervention will aim at facilitating his independence and also putting local community supports in place.'
Diagnostic reasoning (Rogers & Holm 1991)	Brian has been working in acute care for only a few months and has used a hypothesis testing approach to determine the underlying cognitive impairments that are limiting his client's ability to make a cup of tea. 'He presents as really confused, and so I was very cautious in putting everything out on the bench and I didn't have the water in the kettle any hotter than tap water. He started by breaking open the teabag and tipping the tea into the cup. Then he tipped in half the sugar from the sugar pot, played around with this for a while and then filled the cup with milk. Before the session, I was wondering what was going on and whether he had some complex perceptual problems. But over the session it became clear that he has ideational apraxia. This hypothesis fits with the fact that he has left brain damage as a result of the stroke and has quite severe receptive aphasia as well.'
Procedural reasoning (Mattingly & Fleming 1994)	Alex works on a stroke ward. His new client has cognitive and perceptual problems. 'I did a dressing assessment with Mr P this morning and the hypotheses were just flying around my head. He has so many cognitive and perceptual problems but hardly any physical ones … so I just watched him and tried a few things as we went. He looks as if he has a unilateral neglect and some short-term memory problems, as well as complex perceptual problems … but I've got to check for homonymous hemianopia too. I'm just trying to work out which standardized assessments to do … maybe the RPAB [Rivermead Perceptual Assessment Battery] or LOTCA [Lowenstein Occupational Therapy Cognitive Assessment] and the BIT [Behavioural Inattention Test] … but I probably don't have enough time for all three, so maybe just the LOTCA and some confrontation testing to check for neglect versus homonymous hemianopia versus both.'

Continued

TABLE 15.2	Types/Modes of Clinical Reasoning in Occupational Therapy and Other Related Constructs—cont'd	

Interactive reasoning (Mattingly & Fleming 1994)	Dana describes to her fieldwork student some of her interactive reasoning as she gets to know her clients during an initial interview. As Dana will get to know these clients over several months, she reasons that she has this time to use the initial interview to 'go deep'. 'What I do is just start off with the initial interview structure but explore any directions the client's responses take me in. I don't want to limit this opportunity to get to know the client by sticking to the form, as the sooner I can get my head around understanding who this person is and what makes them tick, the better the therapy plans we make will be. I try to keep it light and friendly so the client feels at ease and that it's an open and sharing environment. If there is an opportunity to share a joke I will … or if the client becomes upset or distressed, then I take time to support them through this and slowly we move on. I guess what I'm aiming for is to get the clients to see me as someone who is going to be useful in their recovery and someone they can trust.'
Conditional reasoning (Mattingly & Fleming 1994)	Maryella is reflecting on a session with Joseph, a 5-year-old boy with developmental delay. She started by interviewing Joseph and then undertook Ayres Clinical Observation to examine his motor skills. She completed this assessment about 12 months ago as well. 'I did this assessment last year and I haven't seen Joseph for over 6 months since his family moved away for his Dad's work. Now they're back so I'm just checking on where Joseph is up to with school and socially, and how he feels about coming home and so on. We've had a chat and I can really tell he's made a lot of good gains. He's a bit anxious about starting back at his old school, so I've been reassuring him about that and now I'm just using Ayres Clinical Obs assessment to run through his current performance. He's made some nice gains over the time he's been away; he has more core trunk stability and I can really see changes compared with the last time I saw him in terms of balance, righting reactions and even fine motor coordination. I think we can work on some more advanced goals now with him, such as …'
Ethical reasoning (Rogers 1983, Barnitt & Partridge 1997)	Alan had a head injury and attends a day therapy programme as an outpatient. His therapist, Kate, reflects on the fact that Alan takes illegal drugs (Unsworth 2004b). 'Alan still lives in his parents' house, but he can't stay there much longer, and they want him out. Alan takes drugs and I find it a real dilemma. I have to help him find other housing, but he shares his drugs around, and I'm really worried that if I help him find a group home, then he could be putting other people at risk. I also feel really disappointed because he's made such amazing gains in therapy and he could do so much, but when he takes drugs he just loses all his cognition, basically. He just sits there and misses out on therapy, and it's a real shame. Sometimes I think the therapy I provide is going to waste … should I spend less time with him and more with my other clients who seem to make more gains? I try not to dwell on it but it's a bit disappointing, as if he didn't do drugs, then he could easily be living in a good home and making fantastic progress towards independent living and getting some part-time voluntary work. Anyway, it's his life and I try not to judge him. But I have to think some more about what kind of place he can live in so he doesn't put others at risk as well.'

TABLE 15.2   Types/Modes of Clinical Reasoning in Occupational Therapy and Other Related Constructs—cont'd

Generalization reasoning (Unsworth 2005)

Within the forms of procedural, interactive, conditional and pragmatic reasoning, therapists use generalization reasoning to draw on past experience or knowledge to assist them in making sense of a current situation or client circumstance. The kind of reasoning in force when a therapist thinks about a particular issue or scenario with a client, then reflects on their general experiences or knowledge (i.e., making generalizations) related to the situation, and then refocuses the reasoning back on the client.

Max works in a short-stay residential facility, helping adolescents with intellectual disability to become more independent.

'Kate is making some good gains with her goal of grooming, which includes managing her long hair and doing some basic make-up. So often these kids have a kind of learnt helplessness because their parents have often done everything for them. So with Kate, she asks for help all the time but really she can do it. I think it's more about reassurance and just reinforcing what a great job she's doing. So that's what I'm focusing on with Kate in this session, supporting and reassuring her that she can do her hair and so on and that she's doing a great job.'

Pragmatic reasoning/management reasoning

(Schell & Cervero 1993, Barris 1987, Neuhaus 1988, Fondiller et al 1990, Lyons and Crepeau 2001)

Xui Sing works in community health with elderly clients living at home.

'I really want to be able to provide my client, Mrs Beller, with an adjustable over-toilet frame, as I know her husband is having hip replacement surgery in 6 weeks and he's a lot bigger than her. So if I get an adjustable one, they can both use it. But our centre has just had a major policy change in equipment allocation, and I think I can only provide a seat that is a fixed height and suitable for her. Maybe they can afford to buy an adjustable one now, or maybe we'll have to worry about Mr Beller later when he has his surgery? I'll have to work out the best solution based on their needs now, their budget and what my centre can provide.'

Embodiment/embodied knowledge

(Schell & Harris 2008, Kinsella 2018, Arntzen 2018)

Embodied knowledge is gathered not only from what the client tells us but also from the information gathered through other senses. For example, the occupational therapist; observes the client's body language and positioning, smells any body odours, and palpates a muscle to determine a contraction. Clinical reasoning is 'embodied' because we reason with our whole bodies.

Helen describes how she knows when an autistic child begins to relax and settle into an activity.

'Well, if I describe a typical client, then I could tell you about Paul. Let's say I've started with a warm-up activity outside climbing the rope ladder and swinging on the bars, so it's a gross motor activity using major muscle groups. And that's really helpful, so that when he comes inside I might then start with a large weighted floor puzzle. This kind of "heavy work", with lots of joint compression seems to help kids like Paul to relax. And as he's moving the puzzle, I can see his whole body kind of slows and I can place my hands over his back or at his hips, and feel the tension releasing and his muscles relaxing.'

Continued

TABLE 15.2   Types/Modes of Clinical Reasoning in Occupational Therapy and Other Related Constructs—cont'd

Worldview Wolters 1989, p.15, Hooper 1997	Asher describes his worldview. 'Well, I suppose my worldview makes me who I am, and I guess it colours every-thing I think and do. It's about my faith and what values I hold and my sense of right and wrong. Sometimes I'm aware of it but mostly I'm not. I guess I have to think about what my worldview is, when I'm confronted with it being different from the client's. It's times like these I really have to work at not making judge-ments about the client but try to see it from their point of view or try to accept that it's OK to have that particular worldview. When I have OT fieldwork students, they find this hard at times. Often you can't solve the dilemma for them, but at least you make them aware of what the problem is—in other words, you can at least look at it objectively for what the problem is, and also see that it's normal to have to work at understanding these issues and resolving or making peace with these differences.'
Intuition Defined as the 'knowledge of a fact or truth, as a whole; immediate possession of knowledge; and knowledge independent of the linear reasoning process' (Rew 1986, p.23). Within cognitive contin-uum theory, Hammond (1996) posits that cognition can be ordered on a continuum from intuition to analysis.	Fiona reflects on the development of her intuition and its value in her practice. 'When I first started in mental health, working with depressed clients, I would have done A, B and C as I was taught and expected to do by others in the team. But now I'm 8 years on, and I do so many things differently based on that experience. And I'm really comfortable with what the A, B, C is, and I can see where it will work and where it will need to be changed. And I just trust my intuition. When I was new at this job, I didn't have the same "feel" or gut instinct for clients that I have now. But now I can just sense when something isn't quite right or when the client is going downhill … even if that isn't what they're telling me. And I trust this intuition.'
Reflection (Schön 1983, Alsop & Ryan 1996, McKay 2009) Involves reviewing performance and examining it in detail by relating it to past knowledge and experiences and relating it to future action, to enhance understanding. There are several types of reflection, including reflection about past experiences (reflection on action), reflecting in the present (reflection in action) and looking forward or antici-patory reflection (reflection for action). Reflection is a bridge to link theory and practice.	Akhmed describes the value in setting aside time for reflection in his practice. 'Each week I try to put some time aside on Friday to go back over the week and identify the highlights and low points, and I reflect on what worked well and the problems … both working with clients and with other staff. I don't keep a journal but some of my colleagues do. But I try to make some notes about events and feelings, and use this time to think about doing things differently or better. Then I also have professional supervision once a month, and I identify something from these "Friday reflections" to really go into more detail … and I find these sessions really useful. My mentor really pushes me to think about the issue from so many different angles and I use her approach when I'm thinking back over the week on my own.'

ADL, Activities of daily living; *IADL,* instrumental activities of daily living; *OT,* occupational therapy/therapist.

therapy studies on the differences between novice and expert therapists (Hallin & Sviden 1995, Strong et al 1995, Robertson 1996, Gibson et al 2000, Unsworth 2001, Mitchell & Unsworth 2005). A review in 2016 (Unsworth & Baker) identified 14 studies that investigated 18 the development of professional reasoning in students and the transition of therapists from novice to expert. One of the consistent findings from these studies and from studies of other health professionals is that experts think and reason differently from novices; experts know how (nonpropositional or tacit knowledge) rather than know what (propositional or factual book-learnt knowledge), their knowledge is embedded in action and experience, and much of their knowledge is automatic and intuitive (Dreyfus & Dreyfus 1980, 1986). Occupational therapy research in this area has revealed that, although novice and expert differences may be readily apparent, the differences between the other levels of expertise are not so apparent. Further research is required to help us identify the hallmarks and key reasoning patterns at each of the three mid-phases (advanced beginner, competent, proficient) so we can aid therapists who are 'stuck' at a particular level to move forward on their journey to expertise. Research by King et al (2008) investigated the variables associated with the development of expertise. Their work was able to disentangle expertise from experience and identify six core features of expertise that include knowledge, personal qualities and characteristics, skills and abilities, reputation and achieving superior outcomes with clients, as well as experience. Importantly, this study is one of the first times that researchers adopted a rigorous approach to identify the level of expertise of their participants by using a battery of objective and standardized measures.

One of the goals of an occupational therapy educational programme is to ensure that students exit with the skills, tools, behaviours, attitudes and reasoning abilities needed to be excellent occupational therapists. Therefore, educators use novice–expert research findings to help students and novices to gain insights into expert thinking so they may hasten their journey on this continuum. However, expertise is not a point of arrival but rather a lifelong quest. This is because expertise is heavily context-dependent and a clinician who excels in one field of practice, such as psychiatry, may have novice skills only in working with clients who are recovering from stroke. In addition, therapists who have attained expert status in a particular context must continue to expand and hone skills on their quest for professional excellence. Hence, novices and experts alike can benefit from undertaking an activity that has been shown as a key to enhancing clinical reasoning, and that is reflection.

Enhancing Clinical Reasoning Skills Through Reflection

Reflection, as described in Table 15.1, is concerned with reviewing one's performance, examining it in detail by relating it to past knowledge and experiences, and relating it to future action, to enhance understanding. Reflection is often referred to as the bridge that links theory and practice (Schön 1983, Alsop & Ryan 1996, McKay 2009). It is essential that all therapists, novices as well as experts, have the time and opportunity to reflect on practice both alone and with a supervisor or mentor. Reflective activities designed to enhance clinical reasoning include storytelling, prebriefing and debriefing, reflective questions after working with a client, reflective journal writing, reviewing critical incidents with a mentor, participation in discussion groups, and videotaping and viewing sessions with clients. These activities are commonly used in occupational therapy texts and educational curricula, and all the chapters in this text include reflective learning questions to facilitate imbedding the material in daily clinical practice. Additionally, activities with a reflective partner can also be helpful; together, therapists can note significant similarities and differences between clients with similar disease processes or occupational performance issues and consider how these differences can influence treatment (Alsop & Ryan 1996, McKay 2009). Therapists who take the time to reflect nurture their clinical reasoning skills, thus promoting excellent practice. However, effective reflection requires skilled tuition, and Wong et al (2016, p.478) caution against teaching reflection in a reductionist way that is stripped back of analytic components, instead promoting deep reflection through finding the '…just right level of possible intrusive guidance and the private reflections of the students'.

One activity that can be used to promote reasoning is to structure reasoning prompts around commonly used theories and associated practice models. Explicitly prompting to use the language of clinical reasoning while planning or structuring a therapeutic encounter with a client can assist students or early career practitioners to consolidate what they have learnt and translate this to a clinical environment. Two examples of how this can be used to assist students are provided in Tables 15.3 and 15.4. In Table 15.3, clinical reasoning terminology has been overlaid on the Canadian Practice Process Framework from the Canadian Model of Occupational Performance and Engagement (Townsend & Polatajko 2013). Students are prompted at each stage of the model to use specific types of reasoning and to prompt reflection. These prompts are by no means exhaustive and should be used as a broad guide that is tailored to each individual practice encounter. Similarly, Table 15.4 provides an overview of some of the clinical reasoning prompts that can be used to guide students when using Kielhofner's Model of Human Occupation (Taylor 2017).

TABLE 15.3   Framework for Professional Reasoning: An Example Applied To Canadian Model of Occupational Performance and Engagement (CMOP-E) with the Canadian Practice Process Framework (Adapted From Townsend & Polatajko 2013)

Action points	Key enablement and actions With the person participating and power-sharing as much as possible.	Professional reasoning prompts What am I thinking and how does this underpin what I am working on with this person? Reasoning at each stage may be more scientific (using the language of chart talk), or more narrative (telling the story), depending on the issues being reflected on.
1. Enter/ initiate	The OT's first point of contact with the person. Establish why the person has come to occupational therapy. Detail any requirements for service such as disclosure.	Focus on procedural and pragmatic reasoning • What are the physical, cultural, social and institutional environments in which the occupational therapy service operates, and how will this affect the service I provide? • What do I need to tell the person about this service? • Why has the person been referred? • Who is this person and why have they come to therapy? • What do I need to do more research on/find out more about/ who do I need to consult with, before I meet this person? Your specific reasoning in relation to the person…
2. Set the stage	Work with person to clarify beliefs, assumptions, expectations and desires. Build rapport. Establish any ground rules. Through reading case notes and collaborating with the person, identify possible priority occupations and possible occupational goals.	Focus on interactive, ethical and conditional reasoning • Who is this person and what are their beliefs and spirituality? • Does the person know what occupational therapy is and have they made any assumptions about therapy? • What seems to 'capture' the person in terms of what OT can offer? • How does the person see themselves in the future? What will change? • What are the person's occupational priorities? • Are there any ground rules I need to clarify with the person? Your specific reasoning in relation to the person…

3. Assess/ evaluate	Assess/evaluate person's occupational status, dreams and potential for change. Consult with person and other specialists, and use specialist evaluations where appropriate.	Focus on procedural (diagnostic and scientific) and interactive reasoning
		• What standardized and non-standardized assessments will be appropriate to administer to identify the
		  • person's cognitive, physical and affective strengths and limitations?
		  • self-care, productivity and leisure occupations the person wants, needs or has to perform?
		• What are the findings in terms of strengths and limitations (impairments, activity limitations and participation restrictions)?
		• What environmental resources are there? What social, familial, community and organizational supports are available?
		• Are other referrals needed?
		Your specific reasoning in relation to the person…

4. Agree on objectives and plan for therapy	Collaborate to identify priority occupations, in light of evaluation. Collaborate to negotiate and plan: • Longer-term goals, and • Shorter-term behavioural objectives or SMART goals.	Focus on procedural and interactive reasoning • What are the long-term occupational goals the person wants/ needs/has to achieve? Why? • What are the short-term goals towards achieving the longer-term goals? • Has the person participated in the goal setting? If not, why not? • Do the goals set have a clear plan for action and an approach for measuring outcomes? Your specific reasoning in relation to the person…

TABLE 15.3   Framework for Professional Reasoning: An Example Applied To CMOP-E with the Canadian Practice Process Framework (Adapted From Townsend & Polatajko 2013)—cont'd

5. Implement the plan	Occupational therapy programme is implemented. Person is engaged through occupation. Techniques and strategies used to effect or prevent change as appropriate.	Focus on procedural and interactive reasoning • Is the person engaging with the therapy? • What grading (in relation to task, therapist and environment) do I need to implement to adjust the therapy as we progress? • Is the environment supporting therapy? If not, what needs changing and how will this impact on therapy? Your specific reasoning in relation to the person...
6. Monitor and modify	Monitor occupational therapy programme to enable success: consult, collaborate, advocate and educate.	Focus on interactive and conditional reasoning • Is the therapy unfolding as planned)as outlined in the goals and objectives)? • Are the therapeutic strategies used effective? What modifications are required and why? • Is the person coping with therapy or are changes required? Your specific reasoning in realtion ot the person...
7. Evaluate outcome	Re-assess and evaluate and compare to initial findings. Make recommendations for next steps.	Focus on scientific, procedural, conditional and ethical reasoning • Is the person making progress towards goals and objectives? Why not? • Are new or modified goals and objectives required? Why? Your specific reasoning in relation to the person...
8. Conclude/exit	Communicate conclusion of occupational therapy with person. Ensure co-ordinated transfer to other services, or re-entry to occupational therapy.	Focus on interactive, ethical, pragmatic and conditional reasoning • How will we conclude therapy? Is the person ready for transition? Why not? • What referrals are needed, who will make them? Your specific reasoning in relation to the person...

SMART, Specific, measurable, achievable, realistic and timely.

TABLE 15.4   Framework For Professional Reasoning: An Example Applied to Model of Human Occupation (Modified from Taylor 2017)

MOHO Concepts	Professional Reasoning Prompts

Person
Volition
  - Personal causation
  - Values
  - Interests
	Focus on interactive reasoning and procedural reasoning
	• What motivates this person? What is the individual's personal causation? What are his/her values? What are the person's interests?
	• May consider administering the Volitional Questionnaire (VQ) and the Interest Checklist.
	Your specific reasoning in relation to the person...

Person
Habituation
  - Habits
  - Roles
  - Patterns
  - Routines
	Focus on interactive, procedural and conditional reasoning
	• How does this person organize their occupations? What roles do they value?
	• May consider administering the Assessment of Occupational Functioning (AOF), and Role Checklist.
	Your specific reasoning in relation to the person...

Person
Performance capacity
  - Psychological abilities
  - Physical abilities
  - Mental abilities
  - Lived experience
	Focus on procedural (diagnostic and scientific) reasoning
	• What are the person's capacities and limitations in relation to psychological, physical and mental abilities?
	• What is the person's lived experience and how does this impact on the therapy?
	• May consider administering the AOF, and Assessment of Motor and Process Skills (AMPS), Occupational Self-Assessment (OSA), Assessment of Communication and Interaction Skills (ACIS) and the Interest Checklist.
	Your specific reasoning in relation to the person...

Continued

TABLE 15.4   Framework for Professional Reasoning: An Example Applied to Model of Human Occupation (Modified from Taylor 2017)—cont'd

MOHO Concepts	Professional Reasoning Prompts

Occupational performance
  - Participation
  - Performance
  - Skill
Environment
  - Occupational identity
  - Occupational competence
  - Leading to occupational adaptation
	Focus on procedural (diagnostic and scientific) reasoning; however, all forms of reasoning will come into play
	  • Following the six-step therapy process:
	    1. What questions do I need to ask to guide information gathering?
	    2. What information should I gather with the person? May consider administering the AOF.
	    3. How do I conceptualize this person? What are the strengths and challenges?
	    4. What therapeutic goals and plans will be implemented?
	    5. Implement and review intervention?
	    6. What are the outcomes of therapy, and what assessments may be readministered to examine change?
	  • How does this person's current environment impact on how occupations are motivated, organized and performed?
	Your specific reasoning in relation to the person…

MOHO, Model of Human Occupation.

CASE VIGNETTE

Zelda is a third-year student on professional practice (clinical fieldwork) in a busy healthcare facility offering outpatient rehabilitation. She is finding it difficult to monitor and modify the intervention plans as her clients progress. She reflects that this might be because she saw her clients every day at the last placement and could directly track their progress. However, on this placement, she only sees her clients weekly, and she is finding it hard to anticipate where her clients might be up to when they come to see her. Zelda and her supervisor identified that using some clinical reasoning prompts could support her at Stage 6 of the Canadian Practice Process Framework, as provided in Table 15.3. Reviewing this table, Zelda used the reflective questions, which focused on interactive and conditional reasoning, to touch base with her clients at the start of each session to 'come up to speed' together with progress, to get each client's views on progress made, particularly in relation to the goals set at the last session, and to determine if these have been met or need revision. Zelda could then review her plans for therapy that day against the client's status to determine what they would do next. When Zelda needs to reflect on a problem she is having, there are several other techniques she has learnt as well, and a favourite that she uses most evenings when on fieldwork is to write in her reflective journal where she records her thoughts and works through situations and tests out assumptions and beliefs.

AN OVERVIEW OF JOURNAL ARTICLES ON CLINICAL REASONING IN OCCUPATIONAL THERAPY, 1982–2018

There have been over 155 journal articles, and a further 35 or so book chapters and books on clinical reasoning in occupational therapy written over the past 38 years. The sheer quantity of musings and research in this area reflects the value that our profession places on clinical reasoning and the commitment made to exploring and understanding it. While the reflective discussions and information presented in a lot of the writing on clinical reasoning provide a raft of ideas for research, this section of the chapter provides an overview of the evidence derived from the empirical research published on clinical reasoning in occupational therapy. Occupational therapy practice requires a sound evidence base (Holm 2000). Evidence-based practice may be defined as the judicious use of evidence to make sound decisions about practice. Therefore, decision making, thinking and reasoning are at the heart of putting evidence into practice. Occupational therapy urgently needs more empirical studies on clinical reasoning, so we are confident that we are judicious in putting the best evidence into practice. Hence, research into clinical reasoning where data were collected with occupational therapists and analyzed in some way, either qualitatively or quantitatively, is vital for the profession. As a result of this process, we can more easily identify where work has been done, and clearly see how this can be built upon as we continue the mammoth task of exploring and understanding clinical reasoning in occupational therapy.

In 2016, a review of all the English language clinical reasoning literature in occupational therapy from 1982 to 2014 was undertaken with two aims: to identify the nature and volume of professional reasoning literature, and to review the specific literature in the area of the transition of therapists from novice to expert status (Unsworth & Baker 2016). The databases CINAHL, Embase, Medline, PsychINFO and OTDBase were searched using versions of the terms *reasoning, occupational therapy* and *allied health personnel.* Research examining the scientific decision-making processes of occupational therapists (S2 rather than S1 reasoning) was excluded, such as my own work and work by other occupational therapists such as Harries (e.g., Unsworth 2007, Harries et al 2018, Harries & Gilhooly 2006) and Rassafiani (Rassafiani et al 2006, 2008). Research examining how clinical reasoning can be used to manage a particular area of practice was also excluded (e.g., Fortune & Ryan 1996). At that time, 140 articles were identified, and the thematic review revealed that the key areas that have been examined in relation to clinical reasoning included:

1. Professional reasoning and types of reasoning:
   a. Empirical studies
   b. Nonempirical/discussion
2. Ethics and moral reasoning
3. Methods of studying professional reasoning:
   c. Classroom
   d. Fieldwork
   e. Novice versus expert differences
   f. Scales/measuring student acquisition of reasoning skills
4. Development of professional reasoning (in students)
5. Professional reasoning of occupational therapy assistants
6. Advancing a specific field of clinical practice using professional reasoning.

A detailed examination was also included in the review (Unsworth & Baker 2016) regarding the quality of the literature on 'novice versus expert differences'. Only eight of the 14 papers reviewed were described as strong research, and overall, the research suggests that expertise evolves over time and that not all therapists attain expert status, despite lengthy experience. Expert status appears to be characterized by the ability to process information rapidly, unconsciously and effortlessly, making therapy appear seamless. Very little information or guidance has been written on how to promote occupational therapists to progress through the stages from novice through to expert. A summary of the 10 scales or measurement tools that have been developed to monitor student acquisition of reasoning skills has also been undertaken (Unsworth 2017). Although some of these scales have been developed

and reported in occupational therapy literature, there is significant scope for further work to validate these scales in university settings and determine how the findings can be used to promote clinical reasoning skills among students.

A new search was undertaken on CINAHL, Embase, PubMed and PsychINFO for the years 2015 to November 2018 to review new papers and provide up-to-date commentary on current evidence and any emerging trends in the clinical and professional reasoning literature. The new search revealed a further 15 papers on clinical and professional reasoning literature in occupational therapy, bringing the total to 155 journal papers over a 35-year period. From the 15 new papers, no specific trends emerged; however, two focused on embodied practice (e.g., Arntzen 2018) and two on emotional intelligence and clinical reasoning (e.g., Gribble et al 2018). The other papers covered a range of topics from the development of professional reasoning in student education to examining reasoning in specific areas of practice such as home modification or using tablet devices with clients.

BUILDING A THEORY OF CLINICAL REASONING THROUGH SCHOLARSHIP OF PRACTICE

One of the central aims of the clinical reasoning study funded by the American Occupational Therapy Foundation was to discover the practical theories-in-use of the occupational therapy profession so that this tacit knowledge could be documented and passed on. Mattingly and Fleming (1994) were able to realize this goal because their research adopted a participatory action research approach within an ethnographic framework. The occupational therapists were not studied from a distance, but rather they became part of the research team as they examined their own practice, working with the researchers in what Schön (1983) refers to as a *scholarship of practice.* This term can be defined as 'delivering and generating evidence for practice through a partnership between academia and practice' (Melton et al 2009, p.13).

This approach to describing how theory can be generated from practice is quite distinct from the traditional basic science view that theory is generated before its application in the field. In the past, many occupational therapy writers have identified how occupational therapists seem to have a problem with integrating theory into practice (Kielhofner 2009, Melton et al 2009). It appears that therapists are somewhat disillusioned with the relevance of theory in daily practice. Therefore, the scholarship of practice approach has been identified as a way of growing relevant theory from within practice, to support and promote that practice (Argyris & Schön 1974, Schön 1983, Creek &

Ormston 1996, Schell & Schell 2018). This section of the chapter examines how theories evolve and proposes that clinical reasoning is actually developing into a theory itself through scholarship of practice.

In Chapter 5 of this text and of the previous edition (2013), Duncan describes not only the value and importance of having theory to underpin practice, but also the complexities surrounding our use and misuse of theory terms such as *paradigm, conceptual practice model, frame of reference* and *approach*. Because the idea that clinical reasoning in occupational therapy is developing into a theory in its own right is relatively new (Unsworth 2018, Schell & Schell 2018) and still evolving, it is too early to map out its structure, function and relationships to the core beliefs of the occupational therapy profession. It may transpire that clinical reasoning becomes incorporated into an existing occupational therapy theory, or it may become known as a frame of reference, because frames of reference link theory to practice and reasoning is often described in this way. Because it is premature to use any particular label at this stage, for the purposes of this chapter the term *theory* of clinical reasoning will be adopted and used in its broadest sense.

Theories may be defined as connected sets of ideas that form a base for practice or action. Theories attempt to explain and predict phenomena (Walker & Ludwig 2004), and help us to recognize what we know and to organize what we do (Mitcham 2003). Differing opinions concerning how theory is generated have also been proposed. In occupational therapy, Mitcham (2003) describes the process of theory generation as involving six sequential steps, starting with observation and ending with tested theory.

Steps of Theory Development

1. Observation of the phenomena over time.
2. Recognition that phenomena present themselves in certain ways.
3. Organization of the phenomena into a conceptual framework.
4. Empirical testing of the propositions and concepts that hold the conceptual framework together.
5. Refinement and retesting propositions and concepts.
6. Acceptance of the new theory (modified from Mitcham 2003).

This description of theory development implies a co-ordinated, concerted approach to theory generation. What we know from the definitions of modes of clinical reasoning as presented in Tables 15.1 and 15.2, and the more than 155 papers written about clinical reasoning and summarized earlier, is that the approach to researching and understanding clinical reasoning has been far from co-ordinated.

However, these stages of theory development do fit well with our understanding of clinical reasoning as a contextualized phenomenon that alters depending on the circumstances. In mapping the development of clinical reasoning as a theory against these steps, it is also important to note that the approach adopted here is to build on the foundation of clinical reasoning, as laid by Mattingly and Fleming (1994), rather than fragment research in this area by seeking out new interpretations of this phenomenon (Unsworth 2004a).

The first step in theory development is to observe the phenomena over time and recognize how clinical reasoning presents itself. The occupational therapy literature is rich with descriptive observations and explorations of clinical reasoning and how it is an interactive phenomenon that varies depending on the practice context and the broader social, cultural and political environment. What is required now is more directed effort to organize clinical reasoning into a conceptual framework for occupational therapy practice. Towards this end, models of clinical reasoning can be seen as emerging from the literature. Models describe a phenomenon in a familiar way so as to increase our understanding (Young & Quinn 1992).

Five models are presented here to explain the phenomenon of clinical/professional reasoning:

1. The linear model, as developed by Dewey (1929, 1934) and described by Ryan (1998)
2. Mattingly and Fleming's foundation research on clinical reasoning
3. The model presented by Higgs et al (2000, 2008)
4. Schell's ecological model of professional reasoning (Schell & Schell 2018)
5. Unsworth's occupational therapy model of clinical reasoning (also referred to as a hierarchical model of clinical reasoning) (2004a, 2005, 2018, see Fig. 15.1).

Although Ryan (1998) also describes a narrative model of clinical reasoning, there is insufficient information on its components and definitions to describe it in any detail. Each of these models is outlined below. In these descriptions, note is taken of whether the model has an S1 focus (clinical reasoning), and also an S2 element (decision making). Models reflecting an S2-only approach have not been included in this chapter.

Dewey (1929, 1934): Linear Model of Clinical Reasoning (S1 and S2).
This is a classic description of general reasoning (Ryan 1998). It has many similarities to the hypothetico-deductive model of reasoning used in early medical research. This linear model consists of five stages, including reflecting on ideas, formulating hypotheses, evaluating hypotheses for truths, determining a course of action and formulating a verbal statement to represent the hypothesis (Ryan 1998). The linear

model has been widely adopted in medicine, as it fits well with the problem-solving approach required for medical diagnosis.

Mattingly and Fleming (1994): Two-Bodied Practice and the Therapist with the Three-Track Mind (S1).

Although not articulated as a model, the documentation of the two-bodied practice and the therapist with the three-track mind nonetheless contributes to a developing model of clinical reasoning in occupational therapy. The eloquent description of the two-bodied practice (1994) reassures and supports occupational therapists in the belief that their practice is indeed complex, as it spans both the biomedical culture (in which we use medical talk) and the social, cultural and psychological issues surrounding the meaning of the illness (in which we use narrative reasoning). The notion of the therapist with the three-track mind provides an excellent description of three core modes of reasoning: procedural, interactive and conditional reasoning.

Higgs et al (2000, 2008): Contextualized Model of Clinical Reasoning (S1 and S2).

Higgs and Jones (2000) described an integrated, patient-centred model of clinical reasoning. They depicted an expanding spiral that reflected the clinician's growing understanding of the client and the clinical problem. At the beginning of the spiral was the clinician's encounter with the client and at the end was the final outcome. The tubing of the spiral represented the interaction of the six elements that make up the model: cognition, metacognition, the clinical problem, knowledge, the environment and the client's input. In the third edition of their text, Higgs et al (2008) describe clinical reasoning as a contextualized phenomenon, and add four meta-skills to the model, including the ability to derive knowledge and practice wisdom from reasoning and practice, the location of reasoning as relating to the selected practice model, the reflexive ability to promote personal growth in clients and self, and the use of critical creative conversations to make clinical decisions. This model has not been updated since 2008.

Schell et al 2009, Schell & Schell 2018: The Ecological Model of Professional Reasoning (S1).

Schell describes professional reasoning and the resulting therapy action as the interface of the therapist, the client and the practice context. Each practitioner brings to the therapy situation knowledge and skills that are grounded in life experiences, including personal characteristics such as physical capacities, sensory profile, personality and intelligence profile, as well as enculturated factors such as values, beliefs and preferences. These form a personal self, which is an inescapable lens through which the therapist frames the therapy encounter. Layered over or entwined with this personal self is the professional self, which includes the therapist's professional knowledge from education and experiences from prior clients, and the therapist's therapy beliefs, along with knowledge of specific technical skills and therapy routines available for use in the practice context (Fondiller et al 1990, Törnebohm 1991, Mattingly & Fleming 1994, Burke 1997). The personal and professional selves act in concert to respond to various problems of practice. Clients also come to therapy with their own life experiences and contexts, which also shape the therapeutic encounter. The therapist and client work together in a community of practice that shapes the therapy process in terms of nature, scope and trajectory (Schell & Schell 2018).

Unsworth (2004a, 2005, 2018, Fig. 15.1): Occupational Therapy Model of Clinical Reasoning (S1).

Based on the research foundation laid by Mattingly and Fleming (1994), Schön (1983, 1988), Barris (1987), Hooper (1997) and Schell and Cervero (1993), Unsworth (2004a, 2018) proposed a three-tier structure to depict clinical reasoning, thus sometimes it is referred to as a hierarchical model. At the top of Unsworth's model is worldview (moral beliefs and socio-cultural perspective) (Wolters 1989), which influences and modifies all other modes of reasoning. The middle level of the diagram contains the three main forms of reasoning: procedural, interactive and conditional. The fact that therapists also seemed to use two or three forms of procedural/interactive/conditional reasoning simultaneously is presented using a Venn diagram, and generalization reasoning is included in each of these modes. The last level of the diagram contains pragmatic reasoning (dealing with what can be achieved, given the practical constraints or benefits of the environment). The arrows flow around the model to indicate that these modes of reasoning or influences on reasoning all have an impact on each other. In Unsworth (2004a, 2018) it was stated that this model operates in the client-centred practice of occupational therapy. This model is expanded here in Figure 15.1 to incorporate the practice and contextual elements that also influence clinical reasoning. This updated model includes the client, acknowledging that reasoning is shaped by the interactive nature of the clinical encounter. The client's reasoning is also shaped by their worldview, their thoughts about health status and expectations of what occupational therapy has to offer. Clients also have many practical issues to consider that affect their therapy, such as their finances and family politics. This kind of pragmatic thinking is influenced by the client's life environment, which exists for both clients and therapists. Life environment is concerned with the social, cultural and political systems in which we live. However, a great deal more research is required to test, modify and expand this model into a conceptual framework.

DIRECTIONS FOR FURTHER RESEARCH IN CLINICAL REASONING

The Occupational Therapy Model of Clinical Reasoning, as illustrated in Figure 15.1, attempts to bring together some of the concepts articulated in the other models in a more integrated fashion to begin work on the third step of theory-building, which is to organize the phenomena into a conceptual framework. Research to build this framework is required in the spirit of scholarship of practice. As proposed by Nixon and Creek (2006), we need to construct theory by 'developing collaborative models of thoughtful practice that challenge assumptions and suggest new lines of inquiry'. Areas for research on the model include exploration of the relationship between pragmatic reasoning and worldview. Embodied knowledge is also not explicitly included in the model, and research is required to examine how a therapist reasons with their whole body. Research is also required to test empirically if the components of the model are sound and hold true across different environments and over time. Finally, there is a need for further longitudinal studies of clinical reasoning. Most of the research undertaken by occupational therapists provides snapshots of practice, and what we need now are studies that track therapists, reasoning and, importantly, shifts in reasoning, over time. We need to have a better understanding of the patterns of reasoning that promote the best therapy outcomes and gain further insights into how to share these patterns with novice therapists. The recent systematic review of clinical reasoning literature (Unsworth & Baker 2016) also identified that further research is required as follows: determining the nature and relationships of constructs entwined with clinical reasoning such as embodied knowledge, worldview and intuition; investigating the methods that can be used to research clinical reasoning and identify rigorous qualitative and quantitative approaches to better study clinical reasoning; shared reasoning between therapists and clients and how this shapes therapeutic encounters; research into the way clinical reasoning skills develop from classroom to clinic and how curricular activities can promote this; and finally that further replication studies are conducted to confirm the research that has already been undertaken.

SUMMARY

When visiting clinics around the world, I see occupational therapists striving to provide the best evidence-based therapy possible. This commitment and aspiration to achieve excellence is supported by clinical reasoning. Therefore it is crucial in our profession that we continue to research and write about clinical reasoning. The clinical reasoning of occupational therapists is a multifaceted process and forms part of the central framework of the profession. In daily practice, clinical reasoning results from the complex interactions between the therapist's own worldview, modes of reasoning and life environment, as well as the worldview, life environment and reasoning of the client. This chapter has explored the concept of clinical reasoning in occupational therapy and related factors such as intuition, worldview, expertise and reflection. It is proposed that occupational therapy researchers and writers in the area of clinical reasoning are slowly contributing to the construction of a theory of clinical reasoning. The challenge now is to ensure that the theory is built using a systematic framework and that research undertaken benefits from a scholarship of practice approach.

✳ REFLECTIVE LEARNING

- Use your own words to describe what clinical reasoning is, and differentiate clinical reasoning from clinical decision making.
- Do you prefer the term *clinical* or *professional reasoning*? Why would one be better than the other in different areas of occupational therapy practice?
- Describe two of the most common modes of clinical reasoning you use in practice (or you used in your last fieldwork). Reflect on why you selected these two. Consider what other reasoning modes you might use to enhance your practice in the future.
- Many of the factors that shape our pragmatic reasoning have the potential to impact negatively on what we can do or offer clients. Can you think of an example or scenario that could lead to the kind of pragmatic reasoning that limits delivery of an ideal therapy service? What could you do to counteract the forces that lead to this kind of pragmatic reasoning?
- Identify an episode in your career (or while doing fieldwork) that has been difficult because of discordance between your worldview and something happening in the clinic or with a client. What happened, why and what would you do differently next time?
- Models of clinical reasoning contributing to a theory of clinical reasoning are presented in the text. Describe a research study that you think might add to our understanding of clinical reasoning in occupational therapy and contribute to theory development in this field.

ACKNOWLEDGEMENTS

This chapter is based on research and reflection over many years and through debating ideas with passionate colleagues and students. I thank you all for sharing insights and experiences.

REFERENCES

Alnervik, A., & Sviden, G. (1996). On clinical reasoning: Patterns of reflection on practice. *Occupational Therapy Journal of Research, 16*(2), 98–110.

Alsop, A., & Ryan, S. E. (1996). *Making the most of fieldwork education: A practical approach.* Cheltenham: Stanley Thornes.

Arntzen, C. (2018). An embodied and intersubjective practice of occupational therapy. *OTJR: Occupation, Participation and Health, 38*(3), 173–180.

Argyris, C., & Schön, D. A. (1974). *Theory in practice: Increasing professional effectiveness.* San Francisco: Jossey-Bass.

Barnitt, R., & Partridge, C. (1997). Ethical reasoning in physical therapy and occupational therapy. *Physiotherapy Research International, 2,* 178–194.

Barris, R. (1987). Clinical reasoning in psychosocial occupational therapy: The evaluation process. *Occupational Therapy Journal of Research, 7,* 147–162.

Benner, P. (1984). *From novice to expert. Excellence and power in clinical nursing practice.* Menlo Park, CA: Addison–Wesley.

Benner, P. E., Tanner, C. A., & Chesla, C. A. (1996). *Expertise in nursing practice: Caring, clinical judgement and ethics.* New York: Springer.

Burke, J. P. (1997). Frames of meaning: An analysis of occupational therapy evaluations of young children. *Dissertation Abstracts International, 58*(3), 644.

Creek, J., & Ormston, C. (1996). The essential elements of professional motivation. *British Journal of Occupational Therapy, 59,* 7–10.

Cronin, A., & Graebe, G. (2018). *Clinical reasoning in occupational therapy.* Bethesda, MD: AOTA Press.

Dewey, J. (1929). *Experience and nature.* New York: WW Norton.

Dewey, J. (1934). *Art as experience.* New York: Minton & Balch.

Dowie, J., & Elstein, A. (1988). *Professional judgement: A reader in clinical decision making.* Cambridge: Cambridge University Press.

Dreyfus, H. L., & Dreyfus, S. E. (1986). *Mind over machine: The power of human intuition and expertise in the era of the computer.* New York: Free Press.

Dreyfus, S.E., Dreyfus, H.L., (1980). A Five-Stage Model of the Mental Activities Involved in Directed Skill Acquisition. Unpublished report supported by the Air Force Office of Scientific Research (AFSC). USAF (Contract F49620-79-C-0063), University of California at Berkeley.

Duncan, E. A. S. (2011). An introduction to conceptual models of practice and frames of reference. In E. A. S. Duncan (Ed.), *Foundations for practice in occupational therapy* (pp. 43–48). Edinburgh: Elsevier.

Fleming, M. H. (1994). The therapist with the three track mind. In C. Mattingly, & M. H. Fleming (Eds.), *Clinical reasoning: Forms of inquiry in a therapeutic practice* (pp. 119–136). Philadelphia: FA Davis.

Fondiller, E. L., Rosage, L. J., & Neuhaus, B. E. (1990). Values influencing clinical reasoning in occupational therapy: An exploratory study. *Occupational Therapy Journal of Research, 10,* 41–55.

Fortune, T., & Ryan, S. (1996). Applying clinical reasoning: A caseload management system for community occupational therapists. *British Journal of Occupational Therapy, 59*(5), 207–211.

Gribble, N., Ladyshewsky, R. K., & Parsons, R. (2018). Changes in the emotional intelligence of occupational therapy students during practice education: A longitudinal study. *British Journal of Occupational Therapy, 81*(7), 413–422.

Gibson, D. B., Velde, B., Hoff, T., et al. (2000). Clinical reasoning of a novice versus an experienced occupational therapist: A qualitative study. *Occupational Therapy in Health Care, 12*(4), 15–31.

Goel, V., Buchel, C., Frith, C., et al. (2000). Dissociation of mechanisms underlying syllogistic reasoning. *NeuroImage, 12*(5), 504–514.

Hallin, M., & Sviden, G. (1995). On expert occupational therapists' reflection-on-practice. *Scandinavian Journal of Occupational Therapy, 2,* 69–75.

Hammond, K. R. (1996). *Human judgment and social policy: Irreducible uncertainty, inevitable error, unavoidable injustice.* New York: Oxford University Press.

Hammond, K. R., & Brehmer, B. (1973). Quasi rationality and distrust: Implications for international conflict. In D. Summers, & L. Rappoport (Eds.), *Human judgement and social interaction* (pp. 338–391). New York: Holt. Rinehart & Wonston.

Hardman, D. (2009). *Judgment and decision making: Psychological perspectives.* Chichester: BPS Blackwell.

Harries, P., & Duncan, E. A. S. (2009). Judgement and decision-making skills for practice. In E. A. S. Duncan (Ed.), *Skills for practice in occupational therapy* (pp. 25–39). Edinburgh: Elsevier.

Harries, P., & Gilhooly, K. (2006). Identifying occupational therapists' referral priorities in community health. *Occupational Therapy International, 10*(2), 150–164.

Harries, P. A., Unsworth, C. A., Gokalp, H., Davies, M., Tomlinson, C., & Harries, L. (2018). A randomised controlled trial to test the effectiveness of decision training on assessors' ability to determine optimal fitness-to-drive recommendations for older or disabled drivers. *BMC Medical Education, 18*(27), 1–10.

Higgs, J., & Jones, M. (2000). *Clinical reasoning in the health professions* (2nd ed.). Melbourne: Butterworth–Heinemann.

Higgs, J., Jones, M., Loftus, S. L., et al. (2008). *Clinical reasoning in the health professions* (3rd ed.). Melbourne: Butterworth–Heinemann.

Holm, M. B. (2000). Our mandate for the new millennium: Evidence-based practice. *American Journal of Occupational Therapy, 54,* 575–585.

Hooper, B. (1997). The relationship between pretheoretical assumptions and clinical reasoning. *American Journal of Occupational Therapy*, 51(5), 328–338.

Kielhofner, G. (2008). *Model of human occupation: Theory and application* (4th ed.). Baltimore: Lippincott Williams & Wilkins.

Kielhofner, G. (2009). *Conceptual foundations of occupational therapy* (4th ed.). Philadelphia: FA Davis.

Kielhofner, G., & Forsyth, K. (2002). Thinking with theory: A framework for therapeutic reasoning. In G. Kielhofner (Ed.), *Model of human occupation: Theory and application* (3rd ed.) (pp. 162–178). Baltimore: Lippincott Williams & Wilkins.

King, G., Currie, M., Bartlett, D. J., Strachan, E., Tucker, M. A., & Willoughby, C. (2008). The development of expertise in paediatric rehabilitation therapists: The roles of motivation, openness to experience, and types of caseload experience. *Australian Occupational Therapy Journal*, 55(2), 108–122.

Kinsella, E. A. (2018). Embodied reasoning in professional practice. In B. A. Schell, & J. W. Schell (Eds.), *Clinical and professional reasoning in occupational therapy* (2nd ed.) (pp. 105–121). Philadelphia: Wolters Kluwer.

Lyons, K. D., & Crepeau, E. B. (2001). The clinical reasoning of an occupational therapy assistant. *American Journal of Occupational Therapy*, 55, 577–581.

Mattingly, C. (1994). Occupational therapy as a two-body practice: The body as machine. In C. Mattingly, & M. H. Fleming (Eds.), *Clinical reasoning: Forms of inquiry in a therapeutic practice* (pp. 37–63). Philadelphia: FA Davis.

Mattingly, C., & Fleming, M. H. (1994). *Clinical reasoning: Forms of inquiry in a therapeutic practice*. Philadelphia: FA Davis.

McKay, E. A. (2009). Reflective practice: Doing, being and becoming a reflective practitioner. In E. A. S. Duncan (Ed.), *Skills for practice in occupational therapy* (pp. 55–72). Edinburgh: Churchill Livingstone.

Melton, J., Forsyth, K., & Freeth, D. (2009). Using theory in practice. In E. A. S. Duncan (Ed.), *Skills for practice in occupational therapy* (pp. 9–24). Edinburgh: Churchill Livingstone.

Mitcham, M. D. (2003). Integrating theory and practice: Using theory creatively to enhance professional practice. In G. Brown, S. A. Esdaile, & S. E. Ryan (Eds.), *Becoming an advanced healthcare practitioner* (pp. 64–89). New York: Butterworth–Heinemann.

Mitchell, R., & Unsworth, C. A. (2005). Clinical reasoning during community health home visits: Expert and novice differences. *British Journal of Occupational Therapy*, 68(5), 215–223.

Neuhaus, B. E. (1988). Ethical considerations in clinical reasoning: The impact of technology and cost containment. *American Journal of Occupational Therapy*, 42, 288–294.

Nixon, J., & Creek, J. (2006). Towards a theory of practice. *British Journal of Occupational Therapy*, 69(2), 77–80.

Rassafiani, M., Ziviani, J., Rodger, S., et al. (2006). Managing upper limb hypertonicity: Factors influencing therapists' decisions. *British Journal of Occupational Therapy*, 69(8), 373–378.

Rassafiani, M., Ziviani, J., Rodger, S., et al. (2008). Occupational therapists' decision-making in the management of clients with upper limb hypertonicity. *Scandinavian Journal of Occupational Therapy*, 15(2), 105–115.

Rew, L. (1986). Intuition: Concept analysis of a group phenomenon. *Advances in Nursing Science*, 8(2), 21–28.

Robertson, L. (1996). Clinical reasoning, Part 2: Novice/expert differences. *British Journal of Occupational Therapy*, 59(5), 212–216.

Rogers, J. C. (1983). Clinical reasoning: The ethics, science, and art. *American Journal of Occupational Therapy*, 37, 601–616.

Rogers, J. C. (2010). Occupational reasoning. In M. Curtin, M. Molineux, & J. Supyk-Mellson (Eds.), *Occupational therapy and physical dysfunction. Enabling occupation* (pp. 57–65). Sydney: Churchill Livingstone.

Rogers, J. C., & Holm, M. B. (1991). Occupational therapy diagnostic reasoning: A component of clinical reasoning. *American Journal of Occupational Therapy*, 45, 1045–1053.

Rogers, J. C., & Masagatani, G. (1982). Clinical reasoning of occupational therapists during initial assessment of physically disabled patients. *Occupational Therapy Journal of Research*, 2, 195–219.

Rogers, J. C. (1982). Teaching clinical reasoning in practice in geriatrics. *Physical and Occupational Therapy in Geriatrics*, 1(3), 29–37.

Ryan, S. (1998). Influences that shape our reasoning. In J. Creek (Ed.), *Occupational Therapy New Perspectives* (pp. 47–65). London: Whurr.

Schell, B. A. B. (2009). Professional reasoning in practice. In E. B. Crepeau, E. Cohn, & B. A. B. Schell (Eds.), *Willard and Spackman's occupational therapy* (pp. 314–327). Philadelphia: Wolters Kluwer.

Schell, B. A. B., & Cervero, R. M. (1993). Clinical reasoning in occupational therapy: An integrative review. *American Journal of Occupational Therapy*, 47, 605–610.

Schell, B. A. B., & Harris, D. (2008). Embodiment: Reasoning with the whole body. In B. A. B. Schell, & J. W. Schell (Eds.), *Clinical and professional reasoning in occupational therapy* (pp. 69–87). Philadelphia: Lippincott Williams & Wilkins.

Schell, B. A. B., & Schell, J. W. (Eds.). (2018). *Clinical and professional reasoning in occupational therapy* (2nd ed.) Philadelphia: Wolters Kluwer.

Schön, D. A. (1983). *The reflective practitioner: How professionals think in action*. New York: Basic.

Schön, D. A. (1988). *Educating the reflective practitioner*. San Francisco: Jossey-Bass.

Sox, H. C., Higgins, M. C., & Owens, D. K. (2013). *Medical decision making* (2nd ed.). Hoboken NJ: Wiley-Blackwell.

Stanovich, K. E., & West, R. W. (2000). Individual differences in reasoning: Implications for the rationality debate? *Behavioral and Brain Sciences*, 23(5), 645–726.

Strong, J., Gilbert, J., Cassidy, S., et al. (1995). Expert clinicians' and students' views on clinical reasoning in occupational therapy. *British Journal of Occupational Therapy*, 58(3), 119–123.

Taylor, R. (2017). *Kielhofner's model of human occupation: Theory and application* (5th ed.) Philadelphia, PA: Lippincott, Williams & Wilkins.

Thompson, D. (Ed.). (1995). *Concise Oxford dictionary* (9th ed.) Oxford: Oxford Clarendon.

Törnebohm, H. (1991). What is worth knowing in occupational therapy? *American Journal of Occupational Therapy, 45,* 451–454.

Townsend, E.A., & Polatajko, H.J., (2013). *Enabling occupation ii: Advancing an occupational therapy vision for health, well-being, and justice through occupation* (3rd ed). Ottawa: Canadian Association of Occupational Therapists.

Unsworth, C. A. (1999). *Cognitive and perceptual disorders: A clinical reasoning approach to evaluation and intervention.* Philadelphia: FA Davis.

Unsworth, C. A. (2001). The clinical reasoning of novice and expert occupational therapists. *Scandinavian Journal of Occupational Therapy, 8,* 163–173.

Unsworth, C. A. (2004a). Clinical reasoning: How do worldview, pragmatic reasoning and client-centredness fit? *British Journal of Occupational Therapy, 67,* 10–19.

Unsworth, C. A. (2004b). How therapists think: Exploring therapists' reasoning when working with patients who have cognitive and perceptual problems following stroke. In G. Gillen, & A. Burkhardt (Eds.), *Stroke rehabilitation: A function-based approach* (2nd ed.) (pp. 358–375). St Louis: Mosby.

Unsworth, C. A. (2005). Using a head-mounted video camera to explore current conceptualizations of clinical reasoning in occupational therapy. *American Journal of Occupational Therapy, 59,* 31–40.

Unsworth, C. A. (2007). Using social judgment theory to study occupational therapists' use of information when making licensing recommendations to older and functionally impaired drivers. *American Journal of Occupational Therapy, 61*(5), 493–502.

Unsworth, C. A., & Baker, A. (2016). A systematic review of professional reasoning literature in occupational therapy. *British Journal of Occupational Therapy, 79,* 5–16.

Unsworth, C. A. (2017). An overview of professional reasoning within occupational therapy practice. In M. Curtin, M. Egan, & J. Adams (Eds.), *Occupational therapy and physical dysfunction* (7th ed.) (pp. 90–104). Oxford: Elsevier.

Unsworth, C. A. (2018). Research and scholarship in clinical and professional reasoning. In B. A. Schell, & J. W. Schell (Eds.), *Clinical and professional reasoning in occupational therapy* (2nd ed.) (pp. 477–491). Philadelphia: Wolters Kluwer.

Walker, K. F., & Ludwig, F. M. (2004). In *Perspectives on theory for the practice of occupational therapy* (3rd ed.). Pro-ed, Austin, TX.

Wong, K. Y., Whitcombe, S. W., & Boniface, G. (2016). Teaching and learning the esoteric: An insight into how reflection may be internalized with reference to the occupational therapy profession. *Reflective Practice, 17*(4), 472–482.

Wolters, A. M. (1989). On the idea of worldview and its relationship to philosophy. In P. A. Marshall, S. Griffioen, & R. Mouw (Eds.), *Stained glass: Worldviews and social science* (pp. 14–26). New York: University Press of America.

Young, M. E., & Quinn, E. (1992). *Theories and principles of occupational therapy.* London: Churchill Livingstone.

16

Occupational Science: Genesis, Evolution and Future Contribution

Matthew Molineux, Gail E. Whiteford

OVERVIEW

Throughout its history, occupational therapy has had distinct periods of conceptual and theoretical development that have impacted on the emergence of subsequent models of practice and the implementation of clearly defined intervention strategies. In this chapter, the authors chart the development of occupational science as one of the most prominent developments the profession has witnessed. The chapter presents an overview of the genesis of occupational science alongside a discussion of some of the attendant issues and tensions associated with its subsequent development. Consideration of the value and contribution of occupational science in informing both the epistemological and practice foundations of the profession is covered, before presentation of a research agenda for occupational science in the future. In essence, it is hoped that the reader will gain a clearer sense of how and why occupational science developed; what it has meant to the profession to date; and, finally, what it may contribute to understandings of the complex phenomenon of human occupation through a coherent and focused research agenda.

> ◎ **HIGHLIGHTS**
>
> - Effective occupational therapy practice is founded on an understanding of occupation and its impact on health.
> - Occupational therapists must have a thorough understanding of humans as occupational beings and of the relationship between occupation and health.
> - Occupational science has been one of the most significant developments in the history of occupational therapy.
> - The future of occupational science rests on its ability to generate new and useful knowledge, as judged by its stakeholders.
> - A research agenda for occupational science, which covers all the levels at which occupation is organized, is one way to ensure appropriate knowledge generation and application.

INTRODUCTION

How new knowledge is generated, tested and then infused into practice is a key concern in all disciplines. Whilst information is abundant in our age, how we make sense of it is especially challenging. Like other disciplines then, occupational therapy finds itself in an historic moment in which the need to consolidate the epistemological foundations upon which it is based is of central concern. Unlike other disciplines though, occupational therapy has experienced particular tensions with respect to the relationship between its central philosophical premise, that is, the dynamic interaction between occupation and health, and how this is addressed in practice. To this end, the development of occupational science may be seen as a cogent response, one that has already had significant positive impacts on the practice terrain of occupational therapy and should play an even more important role in the next several decades. In this chapter, we chart the genesis of occupational science and how it has evolved over time. We also posit some suggestions as to how its research agenda can inform the contribution of occupational therapy in a range of practice contexts in the future.

HISTORY AND DEVELOPMENT

Occupational science was first named by Yerxa and colleagues (1989, p.6) as 'the study of the human as an occupational being including the need for and capacity to engage in and orchestrate daily occupations in the environment over the lifespan'. Although what was named occupational science has a long history in the profession, the naming of occupational science in the late 1980s was driven largely by the work of occupational therapy academics at the University of Southern California, who were developing a proposal for a doctoral programme. In doing so, they gave much thought to the focus of that programme, and felt that the profession of occupational therapy would be usefully served by scholars in a science of occupation. The commencement of that PhD programme and the publication of the first paper that proposed occupational science marked the formal recognition of the new discipline. However, examination of the history of occupational therapy reveals that the naming of occupational science was merely the climax of a slow but steady movement within the profession. For this reason, it has been said that occupational science is not merely a chance happening (Clark & Larson 1993).

A science of occupation was first mooted by the National Society for the Promotion of Occupational Therapy in 1917 (Wilcock 2001, Wilcock 2003, Larson et al 2003). The initial objectives of that organization, which later became the American Occupational Therapy Association, proposed that it should concentrate on 'the advancement of occupation as a therapeutic measure, the study of the effects of occupation upon the human being, and the dissemination of scientific knowledge of this subject' (Dunton 1917). As the profession grew, only the therapeutic use of occupation received much attention (Wilcock 2003), despite continued calls for theoretical unity within the profession, which was consistent with the history and philosophy of early occupational therapy (Clark & Larson 1993). Prominent figures such as Meyer, Slagle, Reilly and Ayres had proposed that such unity would be provided by a basic science that focused on occupation (Yerxa et al 1989).

Although occupational science grew out of occupational therapy, when it was formally proposed in the late 1980s it was represented as a distinct entity. The difference between the two, as outlined at that time, rested in the type of science they embodied. Occupational science was seen as a basic science, that is, one that dealt with 'universal issues about occupation without concern for their immediate application' (Yerxa et al 1989, p.4). Occupational therapy, however, was seen as being concerned with the application of knowledge about occupation for therapeutic ends (Clark et al 1991). Furthermore, it has been stressed throughout the history of occupational science that it is not a model or frame of reference, but a social science or field of enquiry (Clark & Larson 1993, Clark 1997, Wilcock 2001, Larson et al 2003). Given the complexity of occupation and its relationship with health, occupational science has always been seen as an interdisciplinary field (Yerxa et al 1989).

The history of occupational science has been characterized by simultaneous acceptance and controversy. No overview of occupational science would be complete without an acknowledgement of this paradox. Although occupational science continues to develop, it has made significant steps towards becoming a well-established discipline. Some of the milestones and achievements include regular occupational science symposia in countries and regions, including the United States, Europe, Canada, Australasia, Japan

and Latin America. The *Journal of Occupational Science* has been in publication since 1993, and a growing number of books exist that focus explicitly on occupational science, on occupation or on understanding humans as occupational beings (see, for example, Zemke & Clark 1996, Wilcock & Hocking 2015, Hinojosa et al 2017, Cutchin & Dickie 2013, Pierce 2003, Pierce 2014, Molineux 2004, Molineux 2017, Watson & Swartz 2004, Whiteford & Wright-St Clair 2005, Whiteford & Hocking 2012, Christiansen & Townsend 2010). Occupational science has also featured in occupational therapy journals for several decades now, and many journals have published entire issues devoted specifically to the field (e.g., Johnson & Yerxa 1990, Molineux 2000b, Zemke 2000, Clark 2001). Furthermore, occupational science is now embedded in the international standards for occupational therapy education (World Federation of Occupational Therapists 2016).

The emergence and continued development of occupational science has been a cause of concern for some occupational therapists. Whereas Mosey (1992) saw that occupational science might prove useful for occupational therapy, she did argue for complete partition of the two. She proposed that separation would allow for a clear distinction to be made regarding the focus and form of enquiry in each field. Her suggestion was that occupational science should concentrate on theory development (focus) through basic research (form), whereas occupational therapy should concern itself with the testing and refinement of frames of reference through applied research. Her concerns were that if complete partition did not occur, an unhealthy co-dependence would develop, it would be unclear what was a discipline and what was a profession, and the research that took place would be poorly focused. Given that she viewed both forms of enquiry as valuable, she encouraged each field to concentrate on the type of research most applicable to its domain of concern (Mosey 1993). In response, Clark and colleagues (1993) from the University of Southern California argued that the differentiation between basic and applied research was not dichotomous, as Mosey (1992) proposed, and so to categorize occupational science and occupational therapy was inappropriate. This was an interesting assertion, given that only a few years earlier the same authors, with others, had proposed occupational science as a basic science (Yerxa et al 1989). Clark and colleagues now saw that such rigid categorization would unnecessarily limit research and stifle potentially useful work (Clark et al 1993, Carlson & Dunlea 1995).

Issues of basic and applied sciences have featured heavily in other debates about occupational science. There has been some question, for example, as to whether or not a basic science of occupation is necessary at all, given that an abundance of knowledge about occupation exists in other disciplines (Kielhofner 2002). What is clear, however, is that although other fields may address issues that might usefully inform an understanding of occupation, these fields do not use the concept of occupation as the focus of enquiry (Clark et al 1993, Carlson & Dunlea 1995, Zemke & Clark 1996, Haggard 2002, Polatajko 2010). As a result, 'the concept of occupation as an organizer of theory and research falls outside the domain of traditional disciplines' (Clark et al 1991, p.305). The relationship between basic and applied forms of research has also stimulated wider debates around approaches to knowledge generation. Although this was first raised by Mosey (1992), it has been more fully examined recently, in particular by proponents of the Model of Human Occupation. Their concern is with the way that knowledge informs practice. They contrast approaches to knowledge generation, which include from the outset concern for how that knowledge can be used by practitioners and those whose concern is knowledge generation without guidance on how to use that in practice. It is argued that using a conceptual model of practice (as defined by Kielhofner 1992, 1997) and related methods such as the scholarship of practice (Braveman et al 2001, Kielhofner 2005) ensures that the dialectic that exists between theory and practice is preserved. This ensures that any knowledge generated not only addresses the concerns of practitioners but also has clear guidance on how that knowledge can be used in practice (Kielhofner 1997, Kielhofner 2002, Taylor et al 2002). This approach can be contrasted with occupational science, which informs practice but may not necessarily provide specific tools or methods to be utilized by occupational therapy practitioners (Clark 1997, Forsyth 2001a, Forsyth 2001b, Molineux 2001).

It can be seen then that occupational science and occupational therapy are closely linked, and that in fact the former emerged from the latter. Indeed it could be said that they were not initially two distinct entities because the National Society for the Promotion of Occupational Therapy recognized the need to understand occupation and the dynamic relationship between occupation and health, and that this sat comfortably alongside the therapeutic use of occupation. However, it is worth noting that occupational science was formally labelled in the early 1990s continues to develop and negotiate relationships with occupational therapy and other fields. Despite its youth, occupational science has much to offer and this will be discussed in the next section of this chapter.

THE VALUE AND CONTRIBUTION OF OCCUPATIONAL SCIENCE

Although there has been much debate about occupational science and related issues such as approaches to knowledge

generation and the relationship between theory and practice, even those who have raised concerns about the new discipline have also seen its potential (Mosey 1992, Mosey 1993, Kielhofner 1997, Forsyth 2001a, Rey 2001, Hinojosa 2003). The value of occupational science has been well documented and includes (Yerxa et al 1989, Clark et al 1991, Clark et al 1998, Clark et al 2004, Clark & Larson 1993, Carlson & Dunlea 1995, Zemke & Clark 1996, Molineux 2000a, Yerxa 2000, Larson et al 2003, Wilcock 2003):

- providing support for what occupational therapists do in practice
- improving current services to clients and developing new approaches for therapy
- understanding humans as occupational beings
- explicating the relationship between occupation and health
- differentiating occupational therapy from other professions
- enhancing services outside of traditional health and social care boundaries.

Of course, the real test of occupational science will be whether or not it stands the test of time and can make a place for itself alongside other academic disciplines. There is little doubt that the debates and discussion will continue, and it will be worth examining those debates to understand their foundation. One such examination (Molke et al 2004) has noted that although the number of occupational science publications in 2000 was much greater than in 1990, the articles were still being published in the occupational therapy or occupational science literature and not in other fields. Although not growing outside of occupational therapy, that same analysis revealed that occupational science has grown within the international occupational therapy community.

It is this growing base of evidence about the power and the potential of occupation that has been one of the most significant contributions of occupational science to date. Whereas generations of occupational therapy researchers had been focusing on the efficacy of specific treatment regimes aimed at reducing impairment, occupational science has refocused attention on the more fundamental concern of the relationship between doing and well-being. Significantly, there has been a very important outcome of this focus on doing and well-being that has subsequently had a subtle but profound impact on occupational therapy practice. This has been the centralization of the person.

Centralization of the person refers to a conceptual and philosophical shift to an appreciation of the client of occupational therapy services as being both the expert with respect to their own occupational history and the most significant agent of change. Correspondingly, the role of the professional is recast as a facilitator, coach, resource conduit and advocate, hence equalizing the power relationship. Viewed thus, we can see that this has represented a shift away from the dominance of biomedicine as a guiding paradigm: a paradigm in which the locus of expertise and authority (and, some would argue, meaning) resided with the professional. Inevitably such a shift has created some tensions. Specifically, these tensions are experienced most overtly by occupational therapists working in acute care settings where the milieu is one in which a truly person-centred approach becomes not just philosophically challenging but, in the views of some, pragmatically almost untenable (Wilding & Whiteford 2009).

Although a full examination of this particular issue is beyond the scope of this chapter, a paradigm tension such as that described earlier does have implications for what sorts of research question should become prioritized in occupational science. Accordingly, the next section presents an exploration of what should be incorporated into a coherent research agenda for the future, alongside a critical examination of some of the philosophical underpinnings of what constitutes valid research.

THE RESEARCH AGENDA OF OCCUPATIONAL SCIENCE

As has been suggested in the previous section, one of the features that characterizes occupation is complexity; indeed, some authors have advocated that complexity theory itself should be the basis for developing understandings of occupation as a multi-dimensional human phenomenon (Pentland et al 2018, Whiteford et al 2005). Such complexity represents a two-edged sword when it comes to research, however. On the one hand, the complex features of occupation make it a rich field of enquiry. On the other hand, the complexity of occupation requires careful consideration of methodological strategies employed to comprehend it best.

Methodologically, discussions and developments in occupational science research to date have highlighted the importance of narrative approaches in understanding occupation. As numerous authors have argued over time, the dynamism of occupation cannot be captured through traditional experimental means. Indeed, because of its context dependence, occupation cannot be reduced to sets of variables that are controlled or manipulated. It is precisely the random and sometimes chaotic environmental interactions that are the everyday fabric of occupational engagement as lived experience. Narrative approaches have been identified as being a more ontologically appropriate means through which to understand how meaning through occupation is developed over a life course (Frank 1996, Molineux & Rickard 2003, Molineux

et al 2014, Wicks & Whiteford 2003), to understand the relationship between occupation and gender (Wicks & Whiteford 2005), and to understand transitions of young transgender individuals (Schneider et al 2018) and the transition between occupation and identity (Christiansen 2004).

As may be evident, the case for narrative ways of knowing and understanding occupation as a situated phenomenon have been well argued and are generally well accepted. There is, however, a broader methodological discussion that still needs to take place with respect to diversity. Understanding occupation in different contexts and at the different levels at which it occurs (micro through to macro) requires a conscious adoption of methodological pluralism. Such pluralism allows diverse research methods and approaches to be used, depending on the nature of the research focus or question. For example, understanding the impacts of living with a chronic illness on patterns and meanings of occupational engagement may predicate a narrative approach, whilst understanding patterns of occupational engagement nationally would require population-level statistical information. Alternatively, attempting to illuminate impacts of, for example, a new industrial development on the occupations of a specific community would require a multi-method orientation using approaches such as focus groups, surveys, time use instruments and individual interviews. Clearly, although this is an arena in which there is still much debate and dialogue to be had, it is of central importance to the ongoing development of occupational science and its research foci. But what are these foci and how do they relate to an overarching research agenda? We do not have the space in this chapter to discuss these in any great depth; however, we will start with a brief description of the current and future research agenda of occupation science as a segue into a presentation of what we, the authors, consider to be the specific foci for future enquiry.

In essence, the future of occupational science and indeed its potential to inform and guide occupational therapy lies in its ability to generate new and useful knowledge as judged by its stakeholders. Relevancy has overwhelmingly become the concern of not just stakeholders but funders, academics and practitioners alike when they discuss research (Durocher et al 2014). This represents a timely and appropriate response when, at worst, many abuses of intellectual and human rights have historically occurred in the name of research and, at best, research has been compromised in its usefulness by a lack of regard for application in real-world contexts. The notion of research as praxis, eloquently argued some time ago by feminist Patti Lather (1986), is based on a requirement for research to be focused on generating knowledge that leads to changes in practice to empower people. And that is exactly what a research agenda in occupational science needs to do. When we consider occupation and its centrality not only in people's lives but in society per se, a research agenda to understand it further must necessarily address those structural issues that enable or preclude people from engaging in occupation, as well as individual ones. This means including consideration of the historic, political and economic factors shaping access and participation for whole groups of people and the discursive traditions that influence policy development. As described, then, it is an ambitious agenda. Accordingly, and to stand as a discipline alongside others, the enactment of this pluralistic research agenda must also be systematic, rigorous and defensible. It must also be one that is as inclusive as possible, reflecting the diverse social, cultural and linguistic identities of persons living in a range of contexts (Magahlaes et al 2018).

As to the specific foci of occupational science research, they are best articulated within a structural framework relating to the levels at which occupation occurs and is organized. These levels are (from micro through macro): the individual, the family, society and population. The rationale for the approach adopted by the authors in this chapter is that focusing on the structural elements that enable and constrain occupation provides us with a more powerful appreciation of causation as it relates to occupation (Pereira & Whiteford 2013, Whiteford et al 2018). That is, it allows us to understand that what people do never occurs in a vacuum. Rather, all human occupation is situated, an essential characteristic that was initially described thus by Whiteford and Townsend (2010) in their work on the Participatory Occupational Justice Framework:

> All occupation takes place in a context. That is, no human action is independent of the social, cultural, political and economic contexts in which it occurs. These contextual forces, to a greater or lesser extent, shape the form and performance of the occupation as well as the meaning ascribed to it by an individual or group (p.10)

Others have stressed that the broader influences on occupational participation must be acknowledged and addressed, noting that

> Contextual influences can also include the prevailing economic ideologies and related policies, cultural and faith-based systems that govern social and occupational behaviour, health and social network supports, educational systems and structures, use of social media, telecommunications and transportation and environmental protections as well as primary resource management (Whiteford et al 2018, p.4).

Developing understandings of this complex rubric within which occupation takes place and the causal relationships that exist and exert a powerful influence not only on form and performance but also on legitimacy and opportunity obviously represents a significant challenge. Such a challenge will not be met through an ad hoc programme of enquiry, which to some extent may be a criticism levelled at occupational science research in the past. One of the areas that has been explored relatively rigorously, however, has been that of individual determinants of occupation.

LEVEL: THE INDIVIDUAL

There are several reasons why research into human occupation has largely been focused at the level of the individual. The first relates to the specific professional history of occupational therapy (where, to date, most occupational science researchers have come from) as being shaped by biomedical concerns with human systems and structures. The second reason is that such an orientation reflects the dominance of traditional Western epistemological concerns with the individual, rather than the collective (Kantarzis & Molineux 2017). This orientation has been criticized as representing a barrier to more culturally diverse ways of knowing and understanding occupation, with suggestions that the claiming of the theoretical basis of occupation as an essentially Western tradition fails to make visible the diverse socio-cultural identities of whole communities of people (Magalhaes et al 2018).

Such criticisms are valid and point strongly to the need for adoption of more inclusive epistemologies, a notion supported by the authors and one of the reasons for creating a schema for research that addresses multiple levels (including collective) through which to understand occupation. This fact notwithstanding, however, the research to date that has focused on occupational development across the lifespan, mind/brain/body and occupational performance, occupation and time use, and individual constructions of meaning relative to occupational engagement has provided some rich understandings. Although such understandings may have limited cultural generalizability, they have enabled a more informed articulation of the centrality of occupation in the lives of people and the relationship to sense of self. In turn, this has led to clearer understandings of the impacts of disruption to forming established and projected patterns of occupational engagement and decision making (Parnell et al 2019). Given current social trends however, some of the areas of future concern at the level of the individual should necessarily include

- an exploration of the relationship between occupation, choice and mental health

- leisure occupations and their contribution to efficacy and identity
- the impact of new technologies on occupational capacities.

Level: The Family

Families may be viewed as a primary vehicle for the development of value systems with respect to chosen and obligatory occupations; it is through people's experiences in families of origin that they learn about what is valuable, important and discretionary (Whiteford 2010). All of us have either experienced or observed family members condone or reject certain occupations and occupational behaviours. From the occupation of paid employment to the more subtle arena of leisure occupations, the influence of family values on choices made by individuals is sometimes overt, sometimes subtle, but usually pervasive. Indeed, in real terms the value accorded to occupations in family groups influences the mobilization of human and nonhuman resources. Of course, family values are also reflective of the social and cultural context in which they occur; the time and effort required by a family to support an Olympic athlete or concert pianist in the making need also to be viewed as relative to the societal value associated with each.

Given the significant influence of families on occupational development, then, it is surprising that relatively little research on this topic with an occupational focus has taken place. Some of the major foci to date have revolved around co-occupations in family units, parenting as an occupation and patterns of occupational engagement in families who have a child with a disability. Certainly though, a stronger orientation to diversity must inform the research agenda of the future in this area. This is especially true in a context in which what defines a family unit has changed dramatically over time (Stagnitti 2005, Kantarzis & Molineux 2014), gender roles have been revised, and families experience increasing levels of stress. Accordingly, research in the future would be well served by addressing, for instance, time use patterns in families (Zuzanek 2009), occupational stressors on families, occupational development of children in families living in resource-poor settings and jobless households, and families with sole- or same-sex couple parents.

Level: Community/Society

Because what constitutes a community has changed in recent times with the emergence of virtual communities, a definition at the outset seems prudent in this section. Perhaps one of the best descriptions comes from Christiansen and Townsend (2004, p.142), who have attempted to analyze communities critically from an occupational perspective:

Human communities consist of groups of people who do things together and individually. People participate collectively through reflection, communication or action in occupations such as labour, sports, intellectual pursuits or home building. Bonds that draw and keep people thinking about each other and occupied together may include shared beliefs, shared geography, shared interests, shared experiences or shared kinship.

As is evident from this definition, the emphasis is on the element of what is common, or shared, between people. However, exactly what it is that is shared will influence the types and forms of occupation that people in communities will be engaged in together. A case in point, for example, is the erosion of geographic communities as a site of common occupations, as evidenced in contemporary cities around the globe. Whereas previously, living near someone meant some commonality in terms of interest or lifestyle, this is no longer the case. Indeed many people fall into the category of finding that they spend more time occupationally engaged with people halfway around the globe than with people who live within a 10-kilometre radius. Clearly, if we think about the dependence of traditional communities located in geographic space, and about the input of those members to build community capacity in some form (for example, through participating in a neighbourhood watch programme or for a working bee in a local playground), then the implications of this development are serious. Who participates in and who gets left out of what people 'do' together in any type of community becomes a key issue. Despite the demographic and technological shifts influencing what constitutes a community and how it is experienced, people do still have an innate sense of belonging and identity relative to space (Mackay 2007), an issue that needs to inform public policy globally.

To date, these issues and others addressing broader political and economic influences on communities have been tentatively explored in the occupational science literature. Specific foci have included, for example, patterns of occupational engagement in communities, social and cultural influences on occupation and occupational role development, political and legislative influences on occupational participation of community members, and occupational alienation and deprivation (Pizarro et al 2018). If we are to serve society best, however, the research agenda in this area must be referenced to the broader discourse of social inclusion, which is the specifically stated orientation of many countries. Social inclusion developed in Europe and the United Kingdom as a response to greater migrant worker mobility, increased population diversity and inadequate welfare supports (Wotherspoon 2002). In essence, social inclusion is concerned with ensuring that people have resources, opportunities and capabilities (Pereira & Whiteford 2013). Clearly these are areas that are (or should be) of interest to occupational scientists, who may focus on, for example, the impacts made on communities by people such as asylum seekers (Suleman & Whiteford 2013) who have been occupationally deprived, understanding whether work creation schemes have an effect and why/why not, and identifying how governments can best build occupation/community capacity to enhance civic engagement within a human rights framework (Hammell 2014).

Level: Population

If you can imagine the levels we have identified here as a lens, starting with the closest focus on the individual, then this is the lens zoomed right out to the broadest level at which we can understand and, hopefully, capture human occupation. It is also perhaps the most contentious, as enquiry into population-related phenomena has traditionally been the province of economists, epidemiologists and statisticians. Although this may be so, Wilcock (2003) argued that in fact occupational therapists, before their inculcation into a biomedical belief system, were largely oriented to addressing the root causes of population ill health. Historical antecedents notwithstanding, bringing an occupational perspective to how we make sense of the many dimensions of population well-being is both cogent and timely when we face a projected population globally of 9.3 billion in 2050.

To date, this relatively small area of enquiry has been concerned with issues relating to population policy, population health status indicators and economic/employment status indicators. Although these foci need all remain on the agenda, the future should also include deepening our understandings of phenomena that are causally more complex but have an underlying occupational dimension—for example, childhood obesity, ill health as a result of loneliness and isolation and the impact of globalization upon occupational participation rates in developing countries (Rushford & Thomas 2016, Laliberte Rudman et al 2018).

In summary, this section has been a presentation and exploration of the research agenda of occupational science. It is not exhaustive, and needs to be read and understood in relation to the ongoing development of occupational science. Nevertheless it has been presented here because understanding occupation from different perspectives and at different levels is crucial to the development of new knowledge. Such new knowledge has the potential to inform not only the development of relevant and appropriate occupational therapy services, but government policy and resource allocation (Whiteford et al 2017). This, however, will not be a passive process. Rather it must be one in which researchers, educators, practitioners, managers and diverse community groups enact a willingness to discuss and debate key philosophical and conceptual issues to ensure change in social practices (Kantarzis & Molineux 2010). Central to this process must be a commitment to highlighting occupation as a unique, guiding paradigm.

SUMMARY

This chapter has provided an overview of the genesis of occupational science and its evolution to date. It has demonstrated that although the discipline was only formally named in the late 1980s, the seeds were sown at the foundation of the occupational therapy profession. Although occupational science has undergone much development, the precise boundaries of the field continue to be tested and negotiated. That occupational science continues to be refined makes this period in the history of the science and therapy of occupation most exciting, with more stimulating debates to come. One of these must be the relationship between occupational science and other disciplines. Occupational science has always been purported to be multi-disciplinary, but it remains the case that most (but not all) occupational scientists are occupational therapists. An issue that occupational therapists must wrestle with further is the nature of knowledge generation in the profession and the relationship between knowledge and practice. For example, although models of practice are undoubtedly useful, it would be worth considering further whether or not they are the only way of translating knowledge into practice.

Occupational science is concerned with furthering our understanding of humans as occupational beings and the relationship between occupation and health. This chapter has provided a brief overview of the research agenda of the field, organized within a framework relating to the levels at which occupation occurs and is organized. These included research into occupation at the level of the individual, the family, communities and whole populations. Although this framework is not inconsistent with occupational therapy, it challenges therapists to maintain an occupational focus and to take a broader view of their contribution to the health of humans. Occupational science continues to provide useful insights into the factors that facilitate and inhibit the ability of individuals to achieve and maintain health through occupation. In addition, occupational science is explicating new concepts (Durocher et al 2014) such as social inclusion and occupational justice, which require further scholarly development as to how they can most powerfully inform practice (Whiteford & Townsend 2010).

REFERENCES

Braveman, B., Helfrich, C., & Fisher, G. (2001). Developing and maintaining community partnerships within 'a scholarship of practice'. *Occupational Therapy in Health Care, 15*(1/2), 109–125.

Carlson, M., & Dunlea, M. (1995). Further thoughts on the pitfalls of partition: A response to Mosey. *American Journal of Occupational Therapy, 49*(1), 73–81.

Christiansen, C. (2004). Occupation and identity: Becoming who we are through what we do. In C. Christiansen, & E. Townsend (Eds.), *Introduction to occupation: The art and science of living* (pp. 121–139). Upper Saddle River: Prentice Hall.

Clark, F. (1997). Overview of theoretical models: Occupational science. In P. Crist, C. Royeen, & J. Schkade (Eds.), *Infusing occupation into practice* (pp. 13–17). Bethesda: American Occupational Therapy Association.

Clark, F. (2001). Occupational science: The foundation for new models of practice [special issue]. *Scandinavian Journal of Occupational Therapy, 8*(1).

Clark, F., & Larson, E. (1993). Developing an academic discipline: The science of occupation. In H. Hopkins, & H. Smith (Eds.), *Willard and Spackman's occupational therapy* (pp. 44–57). Philadelphia: JB Lippincott.

Clark, F., Parham, D., Carlson, M., et al. (1991). Occupational science: Academic innovation in the service of occupational therapy's future. *American Journal of Occupational Therapy, 45*(4), 300–310.

Clark, F., Zemke, R., Frank, G., et al. (1993). Dangers inherent in the partition of occupational therapy and occupational science. *American Journal of Occupational Therapy, 47*(2), 184–186.

Clark, F., Wood, W., & Larson, E. (1998). Occupational science: Occupational therapy's legacy for the 21st century. In M. Neistadt, & E. Crepeau (Eds.), *Willard and Spackman's occupational therapy* (pp. 13–21). Philadelphia: JB Lippincott.

Clark, F., Jackson, J., & Carlson, M. (2004). Occupational science, occupational therapy and evidence based practice: What the well elderly study has taught us. In M. Molineux (Ed.), *Occupation for occupational therapists* (pp. 200–218). Oxford: Blackwell.

Clark, F., Zemke, R., Frank, G., et al. (1993). Dangers inherent in the partition of occupational therapy and occupational science. *American Journal of Occupational Therapy, 47*(2), 184–186.

Cutchin, M., & Dickie, V. (Eds.). (2013). *Transactional perspectives on occupation.* Dordrecht: Springer.

Dunton, W. R. (1917). History of occupational therapy. *Modern Hospital, 8*, 60.

DuRocher, E., Gibson, B., & Rappolt, S. (2014). Occupational justice: A conceptual review. *Journal of Occupational Science, 21*(4), 418–430.

Forsyth, K. (2001a). Occupational science as a selected research priority [letter]. *British Journal of Occupational Therapy, 64*(8), 420.

Forsyth, K. (2001b). What kind of knowledge will most benefit practice? [letter]. *British Journal of Occupational Therapy, 64*(12), 619–620.

Frank, G. (1996). The concept of adaptation as a foundation for occupational science research. In R. Zemke, & F. Clark (Eds.), *Occupational science: The evolving discipline* (pp. 47–55). Philadelphia: FA Davis.

Haggard, L. (2002). Broadening horizons [letter]. *British Journal of Occupational Therapy, 65*(2), 98–99.

Hammell, K. (2014). Participation and occupation: The need for a human rights perspective. *Canadian Journal of Occupational Therapy, 82*(1), 4–5.

Hinojosa, J. (2003). Therapist or scientist – how do these roles differ? *American Journal of Occupational Therapy, 57*(2), 225–226.

Hinojosa, J., Kramer, P., & Royeen, C. (Eds.). (2017). *Perspectives in human occupation: Theories underlying practice.* Philadelphia: FA Davis.

Johnson, J., & Yerxa, E. (1990). Occupational science [special issue]. *Occupational Therapy in Health Care, 6*(4).

Kantartzis, S., & Molineux, M. (2010). The influence of Western society's construction of a healthy daily life on the conceptualisation of occupation. *Journal of Occupational Science, 17*(4) 62–60.

Kantartzis, S., & Molineux, M. (2014). Occupation to maintain the family as ideology and practice in a Greek town. *Journal of Occupational Science, 21*(3), 277–295.

Kantartzis, S., & Molineux, M. (2017). Collective occupation in public spaces and the construction of the social fabric. *Canadian Journal of Occupational Therapy, 84*(3), 168–177.

Kielhofner, G. (1992). *Conceptual foundations of occupational therapy.* Philadelphia: FA Davis.

Kielhofner, G. (1997). *Conceptual foundations of occupational therapy* (2nd ed.). Philadelphia: FA Davis.

Kielhofner, G. (2002). *Challenges and directions for the future of occupational therapy.* Stockholm, Sweden: World Federation of Occupational Therapists, 13th World Congress.

Kielhofner, G. (2005). Scholarship and practice: Bridging the divide. *American Journal of Occupational Therapy, 59*(2), 231–239.

Laliberte Rudman, D., Pollard, N., Craig, C., et al. (2018). Contributing to social transformation through occupation:

Experiences from a think tank. *Journal of Occupational Science, 26*(2), 316–322.

Larson, E., Wood, W., & Clark, F. (2003). Occupational science: Building the science and practice of occupation through an academic discipline. In E. Crepeau, E. Cohn, & B. Schell (Eds.), *Willard and Spackman's occupational therapy* (10th ed.) (pp. 15–26). Philadelphia: Lippincott Williams & Wilkins.

Lather, P. (1986). Research as praxis. *Harvard Educational Review, 56*(3), 257–275.

Mackay, H. (2007). *Advance Australia where?* Sydney: Hachette.

Magalhaes, L., Farias, L., Rivas-Quarneti, N., Alvarez, L., & Malfitano, A. (2018). The development of occupational science outside the Anglophone sphere: Enacting global collaboration. *Journal of Occupational Science, 26*(2), 181–192.

Molineux, M. (2000a). Another step in the right direction [editorial]. *British Journal of Occupational Therapy, 63*(5), 191.

Molineux, M. (2000b). Occupational science [special issue]. *British Journal of Occupational Therapy, 65*(5).

Molineux, M. (2001). Being clear about what is being debated [letter]. *British Journal of Occupational Therapy, 64*(10), 519–520.

Molineux, M. (Ed.). (2004). *Occupation for occupational therapists.* Oxford: Blackwell.

Molineux, M., Strong, J., & Rickard, W. (2014). Living with HIV infection: Insights into occupational markers of health and occupational adaptation. In D. Pierce (Ed.), *Occupational science for occupational therapy* (pp. 121–132). Thorofare: Slack.

Molineux, M. (2017). *A dictionary of occupational science and occupational therapy.* Oxford: Oxford University Press.

Molineux, M., & Rickard, W. (2003). Storied approaches to understanding occupation. *Journal of Occupational Science, 10*(1), 52–60.

Molke, D., Polatajko, H., & Laliberte Rudman, D. (2004). The promise of occupational science: a developmental assessment of an emerging academic discipline. *Canadian Journal of Occupational Therapy, 71*(5), 269–280.

Mosey, A. C. (1992). Partition of occupational science and occupational therapy. *American Journal of Occupational Therapy, 46*(7), 851–853.

Mosey, A. C. (1993). Partition of occupational science and occupational therapy: Sorting out some issues. *American Journal of Occupational Therapy, 47*(8), 751–754.

Parnell, T., Whiteford, G., & Wilding, C. (2019). Differentiating occupational decision-making and occupational choice. *Journal of Occupational Science, 1*(7), 442–448.

Pentland, D., Kantartzis, S., Glasti Clausen, M., & Witemyre, K. (2018). *Occupational therapy and complexity: Defining and describing practice.* London: Royal College of Occupational Therapists.

Pereira, R. B., & Whiteford, G. E. (2013). Understanding social inclusion as an international discourse: Implications for enabling participation. *British Journal of Occupational Therapy, 76*(2), 112–115.

Pierce, D. (2003). *Occupation by design: Building therapeutic power.* Philadelphia: FA Davis.

Pierce, D. (Ed.). (2014). *Occupational science for occupational therapy.* Thorofare: Slack.

Pizarro, E., Estrella, S., Figueroa, F., Helmke, F., Pontigo, C., & Whiteford, G. (2018). Understanding occupational justice from the concept of territory: A proposal for occupational science. *Journal of Occupational Science, 25*(4), 463–473.

Polatajko, H. (2010). The study of occupation. In C. Christiansen, & E. Townsend (Eds.), *Introduction to occupation: The art and science of living* (pp. 57–79). Upper Saddle River: Prentice Hall.

Rey, D. (2001). Resources and research priorities [letter]. *British Journal of Occupational Therapy, 64*(10), 518–519.

Rushford, N., & Thomas, K. (2016). Occupational stewardship: Advancing a vision of occupational justice and sustainability. *Journal of Occupational Science, 23*(3), 295–307.

Schneider, J., Page, J., & van Nes, F. (2018). "Now I feel much better than in my previous life": Narratives of occupational transitions in young transgender adults. *Journal of Occupational Science, 26*(1), 1–14.

Stagnitti, K. (2005). The family unit in post modern society. In G. Whiteford, & V. Wright-St Clair (Eds.), *Occupation and practice in context* (pp. 213–229). Sydney: Churchill Livingstone.

Suleman, A., & Whiteford, G. (2013). Understanding occupational transitions in forced migration: The importance of life skills in early refugee resettlement. *Journal of Occupational Science, 20*(2), 201–210.

Taylor, R., Braveman, B., & Forsyth, K. (2002). Occupational science and the scholarship of practice: Implications for practitioners. *New Zealand Journal of Occupational Therapy, 49*(2), 37–40.

Watson, R., & Swartz, L. (Eds.). (2004). *Transformation through occupation.* London: Whurr.

Whiteford, G. (2010). Occupation in context. In M. Curtin, M. Molineux, & J. Supyk Mellson (Eds.), *Occupational therapy and physical dysfunction* (pp. 135–151). London: Churchill Livingstone.

Whiteford, G., & Hocking, C. (Eds.). (2012). *Occupational science: Society, inclusion, participation.* Oxford: Blackwell.

Whiteford, G., & Townsend, E. (2010). A participatory occupational justice framework. In F. Kronenberg, & N. Pollard (Eds.), *Occupational therapies without borders – volume 2 towards an ecology of occupation-based practices.* London: Elsevier.

Whiteford, G., Townsend, E., Bryanton, O., Wicks, A., & Pereira, R. (2017). The participatory occupational justice framework: Salience across contexts. In N. Pollard, & D. Sakellariou (Eds.), *Occupational therapy without borders* (pp. 163–172). London: Elsevier.

Whiteford, G., Jones, K., Rahal, C., & Suleman, A. (2018). The participatory occupational justice framework as a tool for change: Three contrasting case narratives. *Journal of Occupational Science, 25*(4), 497–508.

Whiteford, G., & Wright-St Clair, V. (Eds.). (2005). *Occupation and practice in context.* Sydney: Churchill Livingstone.

Whiteford, G., Klomp, N., & Wright-St Clair, V. (2005). Complexity theory: Understanding occupation, practice and context. In G. Whiteford, & V. Wright-St Clair (Eds.), *Occupation and practice in context* (pp. 3–15). Sydney: Churchill Livingstone.

Wicks, A., & Whiteford, G. (2003). The use of life histories in understanding occupation across the life span. *Australian Occupational Therapy Journal, 44*(1), 126–138.

Wicks, A., & Whiteford, G. (2005). Gender, occupation and participation. In G. Whiteford, & V. Wright-St Clair (Eds.), *Occupation and practice in context* (pp. 197–212). Sydney: Churchill Livingstone.

Wilcock, A. (2001). Occupational science: The key to broadening horizons. *British Journal of Occupational Therapy, 64*(8), 412–417.

Wilcock, A. (2003). Occupational science: The study of humans as occupational beings. In P. Kramer, J. Hinojosa, & C. Royeen (Eds.), *Perspectives in human occupation: Participation in life* (pp. 156–180). Baltimore: Lippincott Williams & Wilkins.

Wilcock, A., & Hocking, C. (2015). *An occupational perspective of health.* Thorofare: Slack.

Wilding, C., & Whiteford, G. (2009). Practice to praxis: Reconnecting moral vision with philosophical underpinnings. *British Journal of Occupational Therapy, 72*(10), 434–440.

World Federation of Occupational Therapists. (2016). *Minimum standards for the education of occupational therapists.* Forrestfield: World Federation of Occupational Therapists.

Wotherspoon, T. (2002). *The dynamics of social inclusion. Perspectives on social inclusion working paper series.* Toronto: Laidlaw Foundation.

Yerxa, E. (2000). Occupational science: A renaissance of service to humankind through knowledge. *Occupational Therapy International, 7*(2), 87–98.

Yerxa, E., Clark, F., Jackson, J., et al. (1989). An introduction to occupational science: A foundation for occupational therapy in the 21st century. *Occupational Therapy in Health Care, 6*(4), 1–17.

Zemke, R. (2000). Occupational science [special issue]. *Occupational Therapy International, 7*(2).

Zemke, R., & Clark, F. (Eds.). (1996). *Occupational science: The evolving discipline.* Philadelphia: FA Davis.

Zuzanek, J. (2009). Time use imbalance: Developmental and emotional costs. In K. Matuska, & C. Christiansen (Eds.), *Life balance* (pp. 207–222). Thorofare NJ: Slack.

INDEX

Note: Page numbers followed by *f* indicate figures, *t* indicate tables, and *b* indicate boxes.